D0084136

Groups

Applying
the Functional
Group Model

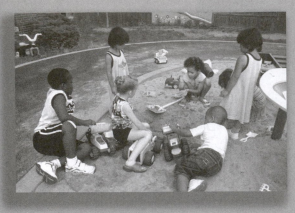

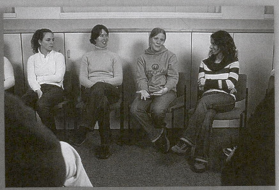

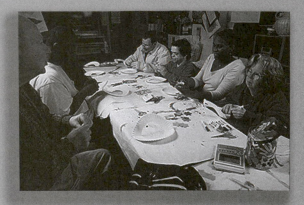

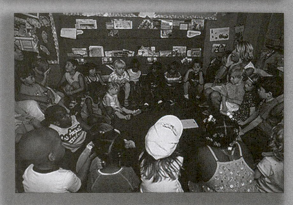

Groups

Applying the Functional Group Model

Sharan L. Schwartzberg, EdD, OTR/L, FAOTA
Professor
Department of Occupational Therapy
Adjunct Professor
Department of Psychiatry
Tufts University
Medford, Massachusetts

Margot C. Howe, EdD, OTR, FAOTA
Professor Emeritus
Department of Occupational Therapy
Tufts University
Medford, Massachusetts

Mary Alicia Barnes, OTR/L
Fieldwork Coordinator
Department of Occupational Therapy
Tufts University
Medford, Massachusetts

F. A. Davis Company
1915 Arch Street
Philadelphia, PA 19103
www.fadavis.com

Copyright © 2008 by F. A. Davis Company

Copyright © 2008 by F. A. Davis Company. All rights reserved. This product is protected by copyright. No part of it may be reproduced, stored in a retrieval system, or transmitted in any form or by any means, electronic, mechanical, photocopying, recording, or otherwise, without written permission from the publisher.

Printed in the United States of America

Last digit indicates print number: 10 9 8 7 6 5 4

Acquisitions Editor: Christa Fratantoro
Developmental Editor: Molly Connors
Manager of Content Development: Deborah Thorp
Manager of Art and Design: Carolyn O'Brien

As new scientific information becomes available through basic and clinical research, recommended treatments and drug therapies undergo changes. The author(s) and publisher have done everything possible to make this book accurate, up to date, and in accord with accepted standards at the time of publication. The author(s), editors, and publisher are not responsible for errors or omissions or for consequences from application of the book, and make no warranty, expressed or implied, in regard to the contents of the book. Any practice described in this book should be applied by the reader in accordance with professional standards of care used in regard to the unique circumstances that may apply in each situation. The reader is advised always to check product information (package inserts) for changes and new information regarding dose and contraindications before administering any drug. Caution is especially urged when using new or infrequently ordered drugs.

Library of Congress Cataloging-in-Publication Data

Schwartzberg, Sharan L.
  Groups : applying the functional group model / Sharan L. Schwartzberg, Margot C. Howe, Mary Alicia Barnes.
       p. ; cm.
  Includes bibliographical references and index.
  ISBN-13: 978-0-8036-1499-4 (pbk. : alk. paper)
  1. Occupational therapy. 2. Group psychotherapy. I. Howe, Margot C. II. Barnes, Mary Alicia, III. Title.
  [DNLM: 1. Psychotherapy, Group. 2. Group Processes. WM 430 S399g 2008]
RM735.S287 2008
615.8′515—dc22   2007023960

Authorization to photocopy items for internal or personal use, or the internal or personal use of specific clients, is granted by F. A. Davis Company for users registered with the Copyright Clearance Center (CCC) Transactional Reporting Service, provided that the fee of $.25 per copy is paid directly to CCC, 222 Rosewood Drive, Danvers, MA 01923. For those organizations that have been granted a photocopy license by CCC, a separate system of payment has been arranged. The fee code for users of the Transactional Reporting Service is: 8036-1499/08 0 + $.25.

Foreword

Group therapy is part of a revolution initiated during the 1880s by Sigmund Freud. In 1905 Dr. Joseph Pratt, working at Massachusetts General Hospital, organized the first groups that were designed to address physical problems. He would present a lecture to his patients at the clinic who were suffering from tuberculosis and then return to his duties while they discussed among themselves what he proposed. His inspirational talks were given to save time in helping patients maintain a wholesome and healthy regimen. He found that the patients who stayed to talk had much better rates of sustaining health than those who left right after his lecture. Pratt also became aware of the patients' sense of belonging, identification with one another, and mutual support. In 1907 Pratt wrote, "The Class Meeting is a pleasant social hour for the members. One confided that the meeting was her weekly picnic....they have a common bond in a common disease and a fine spirit of comradery [sic] has been developed" (p. 14).

Pratt's paper stimulated others with the possibilities of treatment in groups, notably Lazell, who began to utilize the lecture method with schizophrenic war veterans. In an article (1921), Lazell listed the advantages of the group method. Marsh took this a step further by experimenting with the idea of a therapeutic community involving all personnel. At Worcester State Hospital, Marsh utilized radio equipment to deliver mental hygiene courses and lectures to the patients and staff members. Marsh, a former minister, stressed the social and environmental influences of mental illness and stated, "By the crowd they have been broken, by the crowd shall they be healed" (Marsh, 1931, p. 349).

With the expansion of therapeutic tools, treatment of more varied segments of the population has come into demand. Not for adjustment to what is but for enhancement and expansion of what could be. It is no longer thought that patients have to adjust and learn to be satisfied with their limitations. Adaptation to a new set of skills can now allow people to potentiate themselves in different arenas. This volume provides a full and well-organized account on the subject of group work in occupational therapy—the struggle to integrate people with disabilities into the world on an equal footing. Occupational therapists focus on making independence a reality. While complete independence may not occur, depending on the extent of the disability, occupational therapists work with the patient or client to come up with strategies, techniques, or adaptations so that they can be as independent as possible. In the context of occupational therapy, occupation refers to meaningful life activities.

Because of their extensive experience as clinicians and teachers, the authors are able to provide their readers with pertinent and very specific information that illuminates activity-oriented group therapy. The well-integrated chapter headings demonstrate the authors' systematic understanding of the underlying theory. The instructive and very readable chapters are written with great clarity. Every aspect of group work is covered thoroughly and points the way toward a consistent path of working with clients/patients. The book's voluminous references attest to the authors' scholarship and give testimony to their mastery of the field of group work in occupational therapy.

A Concluding Parable

A huge block of marble was being moved into Michelangelo's studio while three boys were playing in a nearby alley. Out of curiosity they went and peeked through the door and saw Michelangelo walking around the big marble piece again and again. The next day the three boys came back, peeked in again, and saw Michelangelo still walking around the hunk of marble. This went on for days. Finally, after many, many days, Michelangelo picked up a hammer and chisel and chipped a small piece out of the marble. The boys just watched. The next day the boys watched as another piece of marble was chipped away. They came back day after day for an entire year to peer into the studio to follow what was happening. Michelangelo was just about finished with his sculpture, and out of curiosity he turned to the boys and asked, "What do you think?" One of the boys responded, "How did you know he was in there?"

References

Lazell, E. (1921). The group treatment of dementia praecox. Psychoanalytic Review, 8, 168–179.

Marsh, L. (1931). Group treatment of the psychoses by the psychological equivalent of the revival. Mental Hygiene, 15, 328–349.

Pratt, JH. (1907). The class method in treating consumption in the homes of the poor. Journal of the American Medical Association, 49, 755–759.

Michael Brook, Ph.D.
Founding Member and Faculty
Center for Group Studies
New York, N.Y.

Preface

Groups are a part of people's experience, not only in "normal" or healthy life but also when life is interrupted by disease and distress. Because of the potential benefits of group work and its versatility, a variety of professionals use this format in settings as diverse as hospitals, schools, businesses, and governmental agencies. Many books have been written about group process, but most have been directed toward psychotherapy, social work, or organizational development. None addressed the unique orientation we hold as occupational therapists that group work is skills-oriented, action-oriented, and here-and-now–oriented until 1986 when two of us published our first book, *A Functional Approach to Group Work in Occupational Therapy.*

Twenty years later, we have written this new book to incorporate changes that have occurred in society, education, practice, and theories about group work itself. Our functional approach to group work, which we call the functional group model, evolved from and combined theory, research, and practice in occupational therapy as well as other disciplines. The functional group model we present today is a model of practice in its own right, based on our experience as educators, researchers, and practitioners as well as our review of the literature and refinements in our theory development. This book is presented from the vantage points of the normal group, the therapeutic group, and the functional group.

It is important for any model to be expanded and evaluated through research and empirical evidence gathered in clinical practice, because this is how the validity of a model is tested. In this book, we present research studies that verify aspects of our theoretical model as well as studies relating to issues of group intervention. The material is organized to lead the reader logically through planning, implementing, and evaluating a functional group. The content is not focused on a verbal, insight-oriented approach to group work; rather, we explain the functional group as a method of aiding individuals in adapting to their life roles and tasks through occupation—the "doing" or "action"—while in a group. The model we propose is an approach designed for people with physical, social, emotional, or developmental problems as well as those wishing to maintain health and well-being. It is an approach that stems primarily from occupational therapy philosophy and practice. We offer you insights from our many years of fruitful professional collaboration and friendship.

Sharan L. Schwartzberg, EdD, OTR/L, FAOTA
Boston, Massachusetts
Margot C. Howe, EdD, OTR, FAOTA
Ashland, Oregon
Mary Alicia Barnes, OTR/L
Natick, Massachusetts

Reviewers

Cynthia Brenner, MA, OTR/L
Associate Professor and Fieldwork Coordinator
Occupational Therapy Assistant
Bristol Community College
Fall River, Massachusetts

Christine DeRenne-Stephan, MA, OTR/L, MEd
Assistant Visiting Professor
Occupational Therapy
University of Puget Sound
Tacoma, Washington

Linda S. Fazio, PhD, OTR/L, LPC, FAOTA
Professor
Occupational Science and Occupational Therapy
University of Southern California
Los Angeles, California

Margo R. Gross, MS, OTR/L
Former Assistant Professor
Occupational Therapy
Redding, Connecticut

Juli H. McGruder, PhD, OTR
Professor
Occupational Therapy
University of Puget Sound
Tacoma, Washington

Georganna J. Miller, MEd, OTR/L
Academic Fieldwork Coordinator
Occupational Therapy
Xavier University
Cincinnati, Ohio

Deborah Walens, MHPE, OTR/L, FAOTA
Clinical Associate Professor
Occupational Therapy
University of Illinois at Chicago
Chicago, Illinois

Acknowledgments

We are grateful to Tufts University for providing us the opportunity to indulge in our passion regarding group work and for bringing us together. Our work with students and the community has enriched our understanding of the need for and potential of group intervention. Specifically, we wish to thank the following people for their support :

- Francine Godfrey and the residents and staff at Jewish Community Housing for the Elderly, Newton, Massachusetts
- Michael Davison, MS, OTR/L, and the clients and staff at New England Sinai Hospital, Stoughton, Massachusetts
- Mary Grace Casey and the children, families, and staff at the Shattuck Child Care Center, Jamaica Plain, Massachusetts
- Noreen Ryan, MS, OTR/L; Craig Fletcher, LICSW, and the clients and staff at the Walnut Street Center, Somerville, Massachusetts
- Generations of occupational therapy students at Tufts University, Medford, Massachusetts
- Our graduate students Camerion Judge, MS, OTR/L; Abigail Canter, MS, OTR/L; Carrie Carmen, OTS; and Jessica Merkin, OTS, OTR/L who so generously gave their time and honest feedback on the manuscript, and last but not least:
- Mona Eklund and our colleagues of the American Group Psychotherapy Association and at Tufts University-Department of Occupational Therapy for their understanding and insights

Also, this work would not be complete without the work of our photographers Julia Nowlan-Sundari Ide, Mark Morelli, and Allison Tarin.

We very much appreciate Christa Fratantoro's genuine interest in and enthusiasm for the work. As editor, she was instrumental to the process. We wholeheartedly thank Molly Connors for her careful attention to detail and feedback about the progression of our work.

Without saying, our deepest thanks go to our families and friends for their dedication and ongoing belief in our capabilities in creating this work.

Contents

 Forms available online at http://davisplus.fadavis.com

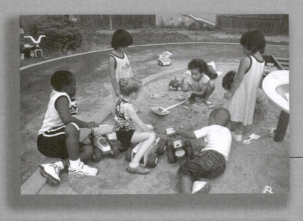

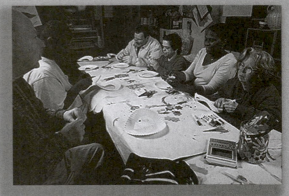

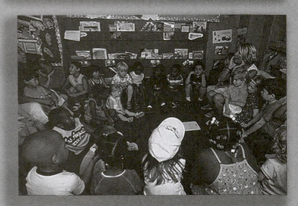

What Is a Group?

Very often we define ourselves through our identification with groups. Questions of belonging or "fitting in" have a powerful role in our sense of self. Most often, we are born into, or begin our understanding of the world in, a family group. Gradually, and somewhat naturally for many, our group membership and worldview expands through our social participation. We become part of groups, such as those found in a neighborhood, by becoming a student in school, through recreational pursuits, and later via career choice or work situations. Concurrently perhaps, group membership or affiliation may occur and evolve through involvement with community activities or service groups and through participation in a spiritual community. Through groups, we avoid isolation and learn about ourselves and other people. As members of groups, we participate in the dynamics of the group's process, even when we are unaware of doing so.

Throughout history, people have considered groups to be essential to survival. Groups can represent sources of support and affiliation or, perhaps, a threat to one's existence. In this way, groups have always played an important role in civilization. Globally, society represents humankind as a group at its largest level. If we consider our global society according to General Systems Theory (Von Bertalanffy, 1968), it is composed of individuals who, viewed as systems, form subsystems as they interact with each other within their larger group context. Similarly, the larger group is a subsystem of its organizational and environmental context. Each system may be embedded in numerous layers of the external environments. In the Ecological Systems Model (Bronfenbrenner, 1979) this layering is referred to as one of microcosms within macrocosms, with the individual at the center of group contexts embedded within contexts gradually representative of some aspects of the larger society. A visual image that most readily depicts this layering is that of concentric rings, somewhat like ripples in a pond. Change in one system may permeate the layers, from the inner layer out, or vice versa. As we learn what defines a group, we also become increasingly aware that subgroups and dynamics, including creative and destructive forces (Nitsun, 1996), can be found at all levels of our existence.

A long-held and common classification of groups according to social scientists has been that of primary and secondary groups (Cooley, 1909). The contacts that occur within a family are often seen as typical of those of a primary group. A primary group displays close, face-to-face relationships. Therefore, this type of contact might be found in family contexts, intimate friendships, or even within community groups such as spiritual congregations or a very close-knit neighborhood. Relationships between people in primary groups are characterized by a sense of interdependence and belonging rather than a sense of individualism. A sense of "we" rather than a sense of "I" prevails. Primary groups remain an important source of nurturing and support for adults; these features may be seen in groups of close friends or small, informal work or social groups where the emphasis is on relationships, informality, and satisfaction of personal needs. In contrast to the primary group, the secondary group is characterized by a more formal relationship between members. Secondary groups may also be small, face-to-face groups, but relations are less personal than in primary groups. School and professional groups, where people relate more formally through their established roles, are examples of secondary groups. The relationships are work- or task-related, entailing a more reasoned, less private, interpersonal style.

In reality, the distinction between primary and secondary, or informal and formal, groups is not as clear-cut. For instance, although a work group may maintain impersonal and formal relations between workers on the job in order to get their work done, the group may be sincerely concerned with the members' feelings about one another as they work together. In this case, the group combines the features of both primary and secondary groups.

In this chapter, we take a closer look at what might conceptually define a group. We begin by identifying various characteristics of groups such as context and climate, open versus closed membership, size, task and emotional functions, and cohesiveness. Variables of group structure and development, including the nature of the group's purpose and goals, group norms, and leader and member interaction, are briefly explored to recognize some of the most common features of groups that contribute to the dynamics that may underlie group process. As you proceed through the material, think about groups to which you belong or have belonged, groups with which you identify, or groups that you have led. As you read, take a moment to reflect on your own experiences in terms of groups. Note the characteristics and other phenomena of groups presented here to which you feel you can relate or that resonate in some way with your experiences in your life in, or perhaps with, groups.

Definition of a Group

As we see, even within determining the larger distinctions of primary versus secondary groups, defining a group very quickly becomes a complex task. However, two features common to all groups are content and process. *Content* refers to the work or task done during the time that the group meets. This includes what is said and discussed, both verbally and non-verbally. *Process* refers to how things are said and done and how the group's goals are accomplished. For instance, does everybody have a chance to talk? Do they seem to enjoy each other's company? These two features appear in every group—be it a meeting of the board of directors or a gathering of friends.

Two types of group behavior contribute to the group process. Group task functions enable the group to get its work done and to achieve its goals. Group-building and maintenance functions contribute to the creation and maintenance of relationships and interconnectedness among group members (Benne & Sheats, 1978). These behaviors can be viewed as functions present in all groups but in varying proportions.

There are many definitions of a group. Perhaps the most basic definition is "an aggregate of people who share a common purpose which can be attained only by group members interacting and working together" (Mosey, 1973a, p. 45). Two features that might characterize a group that has been together for some time are:

1. A "group consciousness, members think of themselves as a group, have a 'collective perception of unity,' a conscious identification with each other" (Knowles & Knowles, 1959, p. 39), and
2. The "ability to act in a unitary manner—the group can behave as a single organism" (Knowles & Knowles, 1959, p. 40).

Certain factors distinguish a group, such as identifiable leadership, members, and a meeting space and time. Taking those parameters into consideration, the following list adds to our understanding of what a group is by describing some of its major characteristics:

Dynamic interaction among members. The group process is diminished when most of the action takes place between the individual member and the leader.

A common goal. The absence of a common goal diminishes group functioning. A shared, clear goal facilitates group functioning.

A proper relationship between size and function. When groups are either too large or too small, they cannot function effectively.

A dependence on volition and consent. A group functions most optimally when its members consent freely to be part of that group.

A capacity for self-determination. The group functions best in a democratic climate (Loeser, 1957).

We can better grasp these characteristics if we examine a specific example. Consider a group of people on a bus. Each of the characteristics listed above could possibly be applied, except for the group's lack of a common goal and self-determination. Even though the riders are aware of other people around them, they are reacting to the bus ride on an individual basis. They are getting off at different stops for different reasons. As long as this is so, they are more accurately called an aggregate or a crowd rather than a group. They would not be called a group until they had an awareness of their dependence on each other to accomplish a goal and an acceptance of the need to interact and meet together to achieve that goal. Should there be a problem that prevents the bus from moving forward, the passengers might shift into a group mode. A process might emerge in which an individual steps forward as a leader to guide the group towards a unified goal of getting the bus going or, if that is not an option, getting the passengers as a group to a destination at which their individual needs (i.e., new form of transportation to where each person or subgroup had intended to get off the bus) could be met.

Characteristics of Groups

As we continue to look more closely at what defines a group, it is important to see beyond the broad features we have thus far identified. Each group exists as an individual entity and is unlike any other. Various combinations of characteristics define a group more precisely. Although these characteristics are often in a dynamic interplay, they consistently include elements of group structure, group cohesion, and stages of group development.

Group Structure

The structure of a group can be defined as the combination of mutually connected and dependent parts of a group that form its existence (Howe, 1968a, 1968b). When we look at group structure, we look at the organization and procedures of the group. We consider not only what type of structure the group exhibits but also how much or how little structure is present or required in order for the group to survive or function. The amount of structure, in terms of how a group is organized and whether the established procedures meet the needs of the group's purpose and members, will influence how and whether a group reaches its goals. For instance, when a group that conducts its business according to Robert's Rules of Order is compared with a group that makes decisions through an informal decision-making process, it is easy to see that the two groups exhibit different structures. In the first group, all communication between members is channeled through the chairperson. One has to address the chairperson if one wishes to speak and follow the highly structured procedures outlined regarding raising and seconding issues to be voted upon. In the second group, communication occurs directly between members without the intervention of a leader. In the latter case, the group may be more spontaneous, but it may also be less efficient. Although the decision-making process of an unstructured or informal group might take a longer time to complete, the members may be much happier with the results because the process allowed for more opinion sharing and participation by the members. Group structure is influenced by a number of elements, including:

- Historical context and climate
- Composition of membership
- Group purpose and member goals
- Leader and member interaction
- Group norms and size

Now consider how each of these elements can contribute to a group's existence and dynamics, be it positively or negatively.

Group Context

If we take a systems theory perspective, we realize that no group exists in a vacuum. Each group takes place in a historical and environmental context. A group may exist because of past history, and this may be openly stated. The historical context, which refers to elements of the social and environmental context outside the group, is a unique factor influencing the structure of the group. The influences of the external context may make it difficult for the group internally. The group may have difficulty restating or altering its goals, broadening or redefining its membership or member roles, or refocusing its activities. Conversely, the prestige or allure of the group for its members may also be related to the historical context. For instance, for some the status of a group's history may be what drives their wish to be a member. For others a newly organized group may be seen as desirable, thereby increasing its attractiveness for present and future members. Other aspects of environmental group context may include the mission of the organization in which the group is formed. An example of this is service groups, such as a Girl Scout troupe in which each member is "sworn in" and each meeting begins by reciting the mission: "On my honor, I will try…" or a group that is formed within a corporate setting or rehabilitation organization. In these examples the mission is clearly stated and visible within the organizational culture via logos, policy statements, and public materials such as posters or brochures, and the expectations of the group members (scouts, employees, clients receiving rehabilitative service) are made known.

Group Climate

Group climate refers to the physical and interpersonal or emotional environment affecting the group. A physical environment that is warm, quiet, and attractive is conducive to informal communication (Fig. 1.1). A seating arrangement permitting face-to-face contact is essential for interpersonal communication. The physical climate may also relate to having the necessary materials the work or activity of the group requires and is often closely related to the emotional climate. The interpersonal climate determines whether members feel accepted, respected, or supported. The climate also determines whether the group can develop a spirit of mutuality between the leader(s) and the members. When considering aspects of physical and emotional climate, one could ask: Does the group seem physically or psychologically

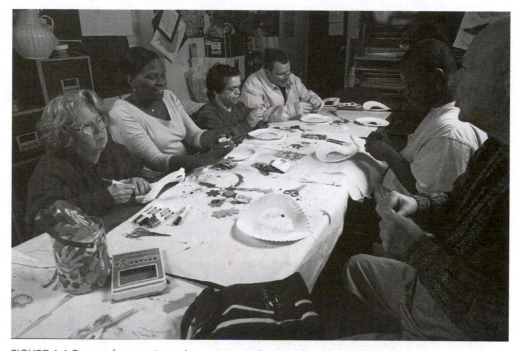

FIGURE 1.1 Face-to-face seating enhances group climate. (Photo by Mark Morelli)

safe? Do members seem relaxed? Comfortable? Willing to express differing opinions or to share personal information? Ideally, the group climate will be somewhat adaptable so that the group can meet the physical and emotional or psychological needs of the members as well as the various requirements of the group's tasks.

External events or forces can also impact group climate. For example, a group can be drawn together through competition with another group. It has been questioned whether the attraction of mutually exclusive rewards—even in the attainment of group goals—is effective in creating an efficient environment for work (Deutsch, 1960). When people undertake a task with an attitude of cooperation and interdependence, they facilitate greater acceptance of ideas, better listening, less possessiveness of ideas and, in general, better communication. In this type of climate, compared with one that stresses interpersonal competition, the group will strive harder to enhance its achievement and build a friendlier atmosphere.

Group Composition

Open Versus Closed Groups. An open group is one in which the membership frequently changes from one group session to the next. A continuous turnover in membership occurs as some people leave the group and new members join. In an open group, a significant amount of time and effort have to be devoted to introducing new members to the group. Each group of individuals develops a unique climate; therefore, the introduction of new members changes the climate and alters member security. Rate of member turnover in open groups can influence the extent to which small groups become cohesive (Hare, 1962).

A closed group is one in which the membership remains constant and no new member(s) can be added. Trust can be maximized in closed groups, and thus the potential for learning and behavior change is increased. However, a stable membership is not always constructive. Over time, closed groups might profit from a change in membership. The experience of seeing members leave the group increases the pressure on the remaining members to do something for themselves. Also, new members joining the group can provide long-standing members with an opportunity to help others and to practice interpersonal skills with the newcomer (Yalom, 1983).

Number of Sessions. The length of time over which a group meets is probably not as important as the total number of hours or sessions. For example, a group may meet three times per week for three weeks or once per week for nine weeks. The total number of hours will be the same. The more frequent sessions, however, may increase the intensity of the group experience for the members. Group leaders have experimented with varying lengths of group time. Workshop formats or extended time sessions over weekends have become popular. Under the pressure of time, the development of the group is accelerated, often catalyzing a more intense experience for members, which may or may not be desirable. It is not unusual for the length of time a group meets to be determined by internal factors as well, such as the time required to complete the chosen task or to meet the group goals. In other settings, such as schools, groups may be timed according to external factors such as the length of a semester or the class schedule.

Voluntary or Involuntary Membership. Group members come together for many reasons, and the motives of the individual members can affect the success of a group in achieving its goals. Voluntary membership means a participant is free to choose whether to join or leave a group. Involuntary membership in a group often signifies a participant is not free to leave a group without permission or consequence. Group attendance may be tied to a legal proceeding or contractual agreement (i.e., terms related to a living, work, or school situation such as floor or task force or project group assignment). Although members may share a common concern, whether members join a group of their own volition can affect the functioning of the group. Group behavior is frequently influenced by the extent to which membership in the group is a result of personal choice or compulsion. Apathy or rebellion may be seen in groups whose membership was involuntary.

Yet, even within less than ideal circumstances, involuntary group membership can offer to meet basic needs for care as well as an opportunity for growth or realization of an important goal. A family experiencing homelessness may be offered placement in transitional housing or at a shelter, provided they agree to attend all group meetings. At-risk youth who broken the law (charged or adjudicated for stealing, assault, etc.) may be mandated to social service or mental health settings that require participation in groups as a condition of being allowed to remain in a less restrictive facility. So even when events that may seem out of members' control or choice result in circumstances of involuntary membership in a group, an effective group can foster a sense that change is possible and empower members to make choices to achieve positive results.

If people are attracted to being a member of a group, they are more likely to accept the responsibilities of membership (Dion, Miller, & Magnan, 1970). Additionally, if group membership is an attraction, members will attend group meetings with more regularity (Back, 1951) and persevere in achieving difficult goals (Horwitz, 1960). Two factors that have been found to attract members to a group are:

1. The group itself is viewed as a desirable object, and
2. Group membership is viewed as a way to satisfy needs that exist outside the group (Cartwright & Zander, 1960).

A group could be deemed attractive because of the activities available in the group, the people who constitute its membership, or both. For instance, a cooking group may be attractive to members because they like to cook and eat the results of their work. On the other hand, the cooking group may be attractive to members because they want to be with the people who are members of that group. The task of cooking is secondary to meeting their interpersonal need or goal.

Members drawn to a group have been found to place greater value on the group goals than members who are not invested or who are forced to attend (Zander & Havelin, 1960). This suggests that benefits are greater from voluntary than from involuntary membership. However, not every compulsory group membership is unattractive. All of us are members of groups whose membership may not have been within our choice or control. Membership in involuntary groups can be a source of security (Lifton, 1961). Ideally, this notion applies to one's family. Involuntary groups, such as family groups, ascribed racial or ethnic groups, and assigned classroom or work groups, may or may not provide us with a sense of belonging, satisfaction, and growth. Outcomes such as these may be dependent upon one's willingness or ability to examine the ways in which membership in such groups might be a source of support or, desirable or not, the underpinnings to one's sense of identity and understanding of self in relation to others.

Group Purpose and Goals

The outcomes of a group are inherently linked to the group's purpose and goals. The purpose and goals for a group may be specific or general. Preferably, the group itself can determine the group's purpose and overall goals. However, aspects of the group's context and climate including someone outside the group may play a key role in determining the group's overall purpose and goals. Authorities other than the group leader may specify and regulate the purpose and task of the group. How a group is formed and who holds authority for the group may dictate whether goals can be changed and by whom. A group may have more than one goal.

Group goals can be a composite of the goals of individual members and an outcome or product the group aims to achieve by working together. Frequently, two levels of goals coexist, personal goals and group goals. While the group is working toward one common goal, members may also be working toward individual goals. When these two levels are compatible, the group will function effectively. When these two levels are incompatible, the individual or group goals will need to be reexamined and modified. Similarly, the group leader may have one set of goals and the membership another set of goals. These two sets of goals may be compatible or in conflict with each other. How the various goals are related will influence the achievement of either or both sets of goals.

Groups fare better when members are clear about the group's purpose and goals as well as their individual goals. Group members who have a clear understanding of the goals are likely to experience greater feelings of group belongingness and be more involved in the process of achieving those goals. The more time a group spends working out agreement on objectives, the more likely members may reach a consensus and the faster the group may reach the agreed upon goals (Raven & Rietsema, 1957). When all members of the group accept a specific group goal, they can become interdependent and improve the quality of group performance through a process of mutual facilitation (Cartwright & Zander, 1960). As a group works to determine its goals, integrate personal goals into group goals, and reevaluate and perhaps change goals, productivity increases. Through working together, group members increase their knowledge of one another and of how they can best work together. Four steps that enable a group to increase its productivity are:

1. A group should have at the outset a well-defined understanding of the goals it wants to reach.
2. The group should be aware of its own process. It should continually evaluate the process and make necessary changes.
3. The group should be aware of and understand the skills, talents, and other resources within its membership.
4. The group should create new tasks as needed and discontinue tasks no longer compatible with the goals (Lippitt, 1961).

Groups need to choose goals they can reach within the limitations of their resources. Groups that are realistic about their aspirations are successful in reaching goals (Atkinson & Feather, 1966). When a group is given a set of alternative goals from which to choose, the group as a whole will select a higher-risk alternative than will an individual group member

(Bem, Wallach, & Kogan, 1965). The collective group feels more empowered to take risks than do individual group members.

Leader and Member Interaction

The pattern of interaction and communication among leaders and group members can differ from group to group. This interaction can be predominantly verbal or physical and activity-oriented. The pattern may be formal and highly structured or informal, spontaneous, and loosely structured. The nature of the group—for example, a work group versus a social gathering—and the type of activity will influence the pattern of interactions. Taking the example of a social gathering further, consider a group of friends who have gathered to prepare a meal. The planning phase will be mainly verbal. After this phase has been completed, members may work individually or in dyads or subgroups while the meal is being prepared. The group's pattern or ways of interacting thus change so that the task is completed effectively. Conversation may occur within the subgroups or flow among all participants. The pattern of interaction may depend on how the layout of the kitchen affects the proximity of people as well as the topics that are raised for discussion. The host may or may not serve as the identified leader in the task, depending on the cooking skills of the group (i.e., host's friend is a chef).

A number of different factors influence communication patterns in groups. For example, persons whose opinions were at the extremes of the existing range of group opinions were found to have 70% to 90% of the communication addressed to them (Festinger & Thibaut, 1951). Interestingly, the effects of the perceived power on the relationships among group members suggests both high-power members (persons having prestige and the ability to persuade others) and low-power members (those who spoke up less and were considered as more conspicuous in their behavior) can be viewed as less liked by other members (Hurwitz, Zander, & Hymovitch, 1960).

Leadership style also influences the pattern of group interactions. In a seminal study on the impact of different leadership styles on group behavior, it was found that, under autocratic leadership, the interaction of members was formal and often hostile; when the leader assumed a democratic style, the interaction patterns of the members were more informal and cooperative (Lewin, Lippitt, & White, 1939).

The purpose and goals of the group, as well as the style of the group leader, will influence the roles members can assume in the group. These roles may be narrowly determined or they may be varied, leaving members free to assume different roles as the need arises. The dynamics of a group's communication and interaction patterns can be further understood by observing the roles group members take in the group. In keeping with their description of group process having group task and group building and maintenance functions, Benne and Sheats (1978) identified three types of roles group members may adopt. First are the group task roles, which assist the group in coordinating its efforts to define and solve common problems. Second are the group building and maintenance roles, which help enable everyone to work together as a group and strengthen or alter the group's processes as needed. Third are the individual roles, which are concerned solely with the satisfaction of individual needs. Specific member roles were identified within each of these three types.

Group task roles assist the work of the group in completing specified task goals. Twelve roles are identified to describe ways in which members function in this capacity:

1. The **initiator-contributor** suggests or proposes new ideas or new ways of viewing the group problems or goals.
2. The **information seeker** asks for clarification of suggestions made and for authoritative information and facts pertinent to the problem being discussed.
3. The **opinion seeker** is less concerned with the facts and looks for clarification of the values pertinent to what the group is doing.
4. The **information giver** offers facts or generalizations that are authoritative or relates his or her experiences to the group problem.
5. The **opinion giver** states a belief or opinion related to a suggestion made or to an alternative suggestion.
6. The **elaborator** makes suggestions in terms of examples and offers a rationale for suggestions made previously.
7. The **coordinator** clarifies the relationships among various ideas and suggestions, tries to pull ideas together, or tries to coordinate the activities of various members or subgroups.
8. The **orienter** defines the position of the group with respect to its goals.
9. The **evaluator-critic** subjects the accomplishments of the group to standards of group functioning within the context of the group task.
10. The **energizer** prods the group into action or decision making and attempts to stimulate the group to a "greater" or "better" activity.
11. The **procedural technician** facilitates group movement by doing things for the group.
12. The **recorder** makes a record of group suggestions and decisions by writing down or recalling for the group the products of discussion.

Group building and maintenance roles focus on maintaining group-centered behavior by building group processes and supportive attitudes. Seven roles comprise this category:

1. The **encourager** praises, agrees with, and accepts the contributions of others. Through these attitudes, he or she indicates warmth and solidarity toward the other group members.
2. The **harmonizer** mediates differences between members, attempts to reconcile disagreements, and relieves tension in conflict situations.
3. The **compromiser** operates from within a conflict in which his or her ideas or positions are involved. The compromiser may compromise by giving up power, admitting error, or in agreeing with the group by altering his or her opinion.

4. The **gatekeeper** or **expediter** attempts to keep communication channels open by encouraging and facilitating the participation of other group members or by regulating the flow of communication in the group.

5. The **standard setter** or **ego ideal** expresses standards for the group to achieve in its functioning or applies norms in evaluating the quality of the group process.

6. The **group observer** or **commentator** keeps records of group process and helps the group to evaluate its own procedures by presenting feedback.

7. The **follower** goes along with the sense of the group, serving as an audience for group discussion.

Individual roles are assumed by individual members of a group to satisfy personal needs that are not relevant to the group task and maintenance functions. When group members exhibit a high incidence of any of the following eight individual roles, the group is experiencing "individual-centered" rather than "group-centered" participation, which suggests that the group is not functioning well:

1. The **aggressor** lowers the status of others; disapproves of the values, acts, and feelings of others; and attacks the whole group or an issue on which the group is working.

2. The **blocker** tends to be negative, stubborn, disagreeing, and oppositional beyond reason.

3. The **recognition seeker** works in various ways to draw attention to himself or herself.

4. The **self-confessor** uses the audience that the group provides to express personal, non–group-oriented communications.

5. The **playboy** displays a lack of involvement in the group's processes.

6. The **dominator** tries to assert personal authority or superiority by manipulating the whole group or selected members of the group. Domination may be in the form of flattery, asserting a superior status, or interrupting the contributions of others.

7. The **help seeker** tries to elicit expressions of sympathy from the group through unreasonable expressions of insecurity or self-deprecation.

8. The **special interest pleader** speaks for special interest groups, usually as a mask for his or her prejudices and biases.

The interaction between the leadership and the membership of the group as well as the group's purpose and goals may determine the extent to which members can assume these different roles. Groups in which members have more access to participation have better morale (Napier & Gershenfeld, 1973). The more open the participation, the better the members' motivation. The roles that members take in the group can influence both the leadership of the group and the potential for conflict.

The pattern of interaction between leader and member(s) may also influence the problem-solving and decision-making capability of the group. A quick decision may fail when the decision is implemented, or the group may be unable to reach any decision at all

Box 1.1   **An Example of Poor Decision Making**

In an after-school group for teenagers, three or four members begin to plan their next group session enthusiastically. They discuss plans to meet at the park. Someone offers to bring a ball. The following week, those particular members are very late in arriving at the after-school program. They say to the other members, "Where were you guys? We were waiting for you at the park." The other members reply, "We didn't plan to go to the park, we never agreed to that, we thought you were just talking about maybe going there."

(Box 1.1). In either case, inadequate discussion of the issues involved in the decision may be responsible for the lack of success. For a group to problem solve and make decisions effectively, members' concerns about the identified problem/task or proposed solution(s) need to be brought forward and discussed openly.

Sometimes, the nature or obligation of the decision is not clearly understood by the group members, and some changes need to be made. Members may have difficulty separating the issues being presented or discussed from the individual(s) or member(s) who proposed them. Interpersonal loyalties or conflicts may impinge on the decision-making process and outweigh the importance of the issues.

A common misconception or error for group decision making is assuming that a vote is representative of the consensus of the group. A vote is often made without the full participation of group members. Discussion typically encourages members who agree, which creates a climate in which hearing from those who have no opinion or who disagree is subtly discouraged or avoided. Factors that facilitate group decision making include:

• A clear definition of the problem
• A clear understanding of who is responsible for the decision
• Effective communication for producing ideas
• An appropriate group size for decision making
• A means for testing different alternative decisions
• A commitment to the decision
• The honest commitment of the leader to the group decision-making process
• Procedures and methods for decision making are agreed upon before deliberations on the issue (Lippitt, 1961)

There are no fixed rules for optimal decision making. However, leader and member interaction that supports member contribution, free expression of opinions, and a unity of purpose may facilitate the process.

Group Norms

Groups often develop patterns of interaction or behavior that, although often seeming implicit, affect the group's process. Seating patterns or configurations, who speaks when, and how one initiates discussion or responds can become part of the normative expectations for behavior in a group. Rules and regulations might be unspoken or unwritten but seem to be unconditionally understood by members. Factors such as prior experiences in similar groups or previous learning or work situations might contribute to the process of a group developing norms. However, group leaders and members need to clarify their assumptions regarding group rules and regulations, which may be contributing to the leader-member interaction. For example, a group member may believe that speaking out of turn or without permission from the leader is not allowed because that was not allowed in the school that person attended or in the member's personal culture such behavior is disrespectful.

Stated or written rules and regulations of membership may also influence the group patterns of interaction. A group contract or group rules may govern attendance, participation, types of acceptable behavior, or the assignment of duties or roles. The leader typically is seen as a pivotal person in terms of establishing group norms and implementing group rules. In some groups, rules and norms are set and agreed on by the members, in which case the group acts as the enforcing body.

Group Size

Group size is directly related to a group's purpose and goals as well as the norms that may emerge and the number of interactions between members. If one of the goals of the group is to get feedback and validation for member behavior, the group must be large enough to ensure a variety of opinions. As more members join the group, the opportunity for people to interact with a variety of individuals increases. However, beyond a certain size, the opportunity that each member has to interact with other group members decreases. Frequently in large groups, only the most assertive members of the group are able to express themselves. In a small group, membership interaction is potentially limited in repertoire, and the leader may need to initiate group activity and interaction.

In a seminal study of task groups of two to seven members, it was found that group size influenced communication patterns. Groups with an even number of members (four or six) had significantly more disagreements and antagonisms and less expression of positive feelings than did groups with an odd number of members (three, five, or seven). An odd number appeared to affect the ability of the group to form competitive coalitions (Bales & Borgatta, 1962). The effects of group size on the number of member-to-member interactions in therapy groups was also studied. When group size reached nine or more members, a substantial reduction in the number of interactions was noted (Castore, 1962). Similarly, another study found larger groups produced lower member satisfaction, and as the size of a group increased, the time available for each member to participate decreased (Hare, 1962). As Yalom and Leszcz (2005) aptly note, "group size is inversely proportional to interaction" (p. 293).

Group Cohesiveness

Group cohesiveness refers to the intensity of feeling that members have for the group, to their sense of solidarity in identifying the group as "our" group (Fig. 1.2). The term cohesiveness also implies a sense of value about the group, the attractiveness that the group has for its members (Frank, 1957) and their wish to defend the group against internal and external threats. Cohesion is seen as the result of all the forces acting on all the members to persuade them to remain in the group (Cartwright & Zander, 1960). Cohesiveness is both determined by, and an effect of, inter-member acceptance. Groups with members who show high mutual understanding and acceptance are, by definition, cohesive (Yalom, 1970). One of the elements that contributes to group cohesiveness is the amount of cooperation, caring, and support that exists between members. Additionally, the amount of group support given to individual members, the encouragement members show each other, group attendance rates, and member punctuality at meetings may also be indicative of group cohesion. The amount of trust and willingness members demonstrate in taking risks to express their opinions and share their points of view can also be seen as a measure of group cohesiveness.

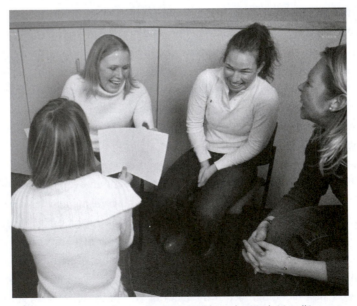

FIGURE 1.2 Power of group cohesion. (Photo by Mark Morelli)

Box 1.2   **Group as a System**

> The notion of a group as a system has its origins in General Systems Theory, developed by Ludwig Von Bertalanffy (1968). A biologist, Von Bertalanffy was concerned with the manner in which living systems were organized and how their constituent parts were interconnected and interrelated. He developed the theory as an alternative to the reductionist scientific trend of the times. He believed that the way to a better understanding of living systems was not to study parts in greater detail in isolation but rather to look at them as parts of a larger system, an organized unit of interdependent parts.
>
> According to this theory, there are two basic kinds of systems: closed systems and open systems. A closed system is usually described as a mechanical system, such as clockworks. An open system is descriptive of a living organism that obtains needed energy from its interaction with its environment. In an open system, the boundaries between the systems and subsystems are permeable, allowing energy and information to move from one part of the system to another. This process permits the system to adjust to changing conditions as needed for continued function.

Stages of Group Development

Groups pass through several stages or phases of development during their existence. This process occurs, in part, because the individuals who form the group are dynamic beings. As mentioned earlier, a group can be viewed as a unit or system, an organized body of interdependent constituent parts. It is the interactive nature of the system that changes in the developmental stages of groups, not necessarily the individual group members, although the processes may be linked (Box 1.2). Complex adaptive systems such as groups are open both internally and externally. The feedback process or interchange between or among their constituent parts may result in changes in the nature of the parts themselves or in the group as a whole.

The developmental stages through which a group must progress do not always proceed in a predictable manner. The progression is often marked with fluctuations. Stages may overlap, or the group may temporarily regress to earlier stages. A group may also plateau for numerous sessions before moving to a different stage or level of functioning. Although patterns in the development of a group may often continue over a number of sessions, each group meeting will also display developmental characteristics. Each group meeting can be seen as a microcosm of a sequence of meetings. An individual group session will begin with a formation period, when members greet each other, establish the climate, and review or establish the goals and norms of the group. The session then proceeds to the working stage and eventually enters the concluding period. Short-term and open groups go through a developmental pattern in individual sessions, even though these developmental periods may be abbreviated and more superficial than in the long-term groups.

The stages or phases of group development have been labeled in various ways according to the theories or frame of reference held by the observers of the group. However, there appears to be remarkable agreement on the basic developmental issues of small groups. In the beginning stages of a group, the members need to get to know each other and to develop a sense of being comfortable in the group. After the group has been meeting for a period, members develop ways of interrelating and working together. The path of development is not a straight line, and frequently groups revert to a previous developmental stage when there is a change in structure or when the group is undergoing stress. Some of the most obvious examples of change are a shift in the size of the group, a change of venue or meeting place, absence of a leader or member(s), or a change in leadership or membership. Any one of these events might be stressful to both the group leader(s) and the group members and thus affect the group as a whole. Other stresses a group may experience may be related to the group understanding or meeting the expectations of the group's task or the group's purpose and goals. Issues may emerge in regard to leader and member communication, leader-to-member interactions, or interactions between members.

A long-held theory regarding the process of group development looks at group dynamics from a psychodynamic point of view, focusing on the tensions experienced by group members and the resolution of these tensions (Bion, 1959). Group members are viewed as coping with and working through their tensions in three stages:

1. Through fighting or fleeing
2. Through dependence and counter-dependence on the leader
3. Through a process of pairing

The pairing in the third stage is seen as a way of creating closer bonds between members and thus overcoming underlying fears and tensions, signifying that the group is moving forward in terms of members' readiness to work together as a group.

Another psychodynamic theory of group development is based on interpersonal needs for inclusion, control, and affection. The inclusion stage involves issues related to belonging or not belonging to the group. The control stage deals with issues of dependence and authority. The affection stage relates to issues of intimacy, closeness, and caring (Schutz, 1960).

Another theory of group development based on studies of group dynamics delineated two major areas of uncertainty for group members. First, they contend with their issues relating to authority and power. Second, they are uncertain about each other. Therefore, according to this psychodynamic perspective, groups proceed along a continuum of development that reflects two stages, within which are subphases:

1. Dependence and power relations
   a. Dependence-flight
   b. Counter-dependence-flight
   c. Resolution-catharsis
   d. Enchantment-flight

2. Group interdependence

    e. Disenchantment

    f. Consensual validation

The group's development through each stage and phase is reflective of the members' attempts to deal with the feelings that emerge as they sort out their issues related to working together as a group. The progression describes member behavior as well as the group as a whole as the group shifts from dependence on the leader to member interdependence (Bennis & Shepard, 1956) (Box 1.3).

A similar theory arose from the discipline of social work, which described five stages of group development (Garland, Jones, & Kolodny, 1965):

1. Pre-affiliation

2. Power and control

Box 1.3   Bennis and Shepard's Phases of Group Development

The first phase of Bennis and Shepard's (1956) developmental model is concerned with dependence and power relations and includes four subphases. Subphase one, dependence-flight, refers to member behavior designed to please the leader in the hope that the leader will ease the member's anxiety and find a goal and task for him or her. Trying to be polite, members engage in "flight" behavior by discussing matters irrelevant to the group. As the leader continues to "fail" the group by not making decisions for the members, expressions of counter-dependence or opposition replace dependence, and the group progresses to subphase two, counter-dependence-fight. Expressions of hostility are more frequent and are also supported by other members. Subgroups emerge and vie for leadership. This chaos leads to a resolution in subphase three, resolution-catharsis. The group members assume leadership roles, and the group becomes unified in its pursuit of a goal. Pairing and involvement in the group task occurs. Then, in subphase four, enchantment-flight, everyone presents as happy. Everyone is amiable, and decisions are unanimous, but the decisions made are related to issues about which no one has strong feelings. An atmosphere of "sweetness and light" prevails, subgroups fuse, and the group becomes ready to move into the second stage.

The second developmental phase relates to group interdependence. The group turns its attention to issues of shared responsibility. The harmony of subphase four soon wears thin, and the group again begins to form subgroups, leading to subphase five, disenchantment. The group divides into subgroups based on the degree of intimacy required for membership. Again, a resolution of the problem occurs under the pressure of having to accomplish a task. The group now reaches the sixth and final subphase, consensual validation, which represents an acceptance of the group in realistic terms, with diminishing ties based on a personal orientation. Group consensus becomes easier to achieve on important issues, and personal ties develop from working together to achieve group goals.

3. Intimacy

4. Differentiation

5. Separation

Again, the developmental issues are those of belonging, control, power, and navigating one's way through the degrees of interpersonal relationship.

Small-group dynamics were investigated and described by Tuckman (1965), who identified five stages of group development:

1. Forming

2. Storming

3. Norming

4. Performing

5. Adjourning

In the first stage, forming, groups have to deal with the issues of coming together to form a group. Members need to get to know each other, their resources and talents, and their tasks. The second stage, storming, is a time of conflict, with disagreement concerning the task and how it should be completed. Conflicts may also arise regarding group leadership. The conflicts of the storming stage are seen as a normal event in the development of a group. By the third stage, norming, these conflicts have been resolved, and the group can develop norms and procedures to carry out its activities. In the fourth stage, performing, a cohesive unit has begun to form. The group is in control of its processes and can work effectively on the task at hand. In the final stage, adjourning, the group comes to a close, and members part due to the fact that the group has accomplished what it set out to do or they must bring their meeting to an end (Tuckman, 1965; Tuckman & Jensen, 1977; Johnson & Johnson, 2006).

Johnson and Johnson (2006) propose that most groups have leaders who are responsible for coordinating and facilitating the group to try to "ensure that the group functions productively" (p. 28). As such, they identify that groups will develop according to seven stages (p. 29):

1. Defining and structuring procedures

2. Conforming to procedures and getting acquainted

3. Recognizing mutuality and building trust

4. Rebelling and differentiating

5. Committing to and taking ownership of the goals, procedures, and other members

6. Functioning maturely and productively

7. Terminating

Group development has also been described in the discipline of occupational therapy according to the group's level of functioning. As members' task or social abilities improved in the group, the leader's role would shift, gradually allowing for more group-centered control of their process and functioning. Five levels of development are defined, based on member capabilities and leader response or actions (Mosey, 1970a):

1. **Parallel:** Members are involved in individual pursuits with little need for interaction. Task as well as social and emotional needs of members are met by the leader. A common example of this is young children at play in a sandbox under adult supervision. Each child constructs his or her own castle with tools, and praise, redirection, or limit setting is provided, as needed, by the adult.

2. **Project:** Members engage in short-term tasks that have common theme and require some interaction, cooperation, or competition (Fig. 1.3). Task completion is the primary focus of the group, and interaction not related to the task at hand is not an expectation. Task selection as well as social and emotional needs of members are still met predominantly by the leader. An example of this is a group of preadolescents (9–11 years old) preparing pizzas for dinner. Each member is to have a role in preparing ingredients, applying toppings, putting pizzas in and taking pizzas out of the oven, cutting and serving the final product, and cleaning the kitchen. An adult facilitates by procuring supplies, delegating tasks, providing praise and encouragement, setting limits, and providing redirection as needed.

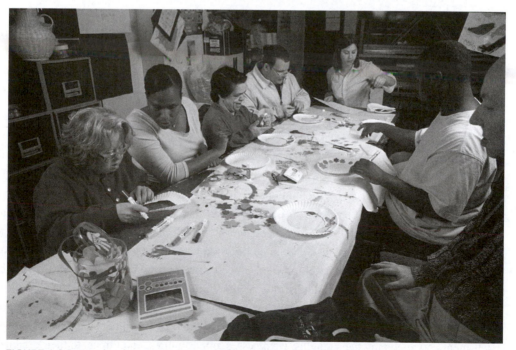

FIGURE 1.3 Project level group interaction. (Photo by Mark Morelli)

3. **Ego-Centric Cooperative:** Group members are able to work together on long-term activity through cooperative interaction. The task is still the primary focus, but members are more capable of responding to each other on a social-emotional level. Members require support and guidance with aspects of the task, and the leader continues to remain a source for satisfying members' emotional needs. An artists' cooperative of adults with developmental disabilities is an example of this type of group level. The artists may be able to respond to each other's needs in terms of basic praise and encouragement as well as sharing of supplies, but leadership is needed in terms of providing emotional support when members experience frustration or anxiety related to their work. Additionally, aspects of either the art task or the business part of the cooperative require leader input and oversight.

4. **Cooperative:** Members are encouraged to address one another's social and emotional needs in concert with activity goals of the group. At this level of group functioning, the leader is primarily an advisor or facilitator and may not need to be present at all meetings. Philanthropic and service groups, such as a Rotary or Lions club or a group organizing a community event or fundraising, are examples of a cooperative group. The members are able to carry on the group's task and mission and meet their needs for social participation and involvement in a meaningful venture without the leader being present.

5. **Mature**: Members balance meeting task and social-emotional roles as the leader is seen as a coequal member of group. A close-knit group of friends who support each other through life events such as a move, divorce, illness, or death and who grow and change in their membership as they integrate their significant others, children, and aging parents could be considered a mature group (Fig. 1.4). Long-time coworkers who know each other well who gather to complete a large project may also be able to function as a mature group. Peer support or self-help groups that have established group cohesiveness may also be examples of a mature group.

It is important to understand that these five developmental group levels are not age-specific and, like the various hypotheses of group development outlined thus far, can likely be identified in a variety of group contexts, from playgrounds to corporate settings.

What appears to be a commonality to understanding stages of group development, regardless of frame of reference, is that as the social and emotional needs of members emerge, a dynamic interplay unfolds as members work through their uncertainty and dependency to build toward interdependence and an ability to balance their individual needs with those of the group. As part of this developmental process, members come to terms with what they are capable of doing and gradually assume responsibility for their actions and interactions at the level to which their chronological age or personal abilities allow (i.e., from toddlers agreeing not to throw sand if they want to remain in sandbox to board members creating a vision statement and analyzing the strengths, weaknesses, opportunities, and threats to their organization to develop a strategic plan that will fulfill the organization's mission).

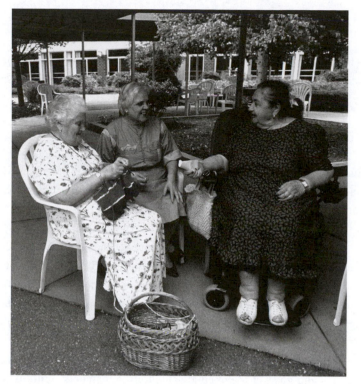

FIGURE 1.4 Mature natural group. (Photo by Mark Morelli)

Types of Groups

Now that some of the basic elements that define a group have been explored, the next step is to look at types of groups. We have thus far looked at characteristics of groups, using examples of natural groups that often form by virtue of common needs, interests, or circumstances, such as families, work groups, spiritual communities, and educational or recreational groups. Additionally, with the ongoing development of technology, the worldwide Web has become another venue where groups form. The rules of engagement, size, and extent to which membership is open or closed, in natural or virtual groups, vary a great deal. In terms of virtual groups, it has been questioned whether a cyber group resembles a large group or if it acts as if it were a small group (Weinberg, 2000).

Many types of groups are conducted in a wide variety of settings. In further classifying types of groups, most groups can be categorized as being one of the following:

• Activity
• Intra-psychic or psychoanalytic

• Social systems
• Growth

These categories are not mutually exclusive. There is considerable overlap, and some groups may be a combination of types. However, each type is examined according to purpose and goals, theoretical perspective, and membership.

Activity Groups
Group Purpose and Goals

Activity groups are small, primary groups in which members are engaged in a common activity or task that is directed toward learning and maintaining occupational performance. It is important to understand that the true purpose of an activity group is "to provide a shared working experience wherein the relationship between feeling, thinking and behavior, their impact on others and on task accomplishment and productivity can be viewed and explored....Task accomplishment is not the purpose of the group but hopefully the means by which purpose is realized. It is seen as the catalytic agent which elicits behavior and interaction, brings into focus both functional capacities and limitations, facilitates collaboration in working through problems and provides a concrete reality factor against which to measure learning and achievement" (Fidler, 1969, p. 45).

Although the goals and activities of activity groups may differ, these groups have inherent structures and goals of therapeutic value for the members. With its focus on the way the group works together to accomplish the task at hand, the activity group closely replicates living in the community or a primary group such as the family. Through recreating this climate and the potential dynamics that may emerge in a primary group while having a concrete activity on which to focus the group's attention, group members are given an opportunity to learn from direct experience and gain increased understanding about their own role(s) and skills in a group situation. Cole (2005) recommends that the activity group process be structured by the leader to ensure that the group members are clear about what to expect and what was learned. She advocates use of a seven-step format that combines many of the properties found in different types of activity groups (Mosey, 1981) (Box 1.4). The purpose of the seven-step format is to allow for "maximum integration of learning by members" (Cole, 2005, p. 3) and consists of:

1. Introduction
2. Activity
3. Sharing
4. Processing
5. Generalizing

6. Applying

7. Summary (Box 1.5)

Clearly, for an activity group, the choice of the activity is of utmost importance. A careful analysis of the activity demands is required to assess the level and variety of skills to complete the task. The activity demands of a task can provide a degree of structure and organization helpful to many group members. However, if the task is too easy or too difficult, the group members will not have a successful learning experience.

Box 1.4   **Mosey's Six Major Types of Activity Groups**

Mosey (1981), an occupational therapist, describes six types of activity groups. These types are not meant to be discrete, because some groups may have the properties of several categories. The description of types is meant to clarify and facilitate communication about the purposes of the group as well as the group's level of functioning on both task and social-emotional dimensions.

1. **Evaluation groups.** Designed to assess an individual's occupational performance strengths and weaknesses within a group setting, evaluating both performance skills and patterns that may affect participation in interpersonal interactions and activities.
2. **Task-oriented groups.** Designed to increase members' awareness of themselves and others through the activity process and in their interactions with other members, exploring the relationships between thoughts, feelings, and actions.
3. **Developmental groups.** Fall along a continuum of leader-dependent to member-driven groups. Designed to teach only group interaction skills, based on the theory these skills are developmentally stage-specific. The developmental level of the group is based on members' needs and abilities.
4. **Thematic groups.** Designed to help members learn the knowledge, skills, and attitudes necessary for accomplishing a specific set of activities. The group is structured to allow members an opportunity to gain knowledge and acquire and practice new skills and/or attitudes. The environment is tailored to member needs to provide elements of challenge or support and allow for feedback to assist with learning.
5. **Topical groups.** Members set goals relating to learning specific skills, knowledge, or attitudes that they identify as wanting or needing to learn, which will be carried out independently in the community. One type of topical group, the anticipatory group, focuses on activities that the group members anticipate doing in the future. A second type, the concurrent group, focuses on activities that the group members are currently doing in the community. The group is designed to help group members share experiences, give each other feedback, and offer suggestions.
6. **Instrumental groups.** Designed to help members maintain their level of functional performance and meet health and wellness needs. Change, although it may occur, is not expected. Activities are selected to meet the goals identified by members related to areas of performance they identify (activities of daily living/self-care, work, education, leisure, social participation, etc.).

Box 1.5   **Cole's Seven-Step Format**

1. **Introduction.** Often a warm-up activity is used to bring the group together, followed by the leader outlining the purpose of the group, expectations, and plans for activity and discussion. The leader is responsible for taking appropriate measures to set the mood for the group. Careful attention is given to the physical space, activity, and the leader's therapeutic use of self in terms of verbal and nonverbal presentation.
2. **Activity.** The activity is chosen to meet therapeutic goals of members and is designed to involve one-third of the group session. The activity is adapted to the performance skill level of group members and should be based on age appropriateness and meaningfulness for members.
3. **Sharing.** Members share the product of their work in the group with each other. Sometimes this process is highly structured by the leader after the activity is completed, whereas at other times it may be incorporated as part of the activity.
4. **Processing.** This step involves eliciting from members how they felt about the group. Members are encouraged to express feelings about the activity as well as member and/or leader actions and interactions, verbal or nonverbal. Covert dynamics are explored and discussed to allow for deeper understanding of issues that may be affecting the group positively or negatively.
5. **Generalizing.** The leader reviews what occurred and identifies general themes or patterns that emerged during the session. Commonalities are viewed and articulated by the leader as "general principles" (Cole, 2005, p.11) to address what was learned during the group.
6. **Applying.** This step builds on Generalizing by looking at how the principles learned in the group may apply to life outside of the group, in order to help members consolidate learning into action. Members are asked what they will do with their newfound knowledge or understanding.
7. **Summary.** This final step emphasizes the key points of the group to assist members with remembering what was learned and how it may be applied to their individual lives. Positive performance or outcomes are acknowledged as well as member participation. It is recommended that members be thanked for their contributions. It is the responsibility of the leader to end the group on time, even if all the steps have not been completed, which can be the content of the summary should this be the case.

The activity goals must be readily understood to facilitate the involvement of the group members. As the group members discover that they have among them the requisite capabilities to meet the expectations inherent in the group's task, their comfort increases, and they are able to assume group roles necessary to fulfill the group's true purpose. Members are given the opportunity to coordinate and use the skills of others available within the group. In this way, people can work on the aspect of the task in which they have greater skill. For example, a person who is shy or who has poorly developed verbal skills may become involved in the group primarily through joining in the actual task. On the other hand, a member who is afraid of the physical demands of the task or who cannot get involved because of physical limitations can participate on the verbal level. Learning occurs in the shared process of *doing* as well as through verbal interaction. In the process of doing, all available skills become important for the completion of the task, and members are drawn together in joining their skills toward accomplishing a single goal. The activity also provides a concrete measure of the progress of the group as a whole toward the achievement of the group tasks and goals. Through their individual contributions, the members may also clearly demonstrate their growth and achievement over time.

Theoretical Perspective

The concept supporting the activity group has its roots in two different theoretical constructs. The first is the principle of group dynamics relating to how the therapeutic factors (Box 1.6) in small groups bring about positive behavioral change. The second relates to the importance of doing—the role of purposeful and meaningful activity in developing and maintaining skills.

Box 1.6   **Therapeutic Factors**

According to Yalom (1975) and Yalom and Leszcz (2005), most groups include many, if not all, of the following 11 therapeutic factors. Different groups may emphasize different factors.

1. **Instilling hope.** When members are in a group with other people who are in the process of changing, their hopes are reinforced. Members in a group usually function at different points on a health continuum. Hope is nurtured when group members with similar problems appear to profit from their interactions in the group.
2. **Universality.** People who seek help may feel that no one else could be as unacceptable as they feel they are and that they are alone in their misery. In a group they learn that others have similar concerns, fears, and experiences. It is reassuring for them to know that they are not so different from other people, even though they may have endured painful experiences in life.
3. **Imparting information.** Members learn a great deal about themselves and others through participation in a group. They also learn about the group process itself. Some groups provide extensive didactic information about growth and development or treatment for specific diseases or states of dysfunction. Other groups teach actual skills and roles. These skills may be practiced in preparation for use outside of the group in contexts such as home, work, or the community.
4. **Altruism.** An important aspect of membership in a group is the opportunity to help others and to be helped by others. Members gain a feeling of self-worth when they are able to help other members and to "make a difference" in others' lives. People need to feel that they are needed. Altruism has traditionally played an important part in the healing rites of primitive cultures.
5. **Corrective recapitulation of the family group.** A closed group can function as a primary group closely resembling the family group. The leader is often perceived as a parental figure. Past familial experiences influence a member's interaction with

(box continued on page 30)

Box 1.6   **Therapeutic Factors** (continued)

other members and with the leader. The therapy group can help a member realize and correct maladaptive behavior that may have characterized relationships in the family group.

6. **Development of socializing techniques.** Socializing techniques, also called social learning or learning social skills, vary in importance and explicitness from group to group. Groups may use learning methods such as role-playing and structured exercises to develop specific social skills. An example is the use of role-playing to practice applying for a job or asking someone for a date. For individuals who lack close relationships, the group may be their only opportunity for accurate interpersonal feedback. This feedback enables them to learn about another person's reactions to their standard behaviors, such as a lack of eye contact when talking or a display of indifference that may mask feelings of caring. Members in long-term groups learn how to listen, to respond to others, and to be less judgmental of themselves and others.

7. **Imitative behavior.** Group members often model their behavior on other members' behaviors. People can learn new behaviors just from watching other people. Additionally, members learn vicariously through the experience of other members who have problems similar to their own.

8. **Catharsis.** The expression and release of feelings are important parts of the healing process in the group. Merely expressing emotion, however, may not be of lasting benefit. Members learn to express feelings and discover that the expression of honest feelings is not as disastrous as they may have feared. People are often surprised to realize that positive and negative feelings toward a person may be present at the same time.

9. **Existential factors.** Personal concerns about isolation, death, and helplessness may be discussed and shared in the group setting. For instance, a group of people who all have a chronic disease may well discuss the limitations imposed by the disease, the areas in which they can still exercise choices, and the responsibilities they must assume for those choices. Often by facing the issues of life and death, people can live life more honestly. The group lends the support needed to face these issues.

10. **Cohesiveness.** Cohesiveness refers to the sense of group belonging. Humans are social beings and need to relate to other people. For some people, isolation is a serious problem. An individual may be separated from familial support systems, where there are few opportunities to share feelings and to be accepted on a personal level. For people who are hospitalized, a group can become a place where sharing experiences and feelings can augment therapeutic aspects of other interventions.

11. **Interpersonal learning.** A group is a microcosm of society in which persons interact in much the same way that they would in society or outside the group. By helping each other to understand their behavior within the group, members get a clearer picture of interpersonal behavior patterns in society at large. Learning in the here-and-now provides individuals with immediate feedback about how others see them. Thus, they learn what behavior brings people closer to them or keeps them at a distance; on the basis of this information, they can decide whether to alter their own behavior. This is a process referred to by some as "reality testing."

Group Membership

Member criteria for activity groups can vary by factors such as age, ability level, and member needs. The activity demands of the group may serve the needs of the members in different ways. In some cases, group members may feel more comfortable working on the task than with interpersonal relationships. These members identify with the group through their involvement in the task elements of the group activity. Other members may be comfortable in the group setting but have difficulty dealing with the nonhuman environment. They need the opportunity to learn how to solve specific problems through participation in a joint activity. For these members, accomplishing the task, rather than the task itself, may be the major goal. For all members, a sense of belonging and partnership can result from the exploration of a shared need to master the activity, be it problem solving the interpersonal aspects or addressing elements of the task related to the nonhuman environment.

Intra-Psychic or Psychoanalytic Groups

Group Purpose and Goals

The general aim of intra-psychic groups is to achieve characterological and personality changes in each group member by "working through" the personal, intra-psychic, and historical antecedents of present maladaptive personality patterns. Intra-psychic refers to the processes and conflicts that occur within the individual. Insight into the unconscious and the self is the goal of psychoanalytic groups. In addition to insight, intra-psychic groups can offer experiences that meet group needs as well as provide ego support for the members (Howe, 1968a, 1968b). Groups of this type focus on working through experiences to move toward more healthy forms of adaptation.

Theoretical Perspective

Intra-psychic groups are based primarily on psychoanalytic theory. The principles of psychoanalytic therapy are applied in the group setting, with the aim being increased insight and understanding of behavior as a source of change in member behavior. The focus of observation and analysis is placed mainly on individual members, not on the group as a whole. Transference is a phenomenon that has particular importance in the intra-psychic group. In transference, members perceive certain qualities in the leader or in their interactions that they associate with individuals from their past or who may be current figures of authority (parent, supervisor, teacher, grandparent, older sibling, etc.). The leader may not actually possess these qualities; rather, they are being projected onto or attributed to the leader by the members. However, in intra-psychic group therapy as developed by Slavson (1950), members work out their preconscious conflicts through activities, and therapeutic results are obtained more through the discharge of tension inherent in the conflict than through insight. In groups using projective media and art, an understanding of object relations theory (Box 1.7) and how

Box 1.7   **Object Relations Theory**

Object relations theory postulates that a newborn child must develop the ability to differentiate external (other person) sources of sensation or gratification versus internal (self). The first step in this process usually involves being able to distinguish the mother or caretaker who provides gratification of basic needs (i.e., hunger), from which the first "love-object relationship" ensues (Fidler & Fidler, 1963, p. 33), which customarily was seen as "characterized by complete dependence on the mother for gratification of all needs" (p. 33). After this occurs, the infant then develops the awareness of his own body and an ability to gratify some instinctive impulses. As the child grows into adulthood and speech-language and abstract reasoning abilities improve, the ability to identify self in relation to others evolves. A positive sense of self is vital to this process to allow the individual to share comfortably and cooperate with others. In healthy object relationships: "People are no longer simply 'used' for immediate gratification....Things will no longer be in themselves the basis for security or ultimate gratification" (p. 33).

Donald Woods Winnicott was an English pediatrician and psychoanalyst who contributed his own perspective to the field of psychoanalysis in the area of object relations theory. He focused on understanding child development in the context of mother-child interaction or parental care as a "facilitating environment" (Winnicott, 1963/1965, p. 239, as cited in St. Clair & Wigren, 2004). Winnicott's work was influenced by the work of other object relations theorists such as Melanie Klein, which seems most evident in his conceptualization of terms such as "good-enough mother," (Winnicott, 1962/1965, p. 57, as cited in St. Clair & Wigren, 2004), "holding environment,"(Winnicott, 1962/1965, p. 61, as cited in St. Clair & Wigren, 2004) and that for which he is most noted, "transitional objects" (Winnicott, 1958).

Object relations theory creates a framework for understanding the potential emotional and symbolic significance of certain objects or relationships in group members' lives or even the group process itself. A poor sense of self/other may contribute to members' inability to share feelings or materials. Members may have difficulty experiencing a sense of the group environment as safe or secure and/or with finding the leader(s) "good enough" to meet their needs as members. Transitions may be hard for the members to manage, whether it involves moving into another phase of the group, close of group sessions, or changes in leadership or membership.

members may relate symbolically with human and nonhuman objects is useful in understanding what may potentially lie beneath or contribute to the group's dynamics.

Group Membership

Members must have a clear ego identity, or sense of self, and specific mental functions, such as the cognitive ability to use the group to develop insight, meaning that they should be able to deal in the realm of the abstract. In these groups, membership criteria may be kept homogeneous in age, gender, and socioeconomic status. A balance of problem areas and characterological style may also be a consideration when selecting group members.

Social Systems Groups
Group Goals and Structure

Social systems groups help participants learn about group processes and dynamics through participation in a collective task experience. When taking a social systems perspective, "attention is directed to how relationships within groups are formed and how these relationships stabilize; how decisions are made; how patterns of behavior emerge; and how parts fit together to form the whole family, team, or group" (Sampson & Marthas, 1981, p. 125). The group's activity and interaction with the environment (Lewin, 1951) is addressed in the moment, focusing on the here-and-now experience of the members.

Theoretical Perspective

The principles of social systems groups are drawn from systems theory and are applied to the concepts of group process and group dynamics. Lewin (1951), a social scientist, described the behavior of individuals in terms of a system of paths, barriers, forces, and goals. He coined the term "life space" to refer to the environment experienced by the individual or the group. Social systems theory acknowledges that a group operates in a milieu within which it plans activities and conducts its business.

Group Membership

A social systems perspective is one that can be applied to groups that are forming or that already exist, such as families or work, educational, or athletic teams or groups, for which there may be a single focus, concern, or goal for the group that keeps the members involved in the group. Ideally, members would have the capacity to process their behavior in the here-and-now, even on the most basic level, in terms of what drives the group and how their behavior might affect the group as a whole. Members' ability to recognize patterns of behavior in the group, as well as their need to do their part to achieve the group goal, may need to be considered or facilitated.

Growth Groups
Group Purpose and Goals

Growth groups are aimed at increasing members' sensitivity to feelings or enhancing members' ability to help themselves through the power of the group. The precise methods by which these goals are accomplished vary from group to group, but all are aimed at personal growth through didactic and action-oriented experiences. The term encounter groups has been used to describe some growth groups in that the encounter group format offers "an intensive group experience that is designed to put the normally alienated individual into closer contact—or 'encounter'—with himself, with others, and with the world of nature and pure sensation" (Shaffer & Galinsky, 1974, p. 211). Peer support groups and self-help groups have been identified as a special category of growth groups (Schwartzberg, 1994) but may have a specific area of focus. In regard to support groups focused on managing chronic illness, it is believed by some that "education has a major role in groups providing support and knowledge to manage chronic diseases (e.g., arthritis and diabetes). During these support groups, patients learn about the disease process and medical management of symptoms, get advice regarding problems related to the chronic illness, and gain support from the group members as they share experiences and attempt problem solving" (Borg & Bruce, 1991, p. 7).

Theoretical Perspective

Growth groups are based on the principles of humanistic and existential philosophy and psychology that seek to fulfill the potential inherent in each person (Maslow, 1962; Perls, Hefferline, & Goodman, 1971; Rogers, 1961; Schutz, 1967). Therefore, growth groups often address issues of the here-and-now and address basic needs of the members. Leadership often emerges from, and is shared by, the group.

Group Membership

Members are individuals who seek a growth experience and will therefore share a desire for growth with others in the group. Commonly, members range in age from adolescence to older adulthood. Ideally, members have the mental functions or cognitive and emotional capabilities to share in the process of problem solving and lending support as well as to make use of the information and support provided.

Conclusion

To define a group, a number of important elements were considered. Being able to observe and identify a group's content versus process as well as the various leader and member roles that contribute to its success or demise are important skills for a leader or a member of a group. To prepare oneself for the role of group leader requires being able to determine needs for or within a group to design a group accordingly. Attending to the vital characteristics of groups enables them to form and function. Variables of group structure, such as the physical and historical or emotional context and climate and membership, can affect a group's purpose and goals. The nature and quality of leader and member interaction can facilitate or stagnate a group's development. Group norms that develop can herald signs of whether a group will be a welcoming and growth-inducing environment or one of hostility and dysfunction.

Issues of group size and composition, as well as the type of group and whether it fits well with group member abilities, must also be a consideration. Groups must grow and develop through a process of building trust and member interdependence in order to become cohesive. A balance of members' and leader's roles will contribute to the group's productivity and survival. Learning to recognize when a group goes through stages of development, and phases of regression under stress, can help to strengthen the bonds of the group and potentially deepen members' understanding of how or when their needs and goals can be met by the group. Realizing the dynamic nature of the group as a system is an important step in learning to trust the process that seems inevitably inherent in groups, small or large, at the level of microcosm or macrocosm.

Now that a working definition of what constitutes a group has been established, the next chapter considers some of the literature that examines the evidence regarding the effectiveness of groups as a therapeutic modality or as offering positive benefits in their outcomes for individuals and populations.

Individual Learning Activities

REFLECTIVE QUESTIONS

1. How might characteristics of group structure affect the possibility of a group achieving specific goals? How could you address group structure if the group were open? If the group was closed? How could you address group structure if group membership were voluntary? Involuntary?

2. What is meant by group cohesiveness or cohesion? How might it be identified in the group?

3. Stages of group development are given many different names. According to Tuckman, what are the developmental stages that a group goes through? What does Mosey describe in her developmental levels? What are some of the issues and key variables at play in these models of group development?

4. How are the purpose and goals of activity and intra-psychic groups similar? How are they different?

LEARNING CHECKPOINTS

Describe how…

• Group size is related to the ability to participate in group activity and member interactions.

• A group's stage of development influences the type of member interactions and leadership roles.

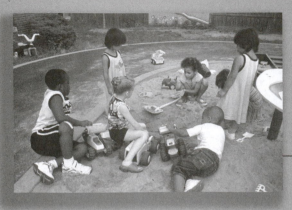

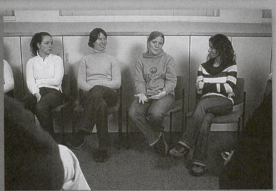

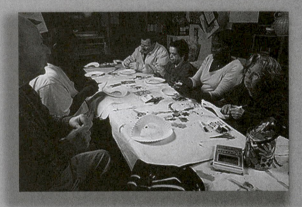

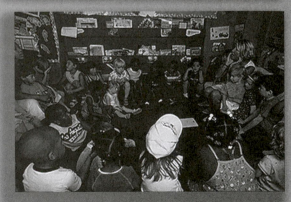

Why Do Groups?

The use of group work, in settings as diverse as hospitals, schools, and governmental and social agencies, continues to grow as the potential benefits and the versatility of the group format gain recognition. Group work is adaptable to a variety of contexts, and there are numerous approaches to guiding the structure and process of groups. Occupational therapists take the perspective of viewing groups in a macrocosm, also taking into consideration historical elements of the existence and functions of group work. Additionally, the fabric of daily life is really constructed of a subset of individual and group activities.

Events affecting health care, group work, and daily life in our global society include ongoing changes in technology, an adult population growing older, and aftereffects of war or acts of terrorism. Additionally, in health care in the United States, reimbursement policies for treatment interventions have created interest groups vying for limited resources as policy makers and administrators aim to control costs. Recently there has been an increased emphasis on client-centered practice as well. This calls for more attention to the contexts surrounding the client that influence performance as reflected in the Occupational Therapy Practice Framework (see Appendix A). Contexts can include the "cultural, physical, social, personal, spiritual, temporal, and virtual" (American Occupational Therapy Association, 2002, p. 630).

Research findings as well as the experiences and observations of group leaders and members about the effectiveness of group intervention add to these complex contexts. This body of knowledge and these perspectives expand understanding both of the nature and process of groups and the benefit of groups to the participants. Occupational therapy developed gradually on the premise of occupation, engagement in purposeful and meaningful tasks and roles that support one's participation in life, as a method of practice (Nelson, 1997). As such, occupation is viewed as both a means and an end product (Trombley, 1995) of occupational therapy services. Group practice has also evolved over the years. However, only in more recent times have group practitioners and researchers begun to explore the use of group activities as a therapeutic procedure. In this kaleidoscope of change, there has been renewed interest in occupation-based and client-centered practice and advances in research and an increased focus on reimbursement and evidence-based practice.

This chapter is titled "Why Do Groups?" Yet most research deals with *how* to do groups, *how* to achieve the best results, and *how* to manipulate the variables in group practice. The research studies provide data on group outcomes, from which *why* there is value to certain group approaches versus other modes of intervention can be inferred. As group leaders build skills and repertoire, clinical reasoning and experience bridge the relationship between the *why* and the *how*.

In reasoning about the procedures for maximizing group outcomes, the *how* to do groups, the leader should be guided by the following reasons as to *why* do groups (Howe & Schwartzberg, 2001):

- Groups provide an occupation-based experience that is reality-oriented and that promotes adaptation.
- Groups are a natural environment that can provide feedback and support for individual and social needs.
- Groups can be structured along a developmental continuum where the nonhuman objects lead the action and the activities are structured to promote group-centered action. Members can learn about their own capabilities in proximity to an externally designated leader, thereby stretching to their higher functional potential.
- Through participating in group activities that promote growth and change, members can learn and practice skills to master and achieve competence in activities required for daily life.
- Groups can be organized in a way to enable the group to lead the doing by giving the members a set of possibilities that empowers the group's capacity for self-direction.
- When groups provide an opportunity for dealing with real-life issues and objects, people can maintain, improve, or enhance their occupational nature to fulfill social demands.
- Postulates and hypotheses support this reasoning not only by a theoretical orientation but also by incorporating the best current research and evidence available as to the effectiveness of intervention approaches. The following discussion examines how evidence might be integrated into reasoning and practice (Fig. 2.1).

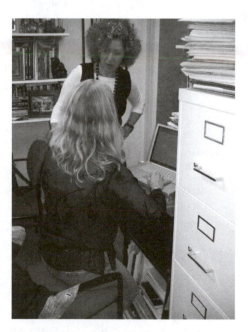

FIGURE 2.1 Evidenced-based practice: Searching. (Photo by Allison Tarin)

Evidence-Based Practice: Find Evidence, Use It, Contribute to It

Evidence-based practice was intended as a means to inform the consumer and provider about the effectiveness of interventions by addressing two main questions:

1. What is best practice?
2. What is the most cost-effective practice?

The process of evidence-based practice involves applying a line of reasoning through formulating questions to "search, evaluate, and use research evidence" (Tickle-Degnen & Bedell, 2003, p. 236) by asking:

"What is possible?"
"Is there a pattern?"
"Is there causality?"
"What is the probability?"

In searching, it is best to formulate a clear and specific question in regard to the:

• Needs of the client
• Possible types of intervention
• Other available options
• Desired outcome(s)

This process of defining what to investigate can be achieved through constructing a question via a structured method that looks at the following information. Remember the acronym PICO:

Person specifics
Intervention that might help (information about diagnostic tests or assessments, prognosis, prevention, therapy, type of occupational performance problem)
Comparison with an intervention (the usual treatment) versus no intervention (a control group)
Outcome(s) the client wants (Box 2.1)

In using evidence to guide practice, it is important to evaluate the level of rigor of the research evidence. The research study must be considered in regard to strength of study design as to size, populations, type of research, and research methodology (Table 2.1).

Although the number of research studies on occupational therapy group work has certainly increased, there are still relatively few that can be ranked highly in terms of levels of

Box 2.1   **Sample PICO Question**

Person:	"In clients who…"; "For a 67-year old woman with…"
Intervention:	"Can…"; "Does the use of…"
Comparison	"Compared with no treatment…"; "As compared with no…"
Outcome:	"Lead to improved [or reduced] symptoms of…"; "Lead to a decrease in… and increase in ability to (function)?"

Adapted from Bailey, D. (2002). Evidence-Based Practice. Tufts University, Medford, MA.

evidence. To be fair, there are many problems that are encountered in conducting research with groups. Standard controls for error are practically impossible to impose. Control groups without intervention cannot be introduced. Intervening variables such as other treatment interventions likely exist, and group functioning varies because each group has a unique membership. The fact that no two groups are alike poses problems of replication. Furthermore, the introduction of research methods can alter group perceptions and behaviors, leading to distorted outcomes as well as possibly affecting therapeutic alliances. Despite these problems, research studies of group work have been published. These studies deserve con-

Table 2.1   **Hierarchy of Levels of Evidence for Evidence-Based Practice**

Level	Description
I	Strong evidence from at least systematic review of multiple well-designed randomized controlled studies
II	Strong evidence from at least one properly designed randomized controlled study of appropriate size
III	Evidence from well-designed studies without randomization Single group pre- and post-test studies Matched case-controlled studies
IV	Evidence from well-designed nonexperimental studies from more than one site or research group
V	Descriptive studies (qualitative research) Opinions of respected authorities Reports of expert committees

Adapted from Evidenced-Based Everything by A. Moore, H. McQuay, & J. A. M. Gray (eds.). (1995). Bandolier, 1(12), p. 1.

sideration because important insights and inferences can be drawn from them, informing group work.

Considering the hierarchy of levels of evidence, strong evidence exists in relation to:

- Group size related to ability to participate in a group activity and interact with members (Howe & Schwartzberg, 2001; Yalom & Leszcz, 2005)
- Cohesiveness related to effectiveness of group intervention (Howe & Schwartzberg, 2001; Yalom & Leszcz, 2005)
- Group composition and cohesiveness in regard to the effectiveness of composing a group with members who have similar performance skills, goals, and abilities (interpersonal, communication, problem solving, decision making) to facilitate participation in activities (Schwartzberg, Howe, & McDermott, 1982)
- Flow state as a means to understanding the need for a balance between the challenges of the activity and the skills and interests of the individuals for enhanced participation (Persson, 1996)
- Choice and control, in that more client satisfaction and participation are seen when group goals are client-centered (Henry, Nelson, & Duncombe, 1984)
- Basic leadership functions in that "the higher the caring and the higher the meaning attribution the higher the positive outcome" (Yalom & Leszcz, 2005, p. 536)

Evidence-based practice can be a guide in terms of choices made in program development and interventions. Although some findings are stronger than others, the weaker findings should not be discounted.

A final important step in evidence-based practice is how findings are communicated to clients, colleagues, administration or management, and stakeholders, including funding sources. To do so, it is helpful to consider the following four steps:

1. Identify to whom research findings are likely to be communicated (client or family member, manager, funding source or payee) and their role in the decision-making process.
2. Identify which decisions can be made collaboratively.
3. Gather and interpret research evidence that is focused on the population of interest and that is the type of information needed by the decision maker(s).
4. Write up findings in a manner that allows all parties involved to have an informed discussion regarding their understanding of the evidence in order to facilitate decision making and a plan of action (adapted from Tickle-Degnen, 2002, p. 223).

As part of finding and using evidence, the literature and topics of interest to group leaders should be investigated continually for new research findings.

Therapeutic Factors:
Client and Group Therapist Views

One of the most relevant places to start looking at evidence-based practice in leading groups is to find out what group intervention might mean for the members and the leader. Through years of study and research, Yalom (Yalom & Leszcz, 2005) identified 11 "therapeutic factors" (pp. 1–2) that may be achieved through group work:

1. Instillation of hope
2. Universality
3. Imparting Information
4. Altruism
5. The corrective recapitulation of the primary family group
6. Development of socializing techniques
7. Imitative behavior
8. Interpersonal learning
9. Group cohesiveness
10. Catharsis
11. Existential factors

In addition to these eleven factors recognized in group psychotherapy, a study done with patients with psychiatric conditions who had been discharged from inpatient care found they identified being engaged in certain activities and developing new skills to be of particular therapeutic value (Eklund, 1997). A study of members' perceptions of "helping factors" in a community-based, occupational therapist–facilitated, peer-developed support group for survivors of head injury found believing in and feeling a part of the group were some of the positive attributes that contributed to a successful peer support group. Members of the group identified that they felt their head injuries to be a problem they all had in common and that, by sharing and receiving information through the group, they were able to validate the effects of the injury in a variety of ways. This process of legitimization, the acceptance of the head injury as real, appeared to be the primary factor that distinguished this group from professionally led groups (Schwartzberg, 1994). A follow-up study (Schulz, 1994) supported these findings with subtle differences in the types of concerns held by the support group members in the two groups studied. The concerns of the group members in the first study seemed more problem-focused, and those of the follow-up study group seemed broader in scope. Differences in research methodologies may account for these results. For example, individual differences in the perspectives of the participant observer in the first study and those of the head injury survivors who participated in the second study may account for the slight variations in the results.

Yalom and Leszcz (2005) reinforce the need to remain client-centered in examining the outcomes and effectiveness of group work, stating: "In research as in clinical work, we do well to heed the adage: Listen to the client" (p. 108). Furthermore, in elucidating the perspectives of clients and group leaders, Yalom and Leszcz (2005) state: "Therapists and their clients differ in their views about important therapeutic factors: clients consistently emphasize the importance of the relationship and the personal, human qualities of the therapist, whereas therapists attribute their success to their techniques. When the therapist-client discrepancy is too great, when therapists emphasize therapeutic factors that are incompatible with the needs and capacities of the group members, then the therapeutic enterprise will be derailed…" (p. 108).

Further research into client perceptions of group leaders showed four important basic leadership functions (Yalom & Leszcz, 2005):

1. *"Emotional activation* (challenging, confronting, modeling by personal risk-taking and high self-disclosure)
2. *Caring* (offering support, affection, praise, protection, warmth, acceptance, genuineness, concern)
3. *Meaning attribution* (explaining, clarifying, interpreting, providing a cognitive framework for change: translating feelings and experiences into ideas)
4. *Executive function* (setting limits, rules, norms, goals; managing time; pacing, stopping, interceding, suggesting procedures)" (p. 536)

These basic leadership functions were found to have a significant relationship to outcome, with greater amounts of caring and meaning attribution functions being directly related to positive outcomes.

Group Format and Group Process

In studying groups, researchers have often been concerned with the relationship between group format and group process. How might one influence the other and vice versa? Research findings come together as three questions regarding a group format's potential effects on variables that are intricately related to group process:

1. What influence does group format have on the *quality and quantity of interaction*?
2. What influence does group format have on the *meaning assigned to the group actions*?
3. What influence does group format have on the *members' functional status*?

Group Format and Quality and Quantity of Interaction

Group format will influence the nature of group interaction. In thinking about the group format, a leader should consider the aims of intervention in terms of the quality and quantity of interaction desired. A study of three group formats on an acute inpatient psychiatry unit of a general hospital sought to identify and analyze patterns in the quality and quantity of verbal interaction in these groups (Schwartzberg, Howe, & McDermott, 1982). The groups studied were a highly structured community group meeting, a moderately structured self-expression group with a combination of task-oriented and process-oriented occupational therapy group treatment, and an occupational therapy group in which the group format was more open, loosely structured to allowed patients to choose from a selection of arts and crafts as well as vocational activities of individual interest. The occupational therapy group that allowed more freedom of activity choice per member's interest showed a significantly greater amount of person-to-person communication and fewer incidences of nonparticipation by members in verbal exchanges (i.e., patients who neither spoke nor were addressed) than the other group formats. It may be inferred from this study that differences in quality and quantity of interaction are related to differences in a group's format.

A corollary hypothesis is that specific levels of group functioning are related in terms of members' age and group level. Using Mosey's (1970a) developmental group levels, children's level of functioning was found to be on a continuum, rather than strictly stage-specific, overlapping with group performance to some degree (Donohue, 2003). A group's ability to function as identified by Mosey is a developmental continuum of parallel (minimum member interaction, highly leader-dependent) to mature (interdependent member functioning with little to no leader input). At the outset, one might set a group format at the most basic level of parallel play for a group of very young children or adults with developmental disabilities. This highly structured group format would require high leader involvement in order for the members to be able to function safely. The parallel level group format would require the group process to be highly structured to support member participation and success. As the age of the children increases or the level of member functioning improves, the group level can be expected to advance to a project level at which more member interaction and less leader dependence are seen. The group format would gradually need to change to facilitate member-to-member interaction to allow the group process as well as the members' functional abilities to evolve.

Group Format and the Meaning Assigned to Group Action

The meaning of group activities is central to the nature of a member's experience. The therapist needs to consider the therapeutic advantages of particular group activities and their meaning for group participants relative to group action as they determine group format. A study of patients with persistent and chronic mental illness, engaged in three different group activities in a community day treatment program, looked at the meaning a patient population assigns to the group activity (Kremer, Nelson, & Duncombe, 1984). Patients were randomly assigned to three occupational therapy groups: cooking group, craft activity group, and sensory awareness activity group. After the group activity, each patient rated the affective meaning of the activity. Results showed some differences in the affective meaning of these three activities. Another study examined the affective responses of subjects to having or not having freedom of choice in engaging in a particular activity (Henry, Nelson, & Duncombe, 1984). In addition, the researchers compared the responses of subjects to completing the activity in an individual versus a group setting. The subjects in this study were college students. The results indicated that there was a significant relationship between choice and affective meaning for activities in the group setting. Subjects in the group with no choice of activity rated themselves as feeling significantly less powerful than those in the group who had a choice.

An exploratory study (Persson, 1996) utilized play and flow theory as a basis for examining whether "attention-focus" could be a means to identify "play/flow" [p/f] and "non-play/non-flow" [np/nf] episodes in an activity group using creative occupations with chronic pain patients. The group participants in each of the sessions were given an activity proposal structured with a different theme. The format of the group sessions was organized to have an introductory phase, an activity phase, and a reflection/discussion phase. Of particular significance were the findings regarding the relationship between task structure and participant states of arousal, curiosity, and attention: "the frustrations of the np/nf states almost exclusively seemed to be due to the challenge presented in the tasks occasionally being experienced as too great in relation to the skills of the participants….periods of the 'in-between state' of the participants, in this study called neutral, were more difficult to demarcate from np/nf states….Between these episodes there was a gradual transition which was difficult to appraise, while the transition from the neutral to p/f episodes shows a sharper qualitative change in behaviour" (Persson, 1996, p. 39).

Group Format and Member Functional Status

The group leader also needs to decide what type of group format to select. The type of format selected will likely influence the outcomes and functional status of members. The widely acclaimed University of Southern California Well Elderly Research Study (Clark, et al., 1997; Jackson, et al., 1998; Mandel, et al., 1999) provides strong support for the effectiveness of group programs on member functioning and quality of life. In this large-scale randomized controlled study, a group program using an occupation-based format was found to be highly successful in influencing the physical and mental health, occupational functioning, and life satisfaction of a culturally diverse population of well elders. The well elderly study program model is a design well suited for replication with other populations.

Interestingly, a large-scale, population-based, 13-year study of the elderly confirmed the importance of social engagement and productive activity in relation to successful aging

(Glass, et al., 1999). Social activity was found to be as responsible for lowering the risk of mortality as were fitness activities. One inference was that activity might confer survival benefits through psychosocial means. Another study conducted with patients who had experienced cranial trauma and stroke showed the feasibility of increasing levels of leisure and social activity via occupational therapy group intervention (Teasdale, Christensen, & Pinner, 1993). Treatment outcomes achieved by individuals with psychiatric impairment who received outpatient group-based occupational therapy were compared with those of a matched group receiving verbal therapy (Eklund, 1999). Results indicated that the occupational therapy group format was helpful for some patients on a variety of outcome variables relating to occupational performance, global mental health, and psychiatric symptoms. One factor that was isolated was effective occupational therapy group programs had a well-articulated frame of reference. In this case, it was inferred that the occupational therapy group program's effectiveness resulted from conscious use of object relations theory that consistently framed the leader's behavior and therapeutic approach.

A study of a group for adults with head injury, again using Mosey's developmental group structure in a controlled social environment, found trends in improvement in memory and social interaction skills (Lundgren & Persechino, 1986). Similarly, a study of groups with healthy older adults found task group structure can have "a significant effect on verbal interaction, nonverbal interaction, and the perception of action in the group" (Nelson, et al., 1988, p. 28). Groups structured in a project format, wherein sharing and interaction are required for successful task completion, elicited more verbal and nonverbal interaction than groups structured in parallel fashion, where each member has his or her own task supplies required for successful task completion. Determining group structure in advance (amount of sharing and creativity required) may foster or inhibit different types of social interaction or affect depending on the needs of members.

In a study of female graduate students it was found that even a moderate limitation in the supply of the essential tools used in a stenciling activity increased group engagement and decreased conflict (Steffan & Nelson, 1987). A collage task introduced as an activity group with the leader assuming the role of nondirective helper versus introducing the collage task as a parallel activity was concluded as possibly causing each group to develop its own character and atmosphere. The activity group interacted in a positive way (talking when finished with activity) and the parallel task format in a less positive way (silence when finished and waiting) (Froehlich & Nelson, 1986).

A study of clients receiving activity therapy versus verbal therapy in a psychiatric day treatment program found greater symptom reduction and an increase in independent functioning in the community in areas such as self-esteem and decision making (Klyczek & Mann, 1986). Little overall difference in community tenure was noted between the two groups (patients with activity therapy were hospitalized significantly more often than those with verbal therapy but for a shorter duration than the verbal therapy group). The effectiveness of a verbal versus an activity group format in relation to improvement in self-perceptions of interpersonal communication skills was compared in another study in psychiatric day treatment (DeCarlo & Mann, 1985). Findings showed "a significantly higher level of [perceived] interpersonal communication skills was attained by the activity group" (p. 20).

A more recent study by Bickes, et al. (2001) furthers knowledge about the effectiveness of verbal and experiential occupational therapy groups as measured by the outcome of functional performance in money management skills. In this study no significant difference was found between the "primarily listening" versus "primarily doing" groups (p. 52). However, overall findings showed that a population of chronically mentally ill individuals achieved improved performance in money management skills through occupational therapy group intervention. The small sample size, lack of control group, and small data set were recognized limitations.

Clinical Reasoning and Program Development

Designing a group program requires selecting activities through searching the literature and utilizing one's clinical reasoning. Clinical reasoning is a dynamic process of inquiry in action that takes place in the context of evaluation and intervention. Through clinical reasoning, the therapist thinks about "what to do and why; how to proceed; what works; and what to change" (Cohn & Czycholl, 1990, pp. 171–172) when working with the client. The clinical reasoning process applies whether the client is an individual or a population in need of group services. Therefore, in developing a group, the reasoning process involves asking the questions:

Who is the population is being served?
What outcomes are expected as a result of the intervention?
Is there evidence that one group format is more effective than another?
How does what is known inform:

- How to interact with the group members
- What procedures to select
- Under what conditions

Assume individuals with Alzheimer's disease or dementia as an example (Fig. 2.2). Start with what is known: Support groups for individuals with mild cognitive impairment that may or may not develop into full dementia are often referred to as "early stage groups." The types of groups used with persons with dementia range from psychotherapy, support, psychoeducational, and therapeutic activity interventions or programs, which include the subset of

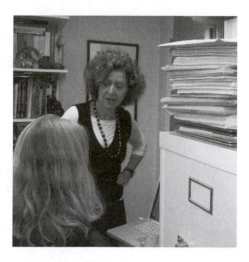

FIGURE 2.2 Evidenced-based practice: Considering. (Photo by Allison Tarin)

intergenerational groups. Another need for these individuals and their families is education and support groups for caregivers and other family members dealing with the losses and devastation of this disease. Outcomes of group treatment that are expected are increased quality of life for clients and their caregivers and improved client functional performance in terms of social participation and task engagement (personal communication, Dementia and Groups, Scott Trudeau, July 12, 2006).

In searching the literature, one discovers that group format is highly important in the selection of activities. In a nursing home for individuals with Alzheimer's type and other dementias, an art-based activity group was effective in being a stimulus to increase residents' ability to identify emotions and socialize with other group members (Bober, et al., 2002). Further searching uncovers support for reminiscence groups for enhancing quality of life for nursing home residents with dementia (Vivero-Chong, 2002), more so than goal-directed crafts or games and unstructured time (Brooker & Duce, 2000). One program outcome study reported Montessori-based activities, using a "rehabilitation approach" of task breakdown, guided repetition, and moving from simple to complex, as more effective with individuals across stages of dementia versus using a variety of activities in the usual individual, small group, and large group activity programs. The program studied produced more active engagement and pleasure for participants when principles similar to the Montessori method of education and those principles guiding occupational therapy approaches were utilized as part of the group format and process (Orsulic-Jeras, Schneider, & Camp, 2000).

These findings, along with generally accepted practice, suggest the type of group programming indicated for clients with Alzheimer's disease and dementia who are in structured settings such as a nursing home. They provide a template for client interaction as one of careful selection of activities to promote outcomes such as social engagement and pleasure.

Using an evidenced-based approach provides information about the value of the interventions to communicate to the group members, family members, program managers, and funding parties as part of the decision-making process of group program design and outcomes measurement.

Conclusion

Although not conclusive, the literature (see Appendix B) does demonstrate that group format has an effect on the quality and quantity of interaction, meaning assigned to the group action, and members' functional status. New and creative ways need to be developed to evaluate the outcomes of different types of group intervention. Descriptive and phenomenological research designs may prove to be better suited for evaluating the complex variables found in group outcome studies. For example, it is important that concepts of "social function," "social skills," and "social cognition" be clearly defined and not used interchangeably to enable accurate measurement and outcome studies. Such clarity will assist evidenced-based practitioners to better select and evaluate intervention programs for social behaviors that are multidimensional (Yager & Ehmann, 2006). A phenomenological study regarding the complexity of occupational therapy group work makes a case for careful study of the clinical reasoning supporting interventions (Ward, 2003). Research can also help describe more accurately the processes within groups. Gaining greater clarification of these concepts will further their being better understood by group practitioners, group members, and researchers. Because of the increasing concern with accountability in the health-care professions, research on the outcomes of various approaches has become especially important. The information generated through research is crucial to enhancing the clinical reasoning abilities of group leaders to make discerning choices among intervention alternatives.

Individual Learning Activities

REFLECTIVE QUESTIONS

1. On a continuum from least evidence to most evidence, where do you imagine further research on group work?

2. How would you introduce information at a team meeting to explain the value of your group intervention?

LEARNING CHECKPOINTS

Describe a type of group (social, exercise, craft, therapy, occupational therapy, etc.) that would benefit the following individuals and the evidenced-based implications:

PICO Question 1

Person: For a 70-year-old woman who is socially isolated

Intervention: Can a (type) group

Comparison: Compared with no intervention

Outcome: Lead to improved sense of well-being and increased social participation?

PICO Question 2

Person: For a 80-year-old man who lives alone

Intervention: Can a (type) group

Comparison: Compared with no intervention

Outcome: Reduce symptoms of depression and increase quality of life?

PICO Question 3

Person: In children who are at risk for delinquency

Intervention: Does participation in an after-school (type) group

Comparison: As compared with no intervention

Outcome: Lead to improved self-concept and reduced at-risk activities?

PICO Question 4

Person: For a client with schizophrenia

Intervention: Can a supportive, reality-focused, and structured group

Comparison: Compared with an exploration and insight-oriented group

Outcome: Lead to improved interpersonal skill functioning and reduced symptoms?

PICO Question 5

Person: For a school-age child with attention deficit disorder

Intervention: Does the use of a closed, small group

Comparison: As compared with an open, large group

Outcome: Lead to improved performance skills (motor, process, and communication) and client factors (attention) as well as enhanced occupational performance in areas of education, play, or social participation?

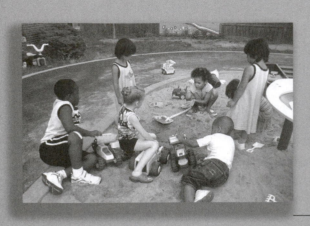

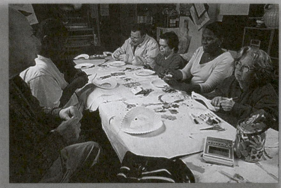

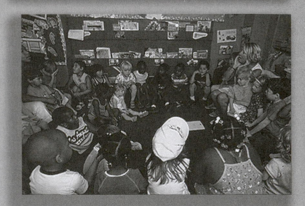

What Does the Leader Do?

Having looked at what might constitute a group and how evidence can guide reasoning, the central questions of this chapter are:

What is a leader?
What do leaders actually do when they are running a group?

Some associate the term leader with followers. To be a leader do you need to have a destination in mind? One definition of a leader is "a person who can influence others to be more effective in working to achieve their mutual goals and maintain effective working relationships among members" (Johnson & Johnson, 2006, p. 168). Perhaps you think leadership is based on natural instinct; either one is born a leader or not. If this is a concern you harbor in wondering if you can be a group leader, rest assured. As you will discover in this chapter, there are definite theories, skills, and strategies one can learn to become an effective leader. In our experience, more effective leaders draw upon a theoretical base for what they do; they reflect on their practice; and they are willing to change direction to enhance the experience of group members.

Theories of Leadership

Social scientists have long been interested in the subject of leadership, and much research has been done on the topic. Researchers have been primarily concerned with identifying specific characteristics that make individuals effective leaders. In approaching this issue, social scientists accepted a number of diverse assumptions about leadership. Consequently, their studies led them in many directions (Hersey, Blanchard, & Johnson, 2001) trying to discern how leaders motivate and mobilize individuals and groups. For our purposes we will briefly discuss some of the most common, or perhaps popular, views of leaders.

One theory focuses on personal traits (Bennis, 1989). A second states that leaders' actions must be seen in context with their constituents, thus having elements that were considered contingency or situational (Fiedler, 1967; Hersey, Blanchard, & Johnson, 2001). A third states that leaders assume styles according to the amount of power and control they can or will allow the group members in the decision-making process (Lewin, Lippitt, & White, 1939; Stogdill, 1948). A fourth identifies with the notion of group task and maintenance functions, looking at the member behaviors that are necessary for groups to successfully satisfy individual as well as group needs and goals (Bales, 1965). More recently, organizational leadership has been promoted as that of a relationship. Viewed as a form of self-development, principles and behaviors have been identified to enable individuals to learn how to be a leader. In this manner, assuming leadership roles is seen as a means to empower others (Kouzes & Posner, 2003).

Trait

For many years, researchers viewed leadership as the combination of personal traits in a particular person. They studied particular traits that they believed a good leader should possess: intelligence, warmth, decisiveness, and assertiveness. This approach yielded little conclusive evidence. There were, inevitably, good leaders who were not decisive, warm, or assertive. This direction of inquiry also proved futile in identifying prospective leaders. Nevertheless, the research results did suggest "that leadership is a relationship that exists between persons in a social situation, and that persons who are leaders in one situation may not necessarily be leaders in other situations" (Stogdill, 1948, p. 65).

Situational

When research into personality traits failed to provide conclusive data, social scientists turned to studying the circumstances in which leadership was present, asking: do leaders emerge from a particular set of group circumstances? The hypothesis was that a leader's behavior in one setting might differ from that of another leader in a different setting. In addition, it was postulated that the behavior of a leader might differ from one group situation to another. This course of inquiry was pursued via a study of groups on a naval vessel during wartime. It was found that leaders changed according to the demands of the situation. When there was little work to be done on board and groups faced inactivity and boredom, individuals who could be entertaining became popular and won recognition. When the ship came to port, those who had knowledge about the port, had been there before, or had contacts on land immediately became the leaders of the group (Homans, 1950). This study seems to emphasize that groups select leaders according to how well an individual's skill or knowledge meets the needs of the situation rather than a skill, or a set of skills, that can be learned or developed. One model of situational leadership promotes the concept that leader behavior needs to be based on constituent readiness (Hersey, Blanchard, & Johnson, 2001). Four categories of leader behavior (telling, selling, participating, delegating) are identified, to be used depending on the follower's willingness or ability to handle a situation. These leader behaviors can also be viewed as styles of leadership if the individual lacks awareness of the need to adjust his or her behavior to the situation.

Styles

A seminal study on leadership styles examined the effects that different leadership behaviors had on groups of 10-year-old boys in a summer day camp. Group leaders were trained to assume three different leadership styles:

1. Autocratic
2. Democratic
3. Laissez-faire (Lewin, Lippitt, & White, 1939)

In the autocratic group, the decision-making power was under the control of the designated leader. In the democratic group, the decision-making power was in the control of the group but under the guidance of the leader. In the laissez-faire group, the decision-making power was left entirely to the individuals in the group.

The autocratic leader dictated rules to be followed and did not discuss problems with the children. He did not participate in the group except when giving instructions and demonstrating how the instructions should be followed. Under democratic leadership, all policies were open for discussion and decision by the group. The leader helped the group to build a decision-making process of its own. The leader acted as a resource person for the group. The laissez-faire leader presented the group members with the supplies they needed for their work and gave them information when asked. Otherwise, this leader took no part in the group.

Five conclusions were reached after evaluating these three groups:

1. The democratic leadership style resulted in a more satisfying, efficient leadership than did the laissez-faire.
2. Autocratic leadership resulted in slightly higher group productivity than did the other two leadership styles but showed a significantly poorer quality of work than did the group with democratic leadership.
3. The autocratic leadership style created hostility and aggression in the group members.
4. There was greater dependency and less individuality in the autocratically led group than in the democratic group.
5. A greater degree of group cohesiveness, a sense of comradeship, and a high morale were seen more in the democratic group than in either of the other two groups.

It is clear that different styles of leadership result in different types of behaviors among group members. You may want to ask yourself, What is my natural inclination? Do you tend to assume more of a democratic, autocratic, or laissez-faire style? As you learn more about yourself as a leader, you may find situations indicate that you modify your style depending on the goals of a group, the population, and setting.

Group Functions: Task and Maintenance

Leadership functions are directly related to group functions. Leadership is viewed as the ability to promote behaviors in members that lead to the satisfaction of group needs or goals. Task and maintenance functions can balance the group process (Benne & Sheats, 1978); these functions were at one time ascribed to leaders (Bales, 1950). In thinking about these functions from the perspective of the role of the leader, the task function relates to how the leader will facilitate the achievement of the group goals or tasks. The maintenance function relates to how the leader helps the group build and maintain a process that enables the group to strengthen itself. In successful groups, a balance of task and maintenance functions is needed to support the ongoing life of the group. Group behavior may address both of these functions simultaneously, but frequently one function may be served at the expense of the other. It is frequently assumed that if a group is called together to perform a task, only what is relevant to the task is important. Yet, when members join a group, they enter as a whole person and do not separate their rational or problem-solving self from their emotional self. For example, a group may be so intent on reaching the task goal that it does not strengthen its decision-making process and depends on one individual (perhaps the leader) to make all decisions. In this case, the group is putting its efforts into task functions while neglecting its maintenance functions. Understanding the task and maintenance functions of the group allows the leader to assume or facilitate member roles to meet both the task and social-emotional needs to bring balance to the group's process.

In most group situations, someone is designated as leader. The leader can facilitate members learning to assume both task and maintenance functions so these roles are shared in the group. The relative importance of group building (maintenance) and goal achievement (task) for any group may change dramatically from early meetings to later stages of development.

Co-leadership

The use of co-leaders in a group is recommended whenever possible, particularly for relatively inexperienced group leaders. You may have had negative experiences working with others and prefer to take charge yourself. This is a time to reconsider the risks of going it alone. Co-leadership has several benefits. It is often difficult, even in a small group of six members, for the leader to attend to both the group process and the content at the same time. These tasks can be advantageously shared between the co-leaders. For instance, one leader may be particularly attentive to what the group members are saying while the co-leader may concentrate on the actions and reactions of the group members. Co-leaders in a group may find opportunities to model interpersonal behaviors for group members in their interactions with each other. This can serve as an encouragement for members to explore new or tentative behaviors.

There are other advantages to a co-leadership arrangement. Both leaders can contribute their observations to the preplanning process and to the post-group evaluation. The planning and analysis will benefit from these dialogues. One of the drawbacks of a co-leadership format is that co-leaders need to set aside time to plan and process the group as well as to review their collaborative processes. Co-leaders need to be clear about:

- Frames of reference and how they influence their actions and interpretations as group leaders
- Leadership style similarities or differences
- How they will balance their leadership in the group sessions
- Their conflict agenda, including personal levels of comfort with conflict and confrontation, ability to tolerate and address issues of transference/countertransference, and skills with, or approach to, limit setting (Box 3.1)

These are important issues to discuss in order to maintain group cohesiveness. If members perceive a notable difference in styles, responses to situations, or how each leader handles certain behaviors or issues, a phenomenon called splitting may occur in the group. This results in certain members seeking out one leader versus another in hopes that this person will ally with them, favoring their agenda or behavior in the group. Subgrouping may occur, which adds to division and lack of cohesion in the group. Splitting or subgrouping can be very detrimental to an effective group process and the group experience for both leaders and members if not monitored and addressed within the co-leadership and the group.

Although co-leadership can add appreciably to the quality of the group, it does require more time, which is not always available. Co-leaders in a group also need to be very sensitive to the amount of the group's time they use, particularly if one of the group goals is increasing member-to-member interaction and socialization skills. For example, in an average group of seven to nine members that lasts 1 hour, there are only 6 to 8 minutes per person of "air" time.

Strategies of Leadership

The structure of the group helps to establish the legitimate group norms, values, and limits of behavior. The group leader has a role in this process, particularly in the early stages. The

Box 3.1   **Position of Strength**

The leader is viewed as the central person or spokesperson of the group, and his or her overt behavior strengthens the norms and values of the group.

leader helps members learn new behaviors that will increase their ability to balance the task and social-emotional aspects of the group. In this way, the group becomes an environment in which members can learn to effectively and appropriately meet other members' needs while achieving group goals. This learning process can occur through direct instruction, group experiences, or a combination of both. Through the group process, leaders facilitate members working toward personal goals and dealing with or addressing their own issues or needs. Leaders need to be highly attuned to key aspects of the group process and utilize leadership strategies and skills to achieve this aim effectively.

Although feelings of chaos may be part of the experience when leading a group, leading a group is not a haphazard process. Although you will find every situation unique, patterns emerge that repeat themselves in leading small groups. There are group processes that are visible, and those that are hidden, or latent. Complex unconscious forces emerge in the leaders, members, and group as a whole. These dynamics can be constructive, or they can be destructive for individuals as well as the group as a whole. Interactive reasoning involves recognizing these dynamic forces and informs what the leader does and how the leader makes decisions about group interventions.

Interactive Reasoning

Interactive reasoning is a collaborative process (Mattingly & Fleming, 1994), and the clinical reasoning behind group process interventions needs to be made explicit (Ward, 2003). Elements of interactive reasoning include:

1. active listening,
2. being genuine and empathic,
3. building an alliance,
4. observing cues and clarifying meaning,
5. giving and receiving information, and
6. "reality testing" (Schwartzberg, 2002, p. 24)

Discoveries in "interpersonal neurobiology" (Siegel, 2001) enhance understanding of how the interpersonal and the neurological are intricately linked. In a well-reasoned group intervention, elements of fostering secure attachments in children can actually serve as a model for interactive reasoning, provided five basic elements are present:

1. Collaboration (p. 78)
2. Reflective dialogue (p. 79)
3. Repair (p. 79)
4. Coherent narratives (p. 79)
5. Emotional communication (p. 79) (Box 3.2)

Box 3.2   **Elements for Fostering Secure Attachments
and Emotionally Attuned Communication**

> *Collaboration*: Attuned communication, often in nonverbal communication
> *Reflective dialogue*: Verbal sharing of internal experiences and meaning-making process through collaborative and reciprocal communication
> *Repair*: Healing of inevitable disconnections in attuned communication through "consistent, predictable, reflective, intentional, and mindful caregiving"
> *Coherent narratives*: The creation of an "autobiographical form of self-awareness, a connection of the past, present, and future"
> *Emotional communication*: Sharing and connecting during positive moments and uncomfortable emotional states. (Siegel, 2001, pp. 78–79)

Carefully implementing these elements of interaction as a leader can allow a meaningful and therapeutic interpersonal exchange and helps foster the transformative potential and healing nature of the group process.

Understanding Transference and Countertransference

An essential task of the leader is to be aware of member transference and personal countertransference in the group. Transference involves members' projection of their inner world of feelings, conflicts, and association onto others. A countertransference response is when the leader's psychological world, unaware and exposed, elicits a reaction to the group process, members, and co-leader. Brown (2003) explains, "members often lack awareness of what is happening and this can lead to feelings of being stuck and accomplishing little, a very uncomfortable and distressing atmosphere. The leader speaks of what is hidden or not understood and the effect of these on the group and its members" (p. 238).

The leader's unexamined countertransference can lead to mistakes in leadership. Unresolved conflicts can create problems, such as managing boundary violations improperly, scapegoating, and creating difficult patients due to poor member selection as norms in the group (Gans & Alonso, 1998). Modern thinking on group process views the group as a "multi-person field" where the leader and member dynamics emerge together (Box 3.3). Bernard (2005) suggests the following self-reflective questions for therapist monitoring

Box 3.3   **Transference/Countertransference: A Modern View**

> Viewing the processes of transference and counter-transference as a co-construction of all parties involved, leader and member(s), has been a useful shift in understanding the potential usefulness and opportunities for working through these dynamics (Bernard, 2005).

and making meaning of their reactions: "What does my experience mean about me and what does my experience mean about one, or a subgroup, or all of the patients with whom I am working?" (p. 153).

Harnessing Destructive Group Forces

Whether you are a beginning therapist or a seasoned one, problems will emerge in a group because of the nature of process and the difficulties members bring to the experience. It is a heavy burden to expect perfection because group process innately has conflict. Engaging the destructive elements is the challenge. Nitsun (1996; 2000) outlines many factors that he calls "anti-group" phenomena that can be harnessed so that creativity emerges in the group. Working to challenge the belief that individual therapy is better than group therapy is one example of countering a negative assumption. By engaging the destructive forces, structuring the group in such a way to promote function, what initially seems negative can become a force for productivity. Care in the selection and planning of group activities is a strategy that can help structure the group in order to maximize its potential.

Selecting and Planning Group Activities

The group leader is initially responsible for planning the group activity. In the early sessions of a closed or ongoing group, the leader must select the group task and decide the duration, number, and types of tasks in each meeting. As soon as possible, the members need to be involved in:

• Selecting tasks
• Formulating and adapting the goals of the group's activity

The process of choosing an activity relies on one's professional knowledge of activities. In selecting a group activity, the following main points need to be considered:

The goals of the activity should have meaning for the group members. The meaning of any activity will vary, depending on the stages of development of the group. The activity should be useful to individual members and related to their culture, interests, life roles, etc.

The group members should be able to participate in choosing or adapting the given activity, to promote a maximal level of self-initiated mental, social, or physical participation.

The activity demands should enable members to take an active role in the group. The task should arouse member interest, and the demands of the task should elicit an adaptive response.

Members' response(s) should suggest an ability to interact with the environment that is supported by neural organization at the subcortical level.

The activity should be chosen according to member skills, ages, and/or performance levels. This includes an awareness of individuals' extent of participation, identification with, relationship to, and role in the group (adapted from Hopkins, Smith, & Tiffany, 1983).

The activity may be play, leisure, social, educational, or work-related. However, regardless of its nature, the tasks involved must facilitate attainment of group as well as individual goals. Group discussion is an activity common to practically all group meetings, but the leader, in consultation with the group, must decide how to balance time spent in discussion with time spent on specific tasks. At the end of the group session, a discussion of the activity experience can generate a realistic evaluation of member participation.

Members of therapy groups often have a limited repertoire of social skills and interests. They may often have met with failure when attempting new tasks, and this failure may discourage their involvement in new experiences. Because of this, the group leader may need to not only plan the activity but also stimulate member interest in the task and structure social interaction. This will require active use of effective leadership skills.

Effective Leadership

Leading a group requires a particular knowledge base and set of skills. The more the leader practices and follows principles of effective leadership, the more likely members will achieve their aims. Nevertheless, the leader cannot expect group outcomes to exceed members' capacities, no matter how optimal the leadership or positive the intentions.

As we proceed with establishing necessary tools of effective leadership, note to yourself both positive and negative reactions you have to the suggested methods. Awareness of such biases will help you to be in more conscious control of your work with a group. Identifying areas of strength and those in need of attention for skill development and effectiveness is also an essential piece of understanding what the leader does.

Ways in which the group leader can increase the effectiveness of the group are to help the group:

- Come to a clear understanding of the goals that it wants to reach
- Become aware of its own procedures
- Understand the skills, talents, and resources within its membership
- Develop group methods of evaluation so that both leader and members can find ways of improving their procedures
- Learn to accept new ideas and members without conflict
- Create new tasks and terminate outdated ones (Lippitt, 1961)

Many of these suggestions strongly resemble the conduct found in the democratic leadership style. The synergistic process of the leader role is to develop and support the processes within the group that enable members to grow and take on greater responsibility for making decisions and reaching group goals. Leaders are in a dynamic relationship with the members. This relationship calls on the interactive reasoning skills and related actions of the leader. In this context, the emphasis is on:

What actions are required by the group members, under various conditions, if they are to achieve their goals?

How can group members best take part in these actions?

When leadership is defined in terms of behaviors that further the goals of the group, it may become difficult to separate the roles of leader and member. Groups with a highly structured, leader-centered process have low membership involvement. Groups with an emphasis on membership involvement have less leadership involvement. The range of possible leadership styles and member involvement can be identified on a continuum ranging from authoritarian, task-focused, leader-controlled behavior to more democratic group-controlled and relationship-oriented behavior (Fig. 3.1) (Tannenbaum & Schmidt, 1958). Your prior experience in working with groups will affect your expectations for leader involvement and your behavior as a leader. Facilitating a group is not the same as being a teacher, for example. The

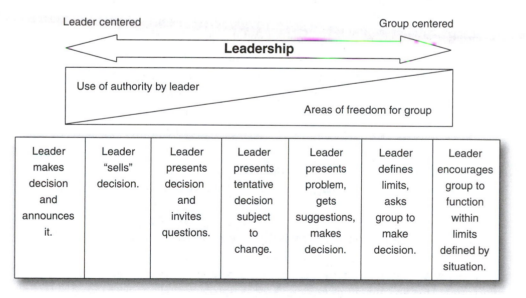

FIGURE 3.1 Leader-member continuum. (Modified from Tannenbaum, R & Schmidt, W. H. [1958]. How to choose a leadership pattern. Harvard Business Review, 36, March-April, 96.)

members are not students for whom you are an authority figure with discrete knowledge to impart. As such, the leader role is not didactic, but rather group-centered and process-oriented.

Working with informal groups in the community, such as family or peer groups, may require a leader approach different from that of a more structured group. The leadership role may be closer to that of a consultant, educator, or resource person. In such cases, leader inter-action with group members may be limited and defined by the members and situation. The family or peer group may wish to retain or need to be supported in their predetermined lead-ership but require assistance with effective communication and effecting change in how it functions or relates as a group.

The theory that leadership varies according to the leader's interaction with the group requires developing the skills necessary for active participation in a variety of group functions and leadership roles. Understanding one's abilities in terms of interpersonal skills and the intrapersonal dynamics at play in terms of how one relates to others may also serve as a measure of the extent to which one's leadership behavior matches one's intended role as group leader.

Genuineness and Empathy

A genuine person is one who can be him- or herself while interacting with other people and remain open to the feelings and attitudes that are experienced. This general principle applies to a group leader (Box 3.4). The term "genuineness" implies an ability to share inti-mate feelings when appropriate. A group leader is conscious of the feelings he or she is expe-riencing and is able to communicate them appropriately to the group members, when necessary. A study of therapy groups found that group members who viewed their leader as "open, accepting, responsive, and confident" did not drop out of the groups as readily as did those members who saw their leader as "distant, neutral, or professional" (Galigor, 1977).

Two characteristics of the genuine person have been identified as spontaneity and non-defensiveness. The genuine person is able to communicate easily about immediate events without being impulsive. When the leader reflects on what has been said in the group, he or she is motivated by a concern for the group members, not by self-protection. He has a feeling for his areas of strength and his areas of deficit in living and presumably is working toward being more effective all the time. When a client expresses negative attitudes, rather than

Box 3.4   **Genuine and Empathic Leadership**

"The basic posture of the therapist to a client must be one of concern, acceptance, genuineness, empathy. Nothing, no technical consideration, takes precedence over this attitude." (Yalom & Leszcz, 2005, p. 117)

becoming defensive, the leader tries to understand what the client is thinking and feeling and continues to work with him (Egan, 1975).

Empathy, often explained as caring for and understanding another individual, is another skill of the effective group leader. In a factor analysis of leader behaviors, it was found that the most effective leaders were rated high in caring (Lieberman, Yalom, & Miles, 1973). Caring was defined as a leadership style that offered members protection, friendship, and affection. Caring leaders provided frequent opportunities for members to receive feedback, as well as praise and encouragement for their behavior. Another quality of caring was careful listening and attending to what was being expressed in the group. Members are reassured when the leader validates their feelings or experience, can identify with or relate to their problem(s) or point of view, and accepts their emotional reactions at face value. Communication that conveys respect and caring is supportive and reduces the potential defensiveness of the other person. Nonverbal communication (gestures, facial expression, body posture/position, nodding, eye contact appropriate to the individual's culture, and other behavioral signs that indicate listening) is also important in expressing empathy and caring.

Communicating

Interpersonal effectiveness depends on one's ability to communicate clearly, convey the desired impression, and influence another person in a specific manner. Leadership effectiveness builds on interpersonal effectiveness and can be improved through developing one's skills in several areas, including:

• How one listens and responds to others
• Giving and receiving feedback
• Using concrete language
• Confrontation, when appropriate, to facilitate adjustment of behavior
• Self-disclosure
• Meaning attribution (Yalom, 1985; Yalom & Leszcz, 2005)
• Reality testing

The following sections consider each of these leadership skills and how they relate to the context of a group's process and dynamics.

Listening and Responding

The way one listens and responds to another person is crucial for building a positive, trusting relationship. In a close relationship, it is important to let the other person know that what was said was both heard and understood. This is also an important skill when building a therapeutic relationship. Active listening is a very important aspect of effective communication. This technique involves reflecting back to an individual what was heard and how it was understood.

One of the major barriers to building close relationships is the tendency to judge, evaluate, approve, or disapprove of a statement that has been made (Johnson & Johnson, 2003). This process can occur almost automatically when someone makes a statement and you "respond inwardly or openly with, 'I think you're wrong,' 'I don't like what you said,' 'I think you are right,' or 'That is the greatest (or worst) idea I have ever heard'" (p. 142). People tend to respond with evaluative statements when strong feelings are involved. The stronger the feelings, the more likely that the individual(s) involved will evaluate the statements according to their own points of view. However, as Johnson and Johnson (2006) wisely note: "Failures to communicate effectively surround us every day, more often bringing problems and discomfort….In fact, breakdowns in communication bring such pain and difficulties that the study of group dynamics pays a great deal of attention to effective group communication" (p. 131).

Learning to be a good listener is an important skill for every group leader. It takes considerable effort and practice to learn to listen accurately and objectively. Below are four suggestions for improving listening skills:

1. Make a firm commitment to listen.
2. Get physically ready to listen and attend (stop what you are doing, face the person with open/relaxed body posture, etc.).
3. Dismiss other concerns from your mind. Concentrate on the other person as a communicator.
4. Give the person a full hearing, avoiding interruption unless absolutely necessary. Impatience can lead to false understanding.

Giving and Receiving Feedback

Stating, or demonstrating nonverbally, one's reaction to another person's behavior is called feedback. The purpose of this technique is to help other people become aware of how their behavior is perceived and how their behavior affects another. Feedback should be given in a manner that is not threatening or demoralizing to the other person. The general rule of stating feedback through the use of 'I' statements is an important aspect of the feedback process. Rather than say, for example, "Your being late for group is an irresponsible thing to do," the leader could say, "I feel frustrated when we delay the start of group because you are late. When members come late to group, sometimes I feel a nonverbal message is being sent about how they feel about being in the group. I am left wondering how you might be feeling or what your thoughts are about being a part of this group." The more defensive individuals are, however, the less likely they will be able to correctly hear and understand the leader's remarks or intent. The remarks may become distorted by their own internal distress or feelings about themselves and be perceived in negative manner or as a personal affront or attack. Clarification may be needed to help convey the message, whether it is one of concern or in fact feedback and limit setting that the behavior is not allowed or acceptable.

In a group, members benefit from feedback about whether what they are doing has a positive as well as negative effect. By knowing not only what is ineffective but also what is effective, they can choose to correct the one and continue the other. Feedback is communicated most successfully when a relationship of trust and confidence has been established in the group. If this is not the case, an atmosphere of anger and blame may be created inadvertently.

Timing is important in giving and receiving feedback. Feedback is generally most helpful if it is connected with a specific incident and is given in terms of objective data about what has just been observed in the group. This gives the recipient of the feedback the opportunity to assess the reactions or gather observations of other members in the group. Sometimes, it is unwise to give feedback right after the incident in question, particularly if strong feelings have been aroused and people need time to calm down. Feedback about a need for a change in behavior is often viewed as criticism. People may react to it by defending themselves through denial, rationalization, or suspicion of the motives of the person giving the feedback. A leader must exercise discretion when providing feedback to members in the group (Box 3.5).

Feedback can be given to a group as well as to individuals. Like individuals, a group can benefit from receiving information about its performance. The group may need to know that the atmosphere seems defensive, that members appear to be having difficulty being heard, or that members are exhibiting too much reliance on the leader. The general guidelines for individual feedback also apply to group feedback. The group may receive feedback from members who have assumed the role of participant observer or leader or who are in the specific role of group observer(s). Forms and questionnaires may be used to elicit group member feedback, either in identified or anonymous formats that can then be reflected back to the group in an aggregate summary.

Using Concrete Language

In some groups, vagueness and superficiality can become a serious problem, leading members to avoid talking about specific issues. If leaders use real and simple examples in their communications with the group members, the members, by imitation, will learn to focus on existing behaviors in their explorations of their own behavior patterns. Learning to be clear and using concrete language can be particularly helpful when leading groups in which avoidance of issues or affect or reality contact (orientation to person, place, time) are problems for certain members.

Box 3.5   **Timing Can Be Everything**

> Timing feedback appropriately can enable people to make necessary changes in their behavior to improve performance and achieve their desired goals.

Successful problem solving also requires becoming progressively more concrete, clearly identifying specific tasks or behaviors that are barriers to or necessary to a solution or successful outcome. When a group is involved in problem-solving tasks, a problem stated simply can more easily be translated into achievable goals. If goals are stated in accurate and realistic terms, members can begin to define the means by which they can reach those goals in terms of needed actions or behaviors. Well-defined goals can be broken down into smaller, more easily achieved subunits. Finally, concrete language can effectively reduce ambiguity, which in turn may lessen the anxiety of group members and thus potentially increase their ability to engage in the group activity and process.

Confrontation

Confrontation has been defined in a positive manner as "A deliberate attempt to help another person examine the consequences of some aspect of his or her behavior; it is an invitation to engage in self-examination. A confrontation originates from a desire to involve oneself more deeply with the person one is confronting, and it is intended to help the person behave in more fruitful or less destructive ways. In ensuring that feedback and confrontations are constructive, it is helpful to differentiate among (1) the behavior being observed, (2) the conceptual framework the observer is using, and (3) the inferences and interpretations made about the person engaging in the behavior" (Johnson & Johnson, 2006, p. 524).

The decision to confront another person is made on the basis of one's relationship with that person. The quality and nature of the relationship is important. The stronger the relationship, the more powerfully the confrontation will be experienced. If the person's motivation to change is low or if his or her anxiety level is high, the confrontation will probably not be seen as an invitation for self-examination but as an attack. In this instance, or in one where there is no reason or desire to increase the intensity of the relationship, a confrontation should not be initiated. Confrontation is best done in a group that has achieved a high level of trust and cohesiveness. Under most circumstances, confrontation is best approached tentatively and with qualifiers that enable the member to accept the message and add to it or to receive it without feeling accused by the leader (Box 3.6).

Self-Disclosure

Letting another person know what one thinks, feels, or wants is called self-disclosure. The term refers to revealing feelings about a present situation and giving information about the

Box 3.6   **Sensitivity Required**

A leader must consider the ability of the person being confronted to receive the input or feedback and respond in a manner that results in taking positive steps to act on the issue.

Box 3.7 **Judicious Disclosure**

Members get to know and understand leaders best when leaders judiciously disclose, after careful titration and evaluation, their own thoughts, feelings, and reaction(s) to present situations occurring in the group.

past if it is relevant to one's understanding of how one experiences the present. Members more easily see leaders who practice self-disclosure as real people rather than as impersonal leaders (Box 3.7). Disclosing past history is helpful only if it clarifies why the leader is reacting in a particular way. If one engages in self-disclosure, one is also taking the risk of being misunderstood or rejected. Therefore, in responding to another person's self-disclosure, it is important to be accepting and supportive. Women seem to find self-disclosure easier than men, and some cultural groups are more accustomed to self-disclosure than others (Jourard, 1964). Self-disclosure and confrontation may encourage and sometimes coerce members to go beyond a level that they feel is comfortable for them, which in turn may cause members to withdraw or even to leave a group.

Meaning Attribution

Effective group leaders are able to provide "meaning attribution" (Yalom, 2005, p. 536). The term refers to the tendency of the group leader to clarify, explain, understand, and interpret what is happening in the group and, in so doing, facilitate members developing a paradigm for change. Effective leaders explain to the members why they (the leaders) did what they did and why they structured the group in a particular way as well as share their perceptions of how members interact with each other at specific moments during the group session (Lieberman, Yalom, & Miles, 1973). A leader's skills in meaning attribution can support members' learning in the group context, as it is "more likely to be retained and internalized in an atmosphere in which leaders (or other members) clarify what they or others are doing" (Napier & Gershenfeld, 1973, p. 34).

Reality Testing

The effective leader also helps the group to achieve its goals through reality testing. Reality testing is the process by which one's understanding of a situation is shared and reviewed with others. Feedback regarding possible distortions of viewpoints, due to one's own prior experiences or beliefs about certain circumstances, is provided along with objective observations regarding what was said or done. The shared experience creates opportunities for reality testing. Furthermore, if the group norms support honest expression, there can be ample opportunities for consensual validation.

Consensual validation is achieved through a comparison of one's own interpersonal evaluations with those of others in the group. Feelings and reactions to a situation can be

shared and discussed. As a result, behavior can be altered or reinforced according to its relation to reality. Recording the group session on audiotape or videotape and replaying the tapes
in the group may enhance reality testing by allowing members to see and review situations as
they actually occurred. Reality testing is essential to therapy groups with most populations
and viewed as reflecting a trusting therapeutic relationship (Yalom, 1970; Rogers, 1959).

In addition to assisting members with getting feedback and testing the accuracy of their
perceptions, the leader can also reality-test his or her impressions of the effects of his or her
behavior within the group. Leaders often become the target of members' feelings and conflicts
regarding persons in authority. These mixed emotions are commonly acted out in behaviors
in the group, often involving a phenomenon called transference. In transference, the member
perceives certain qualities in the leader or certain interactions that are associated with individuals from the member's past or who are current figures of authority (parent, supervisor,
teacher, grandparent, older sibling, etc.). Usually the leader does not actually possess these
qualities; rather, they are projected onto or attributed to the leader by the member.

The effective leader can counter these inaccurate perceptions through reality testing to
clarify a member's beliefs about the leader as an individual. The leader may ask, "How do
you feel about what I just said or did?" or "What did you see me do or hear me say?" Input
from other group members can aid in transforming the experience from idiosyncratic perception to group consensus. It is important that the leader monitor his or her own countertransference response to the member's projection so that scapegoating of the member may be
avoided. Using the technique of bridging (Ormont, 1990) other members into the dialogue by
collecting their views, observations, or reactions may help to diffuse the situation. Staying
open to the member's distress and inviting feedback from the group by asking if anyone else
might have perceived the leader in a particular way may allow an opportunity for more
reality testing to occur.

Modeling Behavior

Another approach to teaching new skills is through the modeling of the desired behaviors.
According to social learning theory (Bandura, 1969), in order to teach group members
through modeling, leaders must first demonstrate the behavior they hope members will learn
as part of their group experience. Additionally, there must be positive reinforcement when
members imitate the behavior that has been modeled (Johnson & Johnson, 2006).

A group member who is relatively unskilled in establishing or maintaining interpersonal relationships may learn by observing the leader as a model. If a group member is taught
to note the consequences of any particular behavior, the member will see that positive results
can be achieved by adapting his or her particular mode of conduct (Box 3-8). In another
instance, a member may know a certain mode of behavior but not know when to apply
it. Therefore, in a group situation, a leader can guide the member in discovering the correct

Box 3.8   **Model Behavior**

> The imitation of leader behavior is followed by positive reinforcement of group members through recognition and approval.

circumstances for certain modes of behavior. In perhaps the most common scenario, a group member may simply watch and copy the leader's behavior. For this reason, leaders must carefully consider the modes of conduct and the responses they may elicit from the group.

A leader must understand the following aspects of the modeling process to teach a certain mode of behavior effectively:

Have the attention of the other person. If he or she is not aware of the leader's behavior, he or she cannot imitate it.

If the other person thinks that imitating the leader's behavior will help to accomplish goals, he or she will be apt to imitate that behavior.

If imitating leader behavior brought success in the past, there is a stronger possibility that leader behavior will be imitated in the present.

If the other person values the leader's friendship, likes the leader, or seeks the leader's approval, he or she is more likely to imitate the leader's behavior.

Others are more likely to imitate the leader's behavior when they are emotionally aroused.

If the other person is unsure about what behavior is appropriate in a given situation and the leader is sure, that person will tend to imitate the leader (Johnson, 1972).

Leaders who wish to help a member develop effective interpersonal skills must demonstrate those skills in the group. Further, they must develop a group climate that is supportive and accepting so that members will risk trying new behaviors in the group. Group members make the most progress in a group in which they feel comfortable and are encouraged to explore new possibilities.

In addition to employing specific leadership skills to guide members in their efforts to achieve specific goals, it may be necessary to use techniques designed to gather information from an entire group (Box 3.9). Gathering and reflecting observations back to the group is a three-step process:

Box 3.9   **Gathering Data**

> Doing a sociogram for 5 minutes at two points during the group session: at 20 minutes and again at 40 minutes can be a useful way to gather data on group communication (Schwartzberg, Howe, & McDermott, 1982).

1. Collecting data regarding what is seen as occurring in the group
2. Reporting this data to the group
3. Collaboratively defining the problem indicated by the data and designing a solution

For this method to be effective, both members and leaders—that is, the entire group—must collaborate in all parts of this process (Bradford, Stock, & Horwitz, 1978). As observers and resource persons, leaders can offer specific concerns for discussion. These are gathered from observations, coupled with analysis or hypothesis of what might be going on with the group's process, which may be based, in part, on leaders' experience. Group members might also be able to assume some of the data-gathering functions. Following are several methods for gathering observations about a group's verbal and nonverbal behavior that can be used in conjunction with the leadership skills already discussed.

Analysis of Group Behavior

A leader can gain an understanding of group behavior by making observations of the nonverbal behavior of the members. Nonverbal communication, such as touching or gesturing while talking or listening, is frequently seen in a group and can reveal how members feel about each other. Posture indicating possible inclusion or withdrawal is another form of nonverbal communication. For example, a member may lean toward the circle of members or away from them. Similarly, posture may indicate interest and attention or boredom. If members of the group are sitting far apart from each other, this may indicate that certain individuals feel isolated in the group. Depending on the cultural norms of group members, eye contact and eye language may signal intimacy or confrontation, and avoidance of eye contact may mean reluctance to get involved. Sweeping eye contact may mean a member is searching for support or feedback (Fig. 3.2).

Other types of member behavior may also be indicative of communication of some type in the group. No behavior is random or accidental. Activities such as eating, smoking, drinking, or visits to the bathroom might be gauges of the level of tension or boredom in the group. Periods of silence also have meanings. Observing how people look during periods of silence—sad, tense, avoidant of eye contact, angry, contemplative—gives the leader clues about the members' feelings. The meaning of the silence may be that it serves as a possible resistance to addressing underlying feelings or issues. The biggest impasse to individuals who isolate themselves is their refusal to identify with others in the group (Ormont, 2004). In working through issues of resistance, it may be useful to understand other ways in which resistance can emerge in the group process. For example, in addition to silence, "frequently-seen resistances are (1) denying responsibility, (2) giving advice, and (3) distorting" (Ormont, 2004, p. 69). Using leadership skills such as feedback, confrontation, or meaning attribution can help members become aware of these patterns of behavior or thinking. Careful use of these skills in conjunction with reality testing or modeling allows members opportunities to learn to communicate more effectively and perhaps stop behaving in ways that create a disconnect with others.

Methods of Observation
Sociogram

A sociogram is an instrument that provides data on the communication patterns in the group. It charts specifically who talks to whom. By using this technique, the observer can follow the flow of the conversation and identify members who speak often, members who speak seldom,

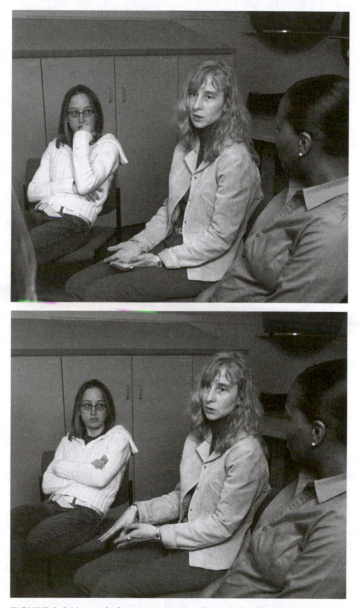

FIGURE 3.2 Nonverbal communication. Top, Ambivalence and anxiety. Bottom, Distrust and avoidance. *(continued)*

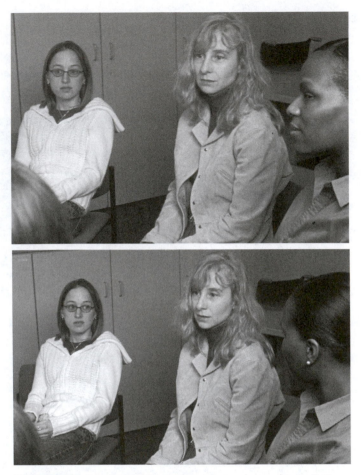

FIGURE 3.2 (continued) Top, Uncertain and searching. Bottom, Approach and guardedness. (Photos by Mark Morelli.)

and members who receive comments or questions. Sociograms can also be useful in identifying specific group members' communication patterns. For instance, a sociogram may reveal that some group members talked only to the leader, perhaps indicating their dependence on the leader or their reluctance or inability to get involved with the other group members.

To use a sociogram, an outline of the group's seating configuration (i.e., circle, rectangle) is drawn, with members of the group marked by first name or initials in their places. Each time someone in the group speaks, a line for each statement or question, indicating the initiator and the recipient, is drawn. Some lines may extend only to the center; these represent statements that were made to the group as a whole and were not directed toward a specific individual. Arrows drawn at both ends of a line indicate that the recipient responded to the statement. Sociograms are commonly used at intervals during the course of a group meeting. Usually the number of statements made during a 10-minute period is recorded (Fig. 3.3).

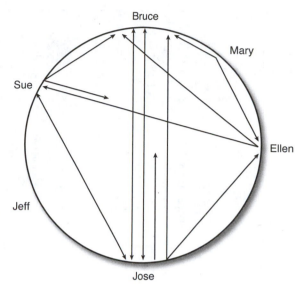

FIGURE 3.3 This sociogram indicates that Bruce received more statements than anyone else and that Mary spoke to two persons, but no one responded to her or addressed a statement to her. Although 15 statements were made during that 10-minute period, Jeff was not involved in any of these communications.

Interaction Process Analysis

A method for analyzing verbal interactions made during a group meeting was developed to observe and note two main points of group process: task issues and maintenance issues (Bales, 1950). This approach is designed to distinguish:

• Communications that give information
• Communications that seek information
• Negative emotional expressions
• Positive emotional expressions
• General nature of verbal content and possible accompanying behaviors (Table 3.1)

This system of communication analysis can augment a sociogram, noting the nature and types of communications that occurred. Analysis of the group interactions in this way can facilitate examination of potential strengths or problem areas in the group process.

Member Role Observation

Information based on group observations can be documented by completing a member role form (Display 3.1). Members' names are placed at the top of the form, and a checkmark is placed in the column corresponding to the role that members appear to take most often in the group. By filling out this form, the different types of roles that were assumed in the group can be assessed. This form also allows any important roles that were not assumed by group members to be noted. If leaders or observers want to record frequency of roles adopted, they can place a check in the column every time the designated member has played that particular role in the group.

Table 3.1   Interaction Process Analysis Chart

Possible Response	Potential Process Area					
	Communication	Evaluation	Control	Decision	Tension	Reintegration
Positive Social-Emotional	Asks for others' ideas & opinions, attentive posture, actively listens	Openly expresses positive feelings about group, peers, activity	Able to compromise, see others' point of view, acknowledge difference in opinion or perception	Agrees or complies, passively demonstrates acceptance or understanding	Uses humor, laughs, relieves tension, expresses satisfaction	Supportive, vocal in offering help or giving praise
Attempted Neutral Task	Gives suggestion, direction	Gives opinion, interpretation, expresses wish or feeling	Gives information, clarifies, repeats what was said, confirms	Willing to go with others' ideas or opinion, not involved in decision-making process	Quietly attentive, nods agreement, indicates willing to "try" activity	Shares material or mild opinion re: what's best for "the group"
Questioning Neutral Task	Asks for information, repetition, confirmation	Asks for opinion, analysis, expression of feelings	Asks for suggestions or direction in terms of possible actions	Acts ambivalent or uncertain, questions if decision is suitable	Asks if there are options in terms of degree of involvement, questions safety	Questions if task and/or process meeting own needs
Negative Social-Emotional	Openly disagrees, devalues others' ideas or suggestions, side-talks	Makes negative comments re: group activity choice, self, or others	Projects negative transferences, unwilling to participate, leaves or arrives late	Disagrees, passively rejecting, formal, withholding	Tense, asks for help or withdraws	Antagonistic, denigrates others, defensive, aggressive in assertions

Adapted from Bales, R. 1950, p. 59.

Display 3.1   **Group Member Roles***

	Member Names							
Task Roles								
Initiator								
Information/Opinion Giver								
Information/Opinion Seeker								
Energizer								
Elaborator								
Evaluator-Critic								
Coordinator								
Procedural Technician								
Orienter								
Recorder								
Maintenance Roles								
Encourager								
Harmonizer/Compromiser								
Gatekeeper								
Standard Setter								
Observer								
Follower								
Individual Roles								
Playboy								
Blocker								
Dominator								
Recognition Seeker								
Help Seeker								
Special Interest Pleader								
Self-Confessor								
Aggressor								

*Benne and Sheats, 1978.

Display 3.2   **Content and Process Analysis**

Content Observations

1. What were the main ideas presented in the discussion?
2. Which ideas were accepted?
3. Were irrelevant ideas and discussion presented?
4. Did the group have the information necessary for making decisions?
5. Did the members talk about ideas and facts or feelings?

Process Observations

1. Describe the tone of the discussion (e.g., friendly, tense, angry, anxious).
2. Is the atmosphere conducive to free expression? Why or why not?
3. Identify any apparent communication blocks (e.g., some members were not listened to; some were not understood; some were not recognized).
4. What factors seemed to keep the group from functioning well? For example, some members appeared uncomfortable physically or otherwise; some could not hear due to noise; some seemed bored; some came late. Did the group seem organized to do the job it was trying to do? Why or why not?
5. What factors assisted the group's functioning?
6. Were there any indications of dissatisfaction with the kinds of decisions made by the group?

Content and Process Analysis

An analysis of the content and process of a group session provides a basis for an evaluation of a group meeting as well. This procedure may be used by group leaders for their own analysis or by all group members for evaluation and discussion. The leader(s), members, or both leader(s) and members should answer specific questions regarding content and process, and a follow-up discussion should be focused on the ensuing information (Display 3.2).

Meeting Evaluations

If members' personal capacities allow, they can be asked to evaluate meetings at the end of a session by completing feedback or evaluation forms (Displays 3.3 through 3.5). Members might be asked to use a brief rating form with which they anonymously provide feedback whether they felt that the meeting was good, fair, or poor and if they were able to express these feelings to the group (Howe, 1968; Knowles, 1970).

Display 3.3   **Meeting Evaluation Form**

Date:
Activity:
Please circle the phrase that best describes how you feel:
1. I think that in this meeting I learned

A great deal	Quite a lot	Some	Very little	Nothing

2. On the whole, today's session was:

Excellent	Pretty good	All right	Disappointing	Terrible

3. I am leaving the meeting feeling:

Enthusiastic	Encouraged	All right	Disappointed	Frustrated

4. At this time, this activity interests me:

Immensely	Quite a bit	Somewhat	A little	Not at all

Comments:
_____
_____
_____

Adapted from Knowles, M. S. [1970]. The Modern Practice of Adult Education. New York: Association Press, p. 233.

Display 3.4   **Group Member Feedback Form: Adult**

1. How would you rate your group experience?
   (please circle as many as apply)

Fun	Boring
Helpful	Not related to my needs
Source of learning	Undecided

   Other (please state):
2. Activities I enjoyed and found meaningful:
   Reasons:
3. Activities I did not like or found demeaning:
   Reasons:
4. Would you recommend this type of experience to a friend?
   Why or why not?
5. What I learned from this experience:

Display 3.5   **Group Member Feedback Form: Children**

1. I thought this group was *(circle as many words you agree with)*
   Fun   Boring
   Helpful   Not really for me
   A time for learning   I'm not sure
   Other (please say what you thought/felt about group):
2. Activities I liked or really meant something to me were:
   I liked them because:
3. Activities I did not like:
   I did not like them because:
4. Would you tell a friend to come to this kind of group in the future?
   Why or why not?
5. What I learned from coming to this group:

Conclusion

The leader of any group is responsible for assisting the group members with achieving their stated goals. Although the definition of a leader is still debated, several techniques aid leaders in carrying out their roles. Not all of these strategies or techniques will be suitable for every leader and every group. The behavior and/or abilities of the group members or the needs of the group as a whole may call for modifications of these techniques and strategies. Each leadership skill and strategy must be adapted to suit the needs and purpose of the group. Having looked broadly at what a leader does, our next step is to introduce a specific approach to group work we have designed, which we call the Functional Group Model. The next chapter outlines the development of this model, briefly outlining its assumptions and theoretical underpinnings. We will then look at each stage of the Functional Group Model, providing both theoretical and practical material in great detail to help you develop your group leadership abilities and deepen your understanding of group process as experienced in a functional group.

Individual Learning Activities

REFLECTIVE QUESTIONS

1. What are the two categories of leadership functions? Why do you need one or both to have a successful group? Are these functions the sole responsibility of the group leader? Which leadership functions are a better fit for you and why?

2. What leadership style might you use for working with groups of young children? Why? What leadership style might be effective for a group of adults with developmental disabilities? Why?

3. How can you gather the information necessary to help you determine the leadership strategies you will need to use? Given your own life experiences, what are elements of yourself that will affect your interactive reasoning and leadership style? (e. g., prior roles in family, community, school, or work).

4. What are the benefits gained from working with a co-leader? Are there any disadvantages? How do you feel about sharing the responsibilities in leading a group? In what ways do you feel vulnerable and secure?

LEARNING CHECKPOINTS

Describe:

• The three leadership styles studied by Lewin, Lippitt, and White

• How a group leader can demonstrate "genuineness"

• What a leader should consider when selecting a group activity

• Circumstances under which confrontation should and should not be used by a leader

• An example of what reality testing entails

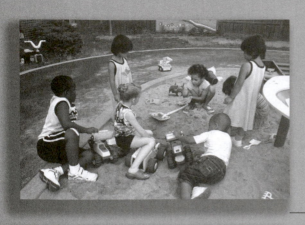

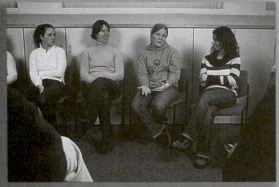

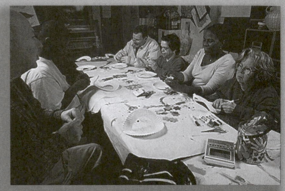

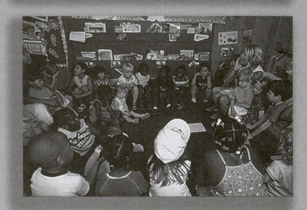

The Functional Group Model

This chapter describes the model developed to incorporate the use of purposeful activity and meaningful occupation into the process and dynamics of group work. The functional group model was first introduced in 1986 (Howe and Schwartzberg, 1986) as an approach to guide occupational therapy group intervention. It is discussed here in greater detail to trace the model's evolution and reflect refinements that have taken place since its inception.

The functional group model is presented in accordance with a framework established for the process of developing practice models (Reed, 1984). Eight elements are identified as fundamental:

1. The frame of reference
2. Assumptions
3. Concepts
4. Expected results of intervention
5. Assessment instruments
6. Intervention strategies
7. Logical deductions
8. Intervention principles

Although based on empirical data, due to the dynamic nature of group work, the model remains in the process of being tested; the final element, intervention principles, continues to need further study and research. Nevertheless, the model has served as a means to organize group practice, education, and research in the field of occupational therapy.

Framework of the Functional Group Model

Frames of Reference

The functional group model is based on research in five areas:

1. Group dynamics
2. Effectance
3. Needs hierarchy
4. Purposeful activity
5. Adaptation

Group dynamics—the domain of social scientists—concerns the interrelationships of persons in a small group. The belief that a psychological field, just as an energy field, acts on and affects the behavior of a group was raised by Kurt Lewin in the 1930s (Knowles and Knowles, 1972). "Effectance" (White, 1959, 1971) refers to the belief that individuals are drawn toward activity and that this behavior is self-motivated. "Needs hierarchy"

(Maslow, 1970) refers to the belief that humans have many needs, which are arranged in order of importance, and lower needs must be filled before higher needs can be met. Purposeful activity can be considered as closely related to satisfaction of needs. Adaptation, either as the process of learning or a person's response to challenge, can occur through engaging in goal-directed or personally meaningful activity or occupations. The desired outcome is the learning or adaptive response that brings about an improved ability to participate more fully in life; e.g., achieving satisfaction in meaningful occupations or more effectively fulfilling life roles (friend, partner, family member, student, worker, citizen, etc.).

Much of the early literature on group dynamics influenced the development of the functional group model. By understanding the normal group, Howe and Schwartzberg (1986) formulated ideas about the therapy group and then the functional group. Concepts central to the beliefs regarding group dynamics were derived from Bales' (1950) work on interaction analysis and Benne and Sheats' (1978) description of group membership and leadership functions. Additional works on group dynamics, such as those on group cohesiveness (Cartwright & Zander, 1968; Yalom, 1970), the phases of group development (Bennis & Shepard, 1956; Garland, Jones, & Kolodny, 1965; Tuckman, 1965), and individual growth through group process (Lifton, 1961), were also used to develop the model.

If it is understood how persons within groups interact, the benefits of group participation for individuals can be increased. Recall several basic principles of group dynamics. Groups:

• Have a common goal and dynamic interaction between members
• Provide multiple types of feedback and support
• Promote independence from an externally designated leader in a developmental progression
• Support growth and change of members
• Have a capacity for self-direction
• Can address individual needs on a task, emotional, and social level (Box 4.1)

Concepts such as "effectance motivation" or the "urge toward competence" (White, 1959, 1971) were central to the development of the functional group model. Simply stated, this theory postulates that exploratory behavior is self-motivated. The term "effectance" describes this motivation, and exploratory behavior is seen as having "adaptive value." When viewed as a dynamic interaction in context: "Effectance motivation must be conceived to involve satisfaction—a feeling of efficacy—in transactions in which behavior has an exploratory, varying, experimental character….The behavior leads the organism to find out how the environment can be changed and what consequences flow from these changes" (White, 1959, p. 329).

Box 4.1   **Principles of Group Dynamics**

- Through use of the information available in a group, members are provided with a "here-and-now" reality orientation that encourages growth and change. Groups can enhance the use of meaningful occupations to help people function independently and/or learn to adapt to their expectations or environment or, if necessary, groups can provide an environment that is modified to support individuals' performance capabilities.
- Groups are designed to give the amount and type of feedback and support that members need. Feedback and support are parts of the process of doing and participating in the group activities selected to meet individual members activity and social needs.
- Group discussions and activities can be structured to encourage group-centered leadership. Structuring activities and the environment so that nonhuman objects lead the action gives members an opportunity to learn about their own capabilities and the effect of the environment or context.
- Through discussion and participation in growth activities, groups can encourage and promote growth and change in members. By selecting activities that permit learning and practicing skills needed to achieve mastery and competency, groups can provide opportunities for member growth and change.
- Groups can be structured or organized to accommodate many levels of human development and functioning. Enabling the group to lead the doing by giving members a set of possibilities empowers the group's capacity for self-direction.

In examining motivation further, the concept of a needs hierarchy emerges. One such theory is that humans are driven by "intrinsic growth tendencies" (Maslow, 1970) that emerge as one tries to meet "basic needs" (Maslow, 1970). These basic needs are organized hierarchically as:

- Physiological
- Safety
- Belonging and love
- Esteem
- Self-actualization (Maslow, 1970)

Unsatisfied needs are thus considered a source of motivation. The individual puts his or her energies into satisfying needs, starting with their physiological survival-based needs such as food, water, etc. The process is sequential, as the individual works through each level of the hierarchy until meeting the most advanced level of need, realizing one's true potential or reason for existence (self-actualization).

A similar needs hierarchy of "health needs" (psycho-physical, security, love and acceptance, group association, esteem, sexual, developmental, and pleasure [Mosey, 1973b, pp. 14–15]) is defined as "inherent human requirements that must be met in order for an individual to experience a sense of physical, psychological, and social well-being" (p. 14). This hierarchy adds to the lens through which we might filter our understanding of individuals and, potentially, their sources of motivation. Therefore, to promote health and well-being, a "need-satisfying environment" becomes an essential backdrop to a program oriented toward change.

Another idea central to the functional group model is purposeful activity. Purposeful activities can be defined as those that encourage an adaptive response (King, 1978). An adaptive response is one in which the activity has elicited adequate sensory processing in an individual to produce functional performance, even at a most basic level (e.g., spontaneity that indicates attention and pleasure such as smiling or laughing, catching a ball, following through with a task or directive, etc.). Purposeful activities or meaningful occupations give direction to goal-oriented behavior (Reed, 1984). Clearly, however, the definition of a term such as "meaningful" is usually subjective. Yet, if many basic needs (Maslow, 1970) are a source of goal-oriented behavior, then "the possible needs or demands which activities could fulfill are physiologic, security, belonging, societal and self-actualizing needs" (Reed, 1984, p. 502). Regardless of the needs they fulfill, all purposeful activities must have intent and be practical in daily living (Reed, 1984).

Further insight into the purpose or value of activity comes from studies regarding intrinsic rewards and motivation (Csikszentmihalyi, 1975, 1990), which assert that people experience a "flow state" when their "skills match with the opportunities for action in the environment" (p. 177). When there is a mismatch, stress, worry, or boredom may result. The flow state increases one's sense of being in control of one's actions. A great sense of enjoyment is often what one feels when in a flow state. This "optimal experience" (Csikszentmihalyi, 1990, p. 3) is that in which there is "a sense that one's skills are adequate to cope with the challenges at hand, in a goal-directed, rule-bound, action system that provides clear clues as to how well one is performing. Concentration is so intense that there is no attention left to think about anything irrelevant, or to worry about problems" (p. 71).

Purposeful action has also been conceptualized as "doing" (Fidler & Fidler, 1978). Doing becomes a means of "enabling the development and integration of the sensory, motor, cognitive, and psychological systems; serving as a socializing agent, and verifying one's efficacy as a competent, contributing member of one's society" (p. 305). Doing is pivotal to the functional group model. "Both the quality and variety of doing is critical for ego development and adaptation" (p. 308). Additionally, intrinsically motivated behaviors are conceived as those that lead to feelings of personal satisfaction (Barris, Kielhofner, & Hawkins, 1983).

All the literature cited above touches on the concept of human adaptation. Ideally, "adaptation through occupation...means the organization and management of occupational activities and tasks in a manner that meets the goal of achieving maximum autonomy or functional independence, actualization or satisfaction and accomplishment" (Reed, 1984, p. 495). In its purest form, occupation can be viewed as "behavior which is motivated by an intrinsic, conscious urge to be effective in the environment in order to enact a variety of individually interpreted roles that are shaped by cultural tradition and learned through the process of socialization" (Burke, 1983, p. 136). The postulate that purposeful activity, or "doing," is primary to adaptation (Fidler & Fidler, 1978; King, 1978) is a cornerstone of the functional group model.

The frames of reference for the functional group model include group dynamics, effectance, needs hierarchy, purposeful activity, and adaptation. A powerful relationship exists among these key ideas (Reed, personal communication, 1986). Additionally, the functional group model assumes a relationship among groups, therapy, and occupation. By examining the normal group (nonspecific), variations in the therapy group (more specific) can then be understood; the concepts will then be applied to the functional group (occupation-specific).

Assumptions

From a review of the literature, Howe and Schwartzberg (1986) formed assumptions that would be inherent to the framework of the functional group model. Assumptions are ideas we accept as valid or true without having scientific proof. Each of us accepts certain assumptions whether or not we are aware of doing so. The assumptions that were made in forming the functional group model are in relation to people (Box 4.2), health (Box 4.3), occupation (Box 4.4), therapy (Box 4.5), social systems (Box 4.6), change (Box 4.7), function (Box 4.8), and action (Box 4.9).

Box 4.2   **People Assumptions**

The functional group model has nine assumptions that relate to people:

1. People are bio-psycho-social systems.
2. People are social beings and therefore exist in groups.
3. People are action- or "doing"-oriented, motivated toward competency.
4. People have needs that can be met through the give-and-take of a social system such as a group.
5. People communicate socially (interact) verbally and nonverbally.
6. People grow and change as an inherent process in life.
7. People are unique, complete individuals, with wholeness or congruence between emotion and action.
8. Groups exist as subgroups of people, which model the social behavior patterns in the larger society.
9. Groups mobilize powerful forces that have important effects on people as individuals. Groups can shape senses of identity. Position in a group effects safety and self-esteem. Group membership may be highly valued or seen as a burden to the individual.

Box 4.3 **Health Assumptions**

The functional group model has four assumptions about health:

1. An individual's state of health involves mind, body (internal), and physical environment—the individual in interaction with the social and physical environment.
2. Purposeful activity supports the health of mind and body in an individual and a collective being.
3. Health involves a state of independence and capacity for self-direction.
4. Health involves a state of interdependence and capacity for relatedness.

Box 4.4 **Occupation-Based Assumptions**

The functional group model has nine assumptions about engagement in meaningful occupation or purposeful activity:

1. Meaningful occupations used in a group experience encourage the person to assume responsibility for meeting individual needs.
2. Purposeful activities involve choice or volition by the individual and group toward a goal or purpose.
3. Purposeful activities, or occupations, used in a group experience are useful in improving the performance level and adaptive behavior of the person and thus increasing the potential for meeting individual responsibilities.
4. Active doing (involvement) in a group encourages social participation and the development, maintenance, and redevelopment of skills in areas of self-care (activities of daily living/instrumental activities of daily living), productivity (work/education), and leisure (play).
5. Through active doing in a group experience, the individual gains a sense of self-worth and self-appraisal.
6. Lack of meaningful occupation or purposeful activity, or idleness, leads to disorientation and breakdown in useful habits and thus threatens the health of mind and body at the level of the individual and the group.
7. Engaging in meaningful occupations or purposeful activities positively influences a person's sense of well-being or state of health.
8. An adaptive response requires:
   a. Active participation
   b. The individual to meet the environmental demands of the tasks and express needs or goals
   c. Subcortical centers to integrate and organize a response that leads to self-reinforcement (King, 1978).
9. An individual's biological, psychological, and social requirements can be addressed through the use of meaningful occupations or purposeful activity as a means to influence change in the person's state of health.

Box 4.5   **Functional Group Assumptions**

Basic principles governing group dynamics are related to the functional group in that groups:

- Have a common goal and dynamic interaction between members.
- Provide multiple sources of feedback and support.
- Promote independence from the leader.
- Support growth and change of members.
- Have a capacity for self-direction.
- Can satisfy individual needs and social demands.

Additional assumptions applying to the more specific therapy group related to a functional group are that groups:

- Provide a here-and-now reality orientation that encourages growth and change.
- Are designed to give the amount and type of feedback and support that members need.
- Can be structured to encourage group-centered leadership.
- Can lead to individual growth and change.
- Can be organized to accommodate many levels of human development and functioning.
- Can address individual needs on a task, emotional or social level and provide learning necessary to fulfill social demands.

The occupation-based nature of a functional group is influenced by the following assumptions:

- Groups can enhance the use of occupations to help people function independently by helping individuals adapt to the environment or adapting the environment to them.
- Feedback and support are part of the process of doing and social participation.
- Structuring activities and the environment allows objects to lead action and permits members to learn about the environment and their own capabilities.
- Activities must be carefully selected to provide individuals opportunities to practice and learn skills to achieve mastery and competence, which can lead to growth and change in members.
- The group leads the doing by giving members a set of possibilities, thus empowering the group's capacity for self-direction.
- Groups can be used to maintain, improve, or enhance individuals' occupational performance by providing members the opportunity to deal with the activity demands and contextual aspects that may influence their participation.

Box 4.6 **Social Systems Assumptions**

The functional group model has six assumptions about functional groups as social systems:

1. Functional groups are not limited to therapy groups. As social systems, they apply to naturally occurring groups in the community such as families or work groups.
2. Functional groups provide a structure to guide the individual's participation. The structure and goals always address the social and emotional needs of the individual and are therefore said to be ego-oriented.
3. Functional groups intrinsically provide therapeutic benefit, because occupational behavior is learned and shaped through a process of socialization.
4. Functional group activities build on strengths of the individual in the group. Therefore, there is interest in the strengths and limitations of each member.
5. Functional groups can parallel and reflect the needs of the individual and the demands of society.
6. Functional groups are assumed to provide benefits to members through mutual help. Groups are therefore structured so that members have the opportunity to help each other, thus enhancing members' perceptions or feelings of self-worth.

Box 4.7 **Change Assumptions**

The functional group model has three assumptions about functional groups as agents of change:

1. Functional groups are structured to motivate members to purposeful and meaningful action.
2. Functional groups are experience-based groups. Experiential learning occurs in the here-and-now in a supportive environment that is structured as a place in which to practice daily living skills.
3. Functional groups attempt to move members from dependence to independence or interdependence and from maladaptive functioning to adaptation.

Box 4.8 **Functional Assumptions**

The functional group model has three assumptions about the nature of the functional group:

1. Functional groups provide a place for members to function in the reality of the present and to learn and practice skills in decision making, judgment, and perception as well as addressing other areas of needed growth.
2. Functional groups are concerned with elements of performance as well as with types of performance in areas such as work, play, social participation, and self-care.
3. Functional groups seek to build group cohesiveness as a certain amount of cohesiveness is necessary to achieve group goals.

Box 4.9   **Action Assumptions**

The functional group model has four assumptions about the action component of the functional group:

1. The goal of the functional group is not the product of the group, even though the group may have a meaningful product, but rather the learning process that occurs through active participation.
2. Functional groups nurture interpersonal and intrapersonal development through activity choice, climate, and goals.
3. Functional groups make use of both the human and nonhuman environment and object relations. Attention is directed to attachments to people and objects, separations from people and objects, and the symbolic nature of attachment.
4. Functional group leaders are cognizant of the individual's need for self-motivation and desire for mastery and guide the activity of the group accordingly.

Concepts

At the heart of the functional group model is a set of concepts that defines the model in precise terms. The basic concepts are adaptation and occupation (hereafter referred to as action). Adaptation is defined as the adjustment of the organism to its environment or the process by which it adjusts (Reed & Sanderson, 1983). Characteristics of adaptation (King, 1978) are inherently related to the functional group model (Table 4.1). Adaptation is brought about through occupation or action. Thus, the functional group model is action-oriented; defined by its use of time, energy, and action designed to promote adaptation. This orientation stems from the belief that behavior is a manifestation of the person as a whole. Therefore, in health, congruence between emotion and action is sought. This belief is based on the view that human beings are action-oriented and, thus, "doing" is basic to human nature.

Action in a functional group manifests itself in four different forms: purposeful action, self-initiated action, spontaneous (here-and-now) action, and group-centered action.

Purposeful action is the means through which the individuals and the group perceive the action or activity in the group as being congruent with their needs and goals (Fig. 4-1). Through purposeful action, "mastery and competence are verified and become obvious in the reality of an end product. When the product resulting from an activity has social and cultural relevance to the individual and to his or her social groups, meaning is enhanced and social efficacy is affirmed" (Fidler & Fidler, 1983, p. 277).

The activity must be suitable to the group members and their available skills. Additionally, the environment and the meaning of human and nonhuman objects related to the activity must be considered. Certain environments and objects may represent attitudes or feelings about one's degree of control, compliance, inclusion, or desirability. People grow from

Table 4.1 **Adaptation and the Functional Group Model**	
Characteristics of Adaptation	**Functional Group Model**
Requires a role that involves active participation	Group empowers maximum involvement through interaction between members, a common goal, and a task. Group mobilizes powerful forces that have important effects on member's sense of individual and group identity.
Requires person to meet the environment demands including needs and safety of other group members.	Group promotes action flow and experience. Group promotes independence and capacity for self-direction through the supportive structure of tasks and goals. Group promotes occupational role performance as well as social participation.
Permits subcortical centers to integrate and organize a response.	Group spontaneously involves members in the action. Group focuses on the here-and-now group task; thus learning occurs through organization of input and output to subcortical centers of individuals.
Leads to self-reinforcement.	Group builds on strengths. Group members' support and feedback provides consensual validation for learning.

From King LJ, (1978). 1978 Eleanor Clarke Slagle Lecture: Toward a science of adaptive responses. *American Journal of Occupational Therapy 32*(7):429–437.

the natural, adaptive response to a proper fit between an individual and a group task: "When there is congruency between individual characteristics and the real and symbolic characteristics of an activity, there is greater likelihood that the doing experience will result in a feeling of pleasure and personal satisfaction, and that the essential learning will be integrated as an adaptive response" (Fidler & Fidler, 1983, p. 277).

Self-initiated action is the manner in which individuals seek to be a part of the group and at some point in the process improve their skills or understanding of themselves on their own volition. Expressions of self-initiation need to be viewed as occurring at the extent to which the individuals are capable. If individuals do not personally choose to join or participate in the group, it is likely they will not view the goals of the group or activity as those they seek to achieve. Thus, forms of self-initiated action must become a focal point in facilitating members understanding or becoming a part of a group.

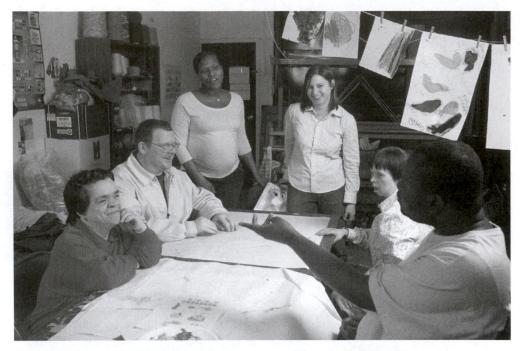

FIGURE 4.1 Purposeful action and the adaptive response. (Photo by Mark Morelli)

Spontaneous (here-and-now) action is essential to a functional group. Functional groups are based on experience. Therefore, experiential learning in the present is optimal to members' participation. Through spontaneous action, members can discover areas of behavior that interfere with or augment adaptation. Functional groups provide a safe and supportive environment, a context to practice skills that enhance or promote one's well-being or ability to carry out tasks and roles in order to function in life. Rather than focus on the past, the group provides a place for members to function in the present and build skills and abilities in decision making, judgment, and perception, as well as other areas (Fig. 4-2). Through spontaneous action, learning in the present is emphasized.

Group-centered action is a distinguishing feature of the functional group. The group structure and goals ought to take into consideration the emotional and social needs of all members. The group leader aims to create an environment that encourages interdependent action through consensus. Group-centered action allows maximal involvement through the interaction of leaders and members working toward a common task and goal. Through group-centered action, powerful forces that have important effects on members' sense of individual and group identity are mobilized (Box 4.10). The process of

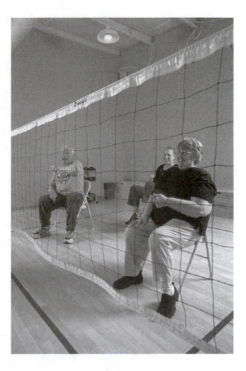

FIGURE 4.2 Spontaneous action and the adaptive response. (Photo by Mark Morelli)

group-centered action can permit, enable, or enhance purposeful, self-initiated, and spontaneous action.

These four types of action underlie members' involvement in action in a functional group. Purposeful action uses goal-directed activity or meaningful occupations of group members, or the exploration of such, and discussion about action with the group as a whole to facilitate the group process. Through purposeful action, members can realize their needs and goals. In so doing, self-initiated action emerges. The here-and-now focus of spontaneous action allows members to participate actively in the tasks and group process to effect interpersonal learning and growth, graded to the level of their abilities. Emphasis is centered on the group as a whole and its interdependence through group-centered action. It is through the dynamic interaction of the four types of action used in a functional group that the group matures and members develop their ability to function.

Expected Results of Intervention

The ultimate goal of the functional group is to promote health or adaptation through purposeful, self-initiated, spontaneous, and group-centered action. A functional group can have multiple goals, incorporating the specific needs and goals of individual members as well as

Box 4.10   **Group-Centered Action**

In an after-school program for 7-year-olds, Joe was disruptive for several weeks. He consistently sought the attention of the leader, unlike the other group members. The leader decided to invite the group to talk about this problem, acknowledging that everyone needs attention. She suggested a sharing time at the end of the group, when everyone took a turn sharing with the group. This, however, resulted in bedlam. After a brief talk with members, sharing time was restructured to a game format, in which each person was required to take a turn.

more general goals and needs shared by all members. The populations served by the functional group can be persons with physical illness or injury, emotional or behavioral disorders, congenital or developmental disabilities, problems precipitated by the aging process, or they can be individuals wishing to increase or maintain their level of adaptation and wellness. A functional group can serve as part of an evaluative process or to provide intervention. Intervention may be at the level of health promotion or maintenance, skill remediation or restoration, environmental or personal modification such as compensatory techniques or adapting one's environment or approach, or prevention. The functional group provides opportunities for observation and evaluation of behavior as well as interaction with the human and nonhuman environment for purposes of identifying performance problems.

Conversely however, a functional group is structured to motivate members to action to facilitate adaptation, prevent deficits, and promote functioning in ways that foster health and well-being. The functional group can be described as providing group experience in which:

• Objects guide action.
• Action is used to enhance individual members' sense of internal control and well-being.
• Talking is used to clarify doing.
• The leader is teaching or empowering members to lead or take ownership of the group to the extent that members are capable.

The functional group may also be characterized by what it is not. First, it is not a leaderless group. The group leader plays an important role in facilitating the group process and planning for the group sessions. Second, it is not group psychotherapy. Although the functional group model is designed to provide therapy for clients with psychosocial problems, it does not focus on, nor is it primarily concerned with, developing insight through surfacing repressed or unconscious material. Third, it is not an activity therapy group. According to Slavson (1950), the founder of activity therapy, the goal of the activity therapy group is to bring about relief of "characterological" (p. 2) pathology. A functional group seeks to enhance occupational behavior and, therein, adaptation. Fourth, the functional group is not focused on etiology. It does not seek to alter the origin of a condition but rather facilitate change in the member's experience of a given condition or symptoms to reduce, whenever possible, maladaptive interference with occupation and adaptation. Emphasis is not on diagnostic categories and symptoms. Individuals who have similar diagnoses or conditions may have markedly different illness experiences manifested in different ways. The expectation by a leader or a group member of a particular set of symptoms or behaviors based on a diagnosis or condition may actually limit the therapeutic progress for the group and the individual members.

Assessment Instruments

Methods of assessment have been developed to collect data for determining whether certain problems exist and what intervention strategy to use (Reed, 1984). The assessment instruments used in the functional group include observation, needs assessment, and content and process analysis. Observation guides (e.g., sociogram, member behavior rating forms, and group evaluation forms) provide a structured approach for initial evaluation and for ongoing assessment of group structure and function. In addition, in a functional group, group members are taught and encouraged to be observers and evaluators of group process and progress towards goals. Even if members are able to understand the evaluation process only at a very basic level, this accountability and feedback loop helps leaders verify the accuracy of their assessment of individual and group potential.

Intervention Strategies

Intervention strategies are the media, modalities, methods, techniques, and equipment used to bring about change in the individual and achieve specific goals or objectives (Reed, 1984). These strategies include defining issues and expectations during the course of the group. Creating a group climate that uses purposeful, self-initiated, spontaneous, and group-centered action to support members' achievement of desired goals is a method for meeting intervention outcomes. Intervention and goal formulation is guided by an in-depth group protocol format.

Logical Deductions

Logical deductions are stated as hypotheses in a question or an answer form (Reed, 1984). If one implements the functional group model, effectively bringing about change and achieving the goals, hypotheses, or logical deductions regarding the group would be:

1. Group members' identified health and wellness needs that were met, and
2. Group members learned skills and behaviors necessary for
   a. Adaptation,
   b. Improved performance in meaningful occupations, and
   c. Increased life satisfaction or quality of life.

Intervention Principles

Generalizations concerning the accuracy of a model must be derived from the results of tests of the hypotheses (Reed, 1984). These generalizations are the intervention principles. Although the functional group model is based on studies that explicitly or implicitly substantiate aspects of the model, evidence is far from complete. As information becomes available and the context of practice changes, new questions need to be raised. Important research studies on group work have been published from which inferences concerning the functional group can be drawn. There is growing evidence in occupational therapy and related literature to support hypotheses (Agazarian & Gantt, 2003; Clark, Carlson, Jackson, & Mandel, 2003; Ward, 2003) and guide intervention principles.

The intervention principles are further strengthened by the use of the functional group model in practice and as applied in theoretical discussions (Barnes & Schwartzberg, 2003; Barnes & Schwartzberg, 2000; Cole, 2005; Schwartzberg, 1993, 1998, 1999; Schwartzberg & Abeles, 1991). Additionally, the functional group model has been used to guide research regarding the effectiveness of group intervention (Clark, et al., 1997; Jackson, et al., 1998; Mandel, et al., 1999). With further study, research questions will serve to test or to validate the assumptions or logical deductions of the model. Furthermore, questions may also elucidate the intervention strategies or principles inherent to the functional group approach. Answers to new or difficult questions can be measured against the statements in the relevant categories of assumptions, logical deductions, or intervention principles. Verification of the functional group model will continue as new questions arise and as a result of the need for evidence-based practice.

Conclusion

The framework presented here guides understanding of the main constructs that serve as the foundation of the functional group model. The subsequent chapters guide you through the process of designing and implementing a functional group. As we proceed, you will build on your knowledge with opportunities for practical application, reasoning, and reflection.

Individual Learning Activities

REFLECTIVE QUESTIONS

1. Why is the early literature on group dynamics important to the understanding of the functional group model?

2. What are some of the principles of group dynamics?

3. What is meant by adaptation, and how does the functional group model propose to effect adaptation?

4. What is meant by a "flow state" and how does it relate to the design of a functional group?

5. What is Mosey's description of a needs hierarchy? How might a "a need-satisfying environment" be created in the design of a functional group?

LEARNING CHECKPOINTS

Describe how.......

• Action is defined in the functional group model.

• The four types of action might be used in a functional group.

• Occupation is the basis of the functional group model.

• Groups can support growth and change.

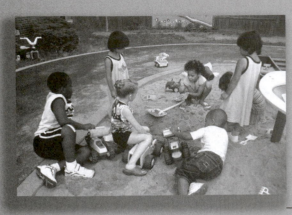

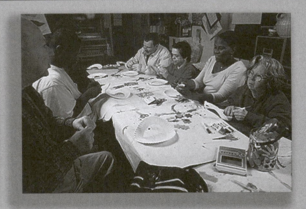

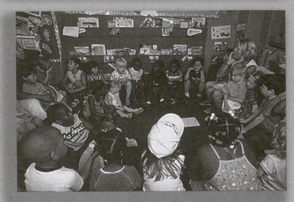

How Is a Functional Group Designed?

Case Study 2: Closed Group in an Outpatient Occupational Therapy Clinic
Case Study 3: Community-Based Group
Individual Learning Activities
Case Studies
Reflective Questions

The complexity of group leadership requires a considerable knowledge base coupled with clinical reasoning abilities. Certainly, both are aspects of group work that develop with study and practice. The functional group model offers an approach that is structured in a way to ensure, whether as a novice or seasoned practitioner, careful attention is given to what drives leaders' thoughts and actions. Part of this learning involves knowing the group member population and context. As this chapter guides you through the **how** of designing a functional group, it will provide you with practical methods to help you consider the contextual elements of:

• **Who** you are working with
• **What** they desire and are capable of
• **When**, in terms of moment in life and best time of day, your group occurs
• **Where,** as in cultural system and physical space

Designing a group according to the functional group model can be particularly useful when working with individuals who have experienced a physical injury or illness; suffer from an emotional, developmental, or congenital disorder; or are dealing with socioeconomic difficulties or the aging process and want or need assistance with changing or adapting to their life situation. Sometimes, more often in community-based groups, the goals of a functional group are to promote or maintain wellness.

Functional groups are designed to progress through three successive, interdependent stages:

1. Formation
2. Development
3. Closure

Beginning with this chapter, cases studies are provided that follow three groups, looking at elements of their design and how they progress through the successive stages of a functional group approach. The first two case studies are groups that meet within a clinical or hospital environment. The third group is held in a community center for senior citizens (see also Appendix C).

Assessing Need and Supports

The functional group model is appropriate for individuals who need:

An evaluation of their ability to function in life roles; including their underlying skills, behaviors, or client factors that are affecting successful performance.
To achieve skills or behaviors deemed prerequisite to functioning in life roles.
To improve or develop the communication and interaction skills necessary to support balanced participation in education; work, play, or leisure; self-care; or social relationships.
To prevent deterioration of skills or behaviors necessary for adaptive performance in meaningful life roles.
Help to facilitate health, wellness, or improved quality of life.

The needs listed here are wide-ranging and include needs of groups as social systems. The emphasis is on quality of functioning in a community rather than on mastery of a given skill or resolution of a specific problem per se. In community-based groups, the clients may be able to identify their goals more readily. Encouraging members to identify their own needs and goals, in whatever manner they can, serves to increase their direct participation in the group.

Prospective group members, depending on why they are seeking help, may be involved in services at various points on the continuum of care in medical or community settings. Therefore, in designing group programming, due to its comprehensive nature, the functional group model can be applicable to a variety of settings such as:

• Acute care units of a hospital
• Specialized medical services or settings
• Rehabilitation hospitals
• Nursing homes
• Outpatient facilities
• Partial hospital or day treatment programs
• Transitional or long-term care
• Schools
• Child care or after-school programs
• (Day) care or housing for elderly individuals
• Client, family, or caregiver education or support groups in the community

There are many populations for whom the structure and format of the functional group model provides a group context that can be adapted to their needs and level of ability. Prospective group members may be experiencing a range of functional impairments or have been diagnosed with certain conditions or disorders. Some examples include:

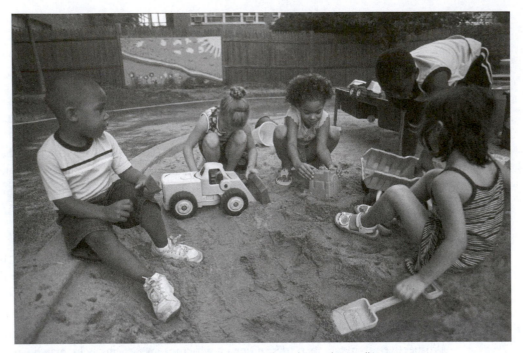

FIGURE 5.1 Design follows population and setting. (Photo by Mark Morelli)

Traumatic brain injury (e.g., head injury, cerebrovascular accident [CVA; more commonly referred to as stroke])

Psychiatric conditions, such as depression, attention deficit disorder/attention deficit hyperactivity disorder, substance abuse, or personality disorder schizophrenia

Dementia disorders, such as Alzheimer's disease

Chronic illness, such as arthritis, fibromyalgia, multiple sclerosis, or chronic obstructive pulmonary disease

Trauma, such as domestic violence, abuse or neglect, acts of terrorism, natural disasters, or physical trauma such as accidents resulting in fractures, burns, or spinal cord injury

Surgery, such as total knee or total hip replacements or mastectomy

The functional group model also offers a structure for groups with those who may be in need of supportive or preventive health services. Group members may also be of varying ages—from a young child to an older adult—and may be from diverse cultural or socioeconomic backgrounds as well as of different educational levels or functional abilities (Fig. 5.1).

The decision to offer a functional group depends in part on a setting's or an institution's aims and the roles and functions of the setting's staff, which may or may not include health professionals. In many settings, those staff or professionals who deliver the services are not necessarily the same people who decide on the programs to be offered. In addition, member needs may not be the most significant factor in a decision due to some of the pragmatics of payment structure or reimbursement, regulatory structure, and scope of practice of the various disciplines involved or agency mission. Other funding sources (i.e., grants, state or federal funding) can also play a role in determining the types of services offered. At times, interdisciplinary overlap in terms of skills or interests may require careful and diplomatic discussion to examine within the staff group how these various individuals will collaborate in terms of service delivery. In discussing inpatient group psychotherapy, Yalom (1983) pointed out, "Decisions about number, types, and frequency of groups are often made on the basis of what will not ruffle the staff rather than of what will be most effective for the patient" (p. 15). Therapists who conduct groups on a private practice basis usually work in collaboration with a referring physician or agency. Self-advocacy and family-centered models may also influence the types of groups offered.

A functional group may be designed to meet the needs of individuals who wish to change the structure of a natural group, such as a family or work group. Because peer groups play an important part in the normal development of adolescents, the functional group is particularly well suited to this age group. Adolescents need strong peer support to feel adequate. They are also developing a sense of self or personal identity and competency through testing a variety of behaviors. The activity and action orientation of the functional group approach match the modes of expression most often used by adolescents to explore their questions of identity and growth.

When a community of individuals who might benefit from a functional group has been identified, it may be beneficial to explore potential resources and present the initial needs assessment and expected outcomes to the various stakeholders (e.g., the client group, families, agency administrators, etc.) (Box 5.1). This is when data from outcome studies or research done in similar groups becomes extremely helpful. Even the outcome data from a few small groups can be of interest.

Methods used to assess or screen prospective group members should be tailored to individual settings and populations. Input from professionals with the appropriate qualifications may be needed to determine what individuals need assistance to maintain or develop performance skills or behaviors to function effectively in their life roles. If a health maintenance

Box 5.1 **Supportive Resources**

Available resources might include:

- Supportive people in the community or institution
- Streams of funding that are readily available
- Additional funding resources
- Data-based information to back up the efficacy and postulated outcomes of the group plan

Box 5.2   **Assessment Data**

The assessment of members of a functional group should include:

- Health
- Behavior
- Member goals
- Member performance and achievements

program is needed, medical screening for member readiness and precautions may be indicated. In evaluating prospective group members and settings, several questions should be asked (Box 5.2):

Are there individuals who need help to meet the expectations of or balance their life roles effectively?

Does the setting have a structure and resources to support programming aimed at outcomes regarding health promotion, improving occupational performance, or quality of life?
Are there political, economic, social, technical, legal, or ethical issues to be considered?
Is there a system in place for documenting member participation and group outcomes? (Box 5.3).

Does the mission of the institution or setting support the aims of a functional group?

Can or does this environment support adaptive behaviors necessary to maintain health or prevent deterioration of skills needed to engage in meaningful life tasks and roles?

Determining Group Goals and Methods

After the need and parameters for a functional group have been identified, group goals and methods must be established. Prospective members' goals may be determined through using one or more of five techniques:

1. Pre-group interview
2. Group history (Display 5.1)
3. Group assessment and plan
    a. Assessment of members and context (Display 5.2)
    b. Functional group protocol (Display 5.3)
4. Session plan (Display 5.4)
5. Session evaluation (Display 5.5)

When completing these protocols and forms, clients should be deidentified so that all data identifying individual members are recognizable only to the leader.

Box 5.3   **Needs Assessment and Documentation**

The ongoing process for goal setting is usually accomplished with the group members. Documentation systems may be agency- or setting-specific or in need of development for recording progress of group members as well as group programs. To help guide this process, the following questions can be asked to determine the best way to proceed:

1. Does there need to be an evaluation process and documentation and progress reporting system to:
   a. document the program's efficacy for the sponsoring agency
   b. document baseline performance of the clients/group members
   c. help guide the leader in structuring the group sessions
   d. determine the clients'/group members' problem areas, goals, and satisfaction with group participation and outcomes
   e. record client/group member participation and track progress
   f. document services in the event of litigation
   g. document the client/program outcomes for purposes of reimbursement?
2. What would you like to know about this group after the initial meetings, midpoint, and at the termination of the group?
   a. How would you gather this information?
   b. Of what importance would this information be to you, to your financial supporters, and to your sponsors?
   c. Is there a need for keeping records of individual change as well as the group's process?

Each technique is best suited to a particular circumstance. For example, taking a group history applies to a setting that has an existing group structure that will be changed to a functional group approach. If the leader chooses to have the group members contribute to establishing the group goals, a tentative first meeting goal may be to offer members an opportunity to state their own needs and goals.

Pre-Group Interview

A pre-group interview can elicit the goals of prospective group members as well as provide general information about members. Several points can be achieved:

Establishing members' level of functioning in areas of occupational performance
Understanding members' self-perceived needs
Developing functional goals
Forming a beginning therapeutic rapport with members
Explaining the nature, processes, expectations, and general purposes of the group to individual members

If someone in addition to the leader is doing the pre-group interview, as sometimes happens in a community-based setting, the information that is needed from and to be communi-

Display 5.1   **Group History**

Name of group:

Date:

General status: How long has the group existed? What is its anticipated duration? How often and for how long does the group meet? What is its general stage and level of development? Who has authority over goals and structure of the group?

Leadership and membership criteria: How was the group leadership and membership determined (i.e., assigned, voluntary or involuntary, referral)? If it is a closed group, what criteria are used to select the members? What was prior group leadership style?

Group structure and current membership: What is the group structure (format, general purpose, methodology)? How stable is the group membership? What is the rate of attendance? Is it an open or closed group? If it is an open group, are there any new members in the group? How long have the new and old members been in the group?

Outcomes: What outcomes have the group as a whole accomplished? What have individual members achieved? In what way has the group or leadership been unsuccessful?

Comments: Are there any other factors pertinent to understanding, assessing, and planning for the group?

---

cated to the members needs to be outlined in a manner that can readily be used to gather and convey the material.

On the basis of initial interviews, the group's general goals and methods can be tentatively outlined before the initial meeting. This process represents the starting point for the group and should be modified in an ongoing fashion, with member input as available and as the group becomes a more cohesive unit. Ultimately, goal setting and program planning should be a collaborative process between group leaders and members as the group moves through the successive stages of formation, development, and closure.

Group History

If an established group exists, the leader(s) can take a group history (see Display 5.1). This history should be a means for understanding the group composition and membership (open vs. closed), how long the group has been together, how stable group membership and attendance have been, and what stage and level of development the group may have achieved. Determining who has decision-making authority regarding group goals and structure, in addition to whether membership is voluntary or involuntary, is important to understanding what may have had an effect on the preexisting group's climate and culture. This information is ideally gathered from group process notes or from setting administrators or staff rather than from interviewing members. Recording a clear statement of former and current goals of both individuals and the group as a whole can help establish a baseline from which to monitor the ensuing progress of the group's process and individual group members. In some instances, the group members or their relatives may interview the group leader and together construct the history and goals. This method is particularly important when the leader is in the role of consultant or facilitator. The group history can be used together with the third technique, which involves the assessment of members and context.

Group Assessment and Plan

Assessment of Members and Context

Once prospective members and a setting have been identified, understanding individual members' abilities in a wide range of areas, as well as contextual elements of the setting, is a crucial next step in designing a functional group. Assessment (see Display 5.2) is a method for outlining information group leaders may find useful. A group leader in a medical setting may be able to gather this information readily; however, a leader of a group outside a medical setting may need to modify what information is gathered. Assessment covers many facets of the members' health status, including:

• Life roles and contexts
• Current performance areas
• Strengths and deficits in motor, processing, communication, and interaction skills
• Possible underlying conditions or impairments related to body structures and functions

This knowledge can help the group leader in planning and helping members with developing realistic goals. Members may identify general expectations for outcomes related to participation in the group, specific goals they might want to achieve in a single group session, or goals they wish to achieve over time as they participate. If possible, description of members' performance and achievements to date should be included.

The setting of the group should be considered to determine if certain contextual aspects will influence the group's goals. Context includes the physical location, the agency mission or philosophy, the emotional environment, and the administrative structure of the setting where the group will be held or of the agency sponsoring the group. Funding sources, required program outcomes, related regulatory bodies, organizational culture, and a general description of the surrounding community (demographics, resources) are also part of understanding larger systems and issues that may affect the group and group members.

After this information has been collected, a set of goals that relate to all group members can be distilled from the many general and specific goals. For the purpose of measuring and reporting progress, goals should be stated in behavioral terms with desired outcome criteria. Although the functional group model does not ascribe to a strictly behavioral frame of reference, goals for the client group (performance skills or behaviors that are to be developed,

Display 5.2   **Assessment of Members and Context**

Assessment of group members: (client profile including range of behaviors, why seeking services, desired goals/outcomes)

General description:

General description of members' expected environment:

Description of current occupational performance:

Education/work:

Self-care (ADLs/IADLs):

Play/leisure:

Social participation:

Strengths and deficits in motor and process skills:

Physical and neuromotor:

Cognitive:

Psychosocial:

What is the significance of these factors with regard to forming the group, setting individual member goals, and/or planning group session(s)?:

Assessment of Group Context (the Facility)

General description of program (mission, administrative structure):

General description of physical environment:

General description of emotional climate:

Frames of reference, purpose, and objectives:

What is the significance of these factors with regard to forming the group, setting individual member goals, and/or planning group session(s)?:

Assessment of Environmental Supports and Constraints

Facilities and materials:

Scheduling:

Group norms and prior therapy group experience (if any):

Do any of the environmental constraints require modification of the group, or could the situation be altered?:

---

improved, increased, or decreased) should be stated in a manner that identifies actions that are observable (Box 5.4).

Goal setting is a continuing process usually done in conjunction with the members. Therefore, initial goals for the group as a whole, and for individual members, may change over time. The criteria for successful attainment of goals in each session should also be stated in behavioral terms. It has been advised that "appropriate goal setting is of crucial importance

Box 5.4   **Goal Setting**

Well-stated goals should either be SMART or meet the criteria of RUMBA:

S - Specific		R - Relevant
M - Measurable		U - Understandable
A - Attainable	Or	M - Measurable
R - Relevant		B - Behavioral
T - Time frame		A - Achievable

to the proper functioning of the small therapy group. Overly ambitious goals impair the effectiveness of the group and lower the morale of the therapist" (Yalom, 1983, p. 62). Depending on the goals, a methodology should then be selected. The methodology should suit the group's general goals, time frame, and structure. Just as group goals need ongoing revision, methods should be regularly adjusted to the pace of the group and its development.

Functional Group Protocol

Once general goals and methods are established, a functional group protocol is developed (Display 5.3). This provides a tentative structure that informs one's reasoning and techniques

Display 5.3   **Functional Group Protocol**

Name of group:

Time/length of meeting(s):

Place:

Group Format: Open ☐ or Closed ☐

Statement of rationale:

General group goals: (depending on group, may include primary and secondary objectives and leader objectives for group and/or individual members)

Rationale for goal selection:

Outcome criteria for successful goal attainment in session(s) (stated in behavioral terms)**:**

Group composition and criteria for selecting members:

Leadership roles and functions:

Characteristics of group contract:

Group methods and procedures to be employed: (briefly describe or list methods, techniques and modalities)

used in interactions within the group. The plan also serves as a guide for program planning while keeping the group working toward its goals. Again, it should be emphasized that the plan and member goals are likely to change as leaders interact with the group and reflect on their observations. Nevertheless, in all circumstances, a specific format is needed. This is especially true for open groups and groups run in acute care settings. Under these circumstances, the leader might have only one or two sessions with a group member. Consequently, each session must have optimal effect.

The functional group protocol sets forth the overall framework for the group, from formation through closure (termination). It presents a detailed statement of: criteria and requirements for group membership, group purpose, objectives as well as leadership roles and functions including group methods, procedures, techniques, and strategies (Box 5.5). The goals presented are long-term and represent what should be achieved by the end of the group series (closed group membership) or by an individual member's departure from the group (open group membership). The methods listed are procedural guides for planning and implementing specific techniques and modalities to achieve group goals. Because of its detail, the functional group protocol is usually based on a group history or assessment of group members and context. If these methods of assessment are not possible, initial group sessions may focus on assessment to develop a detailed plan.

When a group is being designed for the first time, the functional group protocol will probably have to be reformulated following the first meeting of the group when the pertinent information becomes available. However, it is important for the group leader to have a plan for the first session, which includes alternative plans for adapting to member abilities or needs and interests. A session plan should be developed for each session. A session evaluation is used as a method to review and reflect on the group's progress and to aid in reformulating the group or member goals and session plans as needed.

Session Plan

The session plan (Display 5.4) establishes the specific framework for each session (or unit of sessions) designed to fulfill specific aspects of the functional group protocol. Goals are short-term and indicate the anticipated group achievement for the specific session or unit. The session plan also includes what the specific techniques and modalities will be for each group session or meeting.

Box 5.5   **Sharing the Plan**

> The general group plan protocol should be made available to all those involved in the care of a group member.

Display 5.4   **Session Plan**

Name of group:

Date:

Specific goals for the group session:

Specific goals for group members: (if different from previously established goals for each member)

Description and rationale for methods and procedures:

Description and rationale for leadership role:

List material and equipment needed:

Time and sequence outline for sessions, including what you will do and say as leader and what group is expected to do (consider both content and process)**:**

Other information pertinent to this specific session (e.g., will there be any new members, co-leaders, or guests? is there an unusual tone in the unit or special event that is about to occur or just occurred for the individual member or group?)**:**

Session Evaluation

A Session Evaluation (Display 5.5) is a means to determine the group's as well as individual member's progress toward long-term and short-term goals. Information is gathered on whether or not the selected techniques and modalities are appropriate for the group and the effect of leader behavior on the group. This process of reflecting on the overall group process and outlining member progress can be useful in identifying needed changes in leader style or group structure. The information collected can also be used to modify the Functional Group Protocol and, later, Session Plans.

Group Member Criteria

The range of individuals who may be suited to a functional approach indicates that the essential criteria qualifying individuals for the group seem broad. However, to ensure member readiness for participating in a group, there are five general criteria. Each member should be able to do the following:

1. Communicate verbally or nonverbally in a simple manner.
2. Understand basic communications, such as instructions (written, verbal, or demonstrated).

3. Be able to participate in structured tasks in the presence of two other group members for a minimum of 30 minutes. This time may be different for children or others when the group is planned with a short attention span in mind.

Display 5.5 **Session Evaluation**

Name of group:

Date:

Were the goals accomplished? (state outcome and give rationale):

Was the session helpful in accomplishing short- and long-term group and individual member goals? (explain):

Do you have any information that indicates the session(s) has/have been helpful to the members' functioning (adaptation) outside of the group? (explain):

Was the group structure adequate for accomplishing the goals? (give rationale, taking into consideration: leadership; time/length of meeting; open- versus closed-group format; time, sequence, methods, and procedures; media/modalities/techniques employed; norms/behaviors reinforced implicitly or explicitly; methods of reinforcement; and stage of group's development):

Did the structure provide for "optimal experience" or a "flow state" to occur? (explain):

Did the structure provide optimal purposeful, self-initiated, spontaneous, and group-centered "action" to allow meaningful interaction, enhanced performance skills, and/or adaptation to occur through "occupation"? (explain):

Did the structure provide for new learning or reinforcement of current level of role functioning or occupational performance, or did it reinforce functioning below current level of ability? (explain):

Did the structure provide an opportunity for evaluation and feedback regarding the group procedures, process, and member progress? (explain):

What changes would you make regarding group goals and structure for the next session or if you were to lead this session again?

Were you adequately prepared for the session? (give rationale, taking into consideration time, place, materials, and physical and emotional environment):

How did you function as leader? (give rationale, taking into consideration how your behavior and role affected the group, what you did that was effective, leadership opportunities missed, what you learned about yourself as group leader):

Was the group interaction as you anticipated? (explain; if problems occurred, what you can identify as a basis for understanding the problems):

In the future, what might you do differently as group leader? (give rationale):

4. Understand the general purpose and nature of the group, the roles of the members and leader, and the group rules and expectations regarding safety.

5. Tolerate the stimulation of interpersonal contact.

After considering an individual's general qualifications for membership, other factors need to be considered. The group must be formed so that members can work together in some reasonable order. The number of possible members, and the range of problems and goals that can be dealt with, is therefore limited. When designing a particular group, composition and size must be considered.

Group Composition

The composition of a group can be determined according to extent of member similarity or difference. Members may be selected who are alike, who have very similar problems or needs such as skill deficit, role disorder, developmental disability, illness or injury, diagnosis, age, and so on. Another option is to select members who have the same type of problem but in varying degrees. Membership selection may consider individuals who have a variety of issues but may be united in their need or desire to improve their ability to function. Regardless of membership criteria and group composition, the group needs to be composed in a thoughtful manner so that it can potentially become a cohesive one. Yalom (2005) proposes that cohesiveness be the primary guideline in member selection and group composition. In terms of member homogeneity or heterogeneity "heterogeneous groups have advantages over homogeneous groups for intensive interactional group therapy" (Yalom, 1970, p. 193).

In composing a group, membership selection should be based on individuals who not only have similar goals, abilities, or needs but who also will be able to function together in a particular action or activity. It is unlikely, therefore, that on a rehabilitation unit, a patient recently admitted post cerebrovascular accident (stroke) would be assigned to a group of patients several weeks post stroke who are preparing for imminent discharge. The member goals and functional abilities would be too diverse. By contrast, two patients in outpatient services, one with an upper extremity fracture and one with joint inflammation from arthritis, who have identified their need to resume their homemaker role might be quite compatible members of a group. Thus, the goals of the group and the chosen modality, intervention, or activity process need to be carefully considered when members are selected for a specific group.

Group Size

The size of a group will influence how the members relate to each other as well as other facets of the group experience. No strict rule dictates size. Five to ten members is an acceptable number for an "interactional therapy group" (Yalom, 1970, p. 215), with seven considered ideal. Seven members can work together effectively in the activity of a group and participate fully in its process. If a group has fewer than five members, the opportunity for maximal member interaction decreases, and the therapy becomes more leader-centered (Yalom, 1970). When the group size increases beyond 10, there is less time for individual members to fully participate (Fig. 5.2).

Size should be based in part on members' attention spans, functional abilities, and ability to delay gratification. If members have problems in these areas, groups for these individuals should have fewer than five members. However, in some instances, if following Yalom's (1970) axiom of seven as an ideal number, it might be wise to compose a group with two more members than the desired size. One or two members may drop out at the beginning and, therefore, having the two additional members can ensure that overall size does not fall below the minimum needed. Special problems related to settings may affect decisions about group size. In acute care settings, member turnover is high because of the length of stay being relatively short and members being discharged quickly. The size of the group should be large enough to absorb sudden changes in membership.

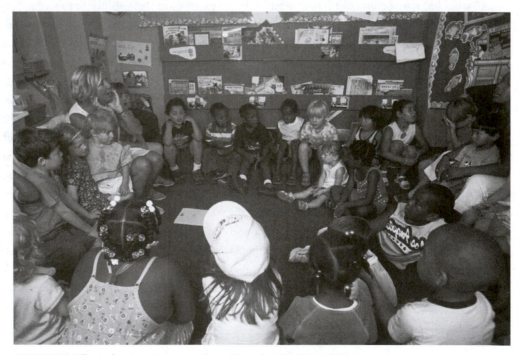

FIGURE 5.2 Effect of group size on process. (Photo by Mark Morelli)

Structuring the Group and the Tasks

The group, including elements of the group environment, should be structured to facilitate specific aspects of working in a group toward the goals. Therefore, the group should be designed and the group environment (to the extent possible) arranged to achieve:

• Maximal involvement of members through group-centered action
• Maximal sense of individual and group identity
• A "flow experience"
• Spontaneous involvement
• Member support and feedback

The task of designing the group involves planning a "structure for the group by delineating clear spatial and temporal boundaries; by adopting a lucid, decisive, but flexible personal style; by providing an explicit orientation and preparation for the patient; and by developing a consistent, coherent group procedure" (Yalom, 1983, p. 108).

Maximal Involvement

Maximal involvement can be achieved through four steps. Each step must be clear to set the pace of the group for the members.

Step One: Orient the Group to the Design. The plan should include introductory remarks that will explain the nature of the group and purpose of the session(s) and, to the extent possible, make leader and member roles explicit. The plan should make sense in terms of the group members' specific needs, perceptions, and abilities to process the information. Reviewing or developing group rules to guide member behavior and possible leader actions as well as to design or refine group goals should occur as part of this introduction.

Step Two: Explain Procedures to Group. Explain the following (in a manner consistent with members' ability to understand):
  • Group purpose
  • Session agenda
  • Group methodology, i.e., specific tasks or procedure(s) to be used in the session(s), and the sequence of activities

Step Three: Set Up the Task or Activity. Depending on the nature of the group and the abilities of the members, the plan may include involving the group in setting up the task or planning time prior to the group session to do this for the group. The group plan may also involve allotting time for members to participate in the clean-up period, if they are able, after the activity has ended.

Step Four: Follow-Up. The plan needs to allow time after the group participates in the task or activity for the group to assess the experience. A format that guides the group in connecting the task and social experience to the group and individual member goals may be needed. This processing time can be used to elicit exchange of feedback and input regarding plans for future sessions, if applicable. Additionally, by planning an opportunity for follow-up within the session, members may be able to realize implications of their behavior in terms of effective task or social performance. If their functional capacity allows, the follow-up period may facilitate members gaining insight as to how their behavior in the group relates to how they behave or interact with others in their daily lives.

Maximal Sense of Individual and Group Identity

A climate of safety is created within the group through support and genuine caring. In planning for the group, the tasks and, if necessary, social interaction can be structured so members feel in control of the process. Plans that involve the members in setting goals, selecting and implementing tasks, and engaging in follow-up as part of the close of the group must be designed at the level of the members' abilities. An open group may require the leaders to structure these procedures highly to create a safe holding environment (Winnicott, 1958) for the group members.

Flow Experience

Structuring a group to facilitate flow experience involves creating an environment that stimulates curiosity and the desire to achieve through opportunities or challenges for action. Csikszentmihalyi's (1975) model of the flow state should serve as a guideline: "When a person believes that his action opportunities are too demanding for his capabilities, the resulting stress is experienced as anxiety; when the ratio of capabilities is higher, but the challenges are still too demanding for his skills, the experience is worry. The state of flow is felt when opportunities for action are in balance with the actor's skills; the experience is then autotelic. When skills are greater than opportunities for using them, the state of boredom results; this state again fades into anxiety when the ratio becomes too large" (p. 49).

Designing a group that will enable the members to achieve a flow state should include only those tasks that are culturally acceptable to the members and that can produce personal satisfaction. In a study of play and flow in an activity group, it was concluded that, in spite of cultural expectations, there appeared to be a developmental progression. Nonverbal expression (such as painting) and non-play/non-flow seemed to be a prerequisite to play/flow states in an activity group (Persson, 1996).

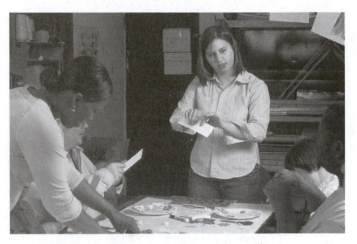

FIGURE 5.3 Leader as model. (Photo by Mark Morelli)

Spontaneous (Here and Now) Involvement

The design of the group needs to guide the group toward discussion and action in the present. This can be achieved through modeling behaviors and feedback (Fig. 5.3). In addition, activities should be planned and structured so that action is required. The leader, in turn, may verbally reflect back to the group how the group's and individual members' behaviors might relate to the purpose of the session(s).

Member Support and Feedback

Leader(s) should plan to demonstrate specific modes of support to encourage members' participation in accordance to these basic principles:

Point out what may be perceived as universal elements, needs, concerns, and reactions to
   group members or the group as a whole
Members are never criticized, blamed, or made to feel isolated
Activities are structured according to the range of members' abilities
Empathize and aim to teach members how to give feedback constructively

Leader Emotional Response

Designing a functional group may elicit mixed feelings for group leaders. In starting a new venture, feelings of anxiety and excitement related to the challenges ahead may surface regardless of whether the group is previously established or newly created. If a group is previously established, someone other than the new leader selected the membership. Member-

Box 5.6   **Self-Reflective Leader Questions**

Ask yourself the following questions:

Will the plan be effective?
Will there be a sufficient number of members?
What are my reasons for working with this group?
Am I being realistic in my expectations of myself? Of the group members?
What are my concerns about acceptance?
How can I monitor that my emotional, social, and spiritual needs are met outside
   of my role as group leader?
Will there be attrition? What are my feelings or concerns about loss?
Will I get paid or adequately compensated? What are my concerns about acknowl-
   edgement?
What are my concerns about my own competence? Are these concerns accurate?
   Who can help me assess my strengths and areas for growth?
What learning resources or persons are available for support, supervision, or mentoring?

ship selection may have been done by an administrator or supervisor or by virtue of a natural group existing in a setting. In such instances, there may be concern about whether there is a good match between leader skills and members' needs. Feelings of insecurity may arise if the existing group had a positive attachment to a prior leader. Likewise, if a previous leader had negative or resistive relationships, this may be of concern. In this instance, more extreme feelings, such as a sense of panic, may be experienced. As a group leader it may be useful to explore one's own expectations, wishes, or even fantasies of rescuing the group from failure or saving members from their plight. If the group is newly created, anxieties concerning whether there will be enough members, sufficient reimbursement, and adequate means to market the program may emerge. The area of highest anxiety in starting a new group is often the fear of "getting off on the wrong foot." In planning the group's initial sessions, remembering that it is common not to find total group participation may be key; "maximal involvement" is a more realistic goal. In designing a functional group, examining one's emotional responses and identifying patterns in reactions is an important aspect of the planning process. Self-reflective questions can aid this analysis (Box 5.6).

Conclusion

Care in the design of a functional group is of critical importance to the group's ultimate success. Assessing the need for a group and group members and context are critical to establishing the group purpose and goals. Subsequently, the development of a plan, selection of group members and methods, and planning the structure of the group and its tasks are all part of how a functional group is designed. In developing a group plan, the aim is to create a structure that facilitates purposeful, self-initiated, spontaneous, and group-centered action. Contingency or alternate plans may be necessary. The initial plans are preliminary. The group structure and format may need to be adapted once the group begins or to flex according to the needs of the members as the group proceeds through the various phases of development.

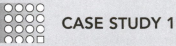

CASE STUDY 1

Open Group on an Inpatient Psychiatry Unit

● **Leaders: Lauri Levy, OTR/L, and Jack Jones, MHC**

This group has existed as part of the program of service delivery on a psychiatric inpatient unit for 3 years. The unit is a 15-bed acute care psychiatric service with an average length of stay of 3–5 days in a private, nonprofit general hospital. Regulatory bodies include the Joint Commission on Accreditation for Hospital Organizations and the state's department of Health and Human Services. The interdisciplinary staff consists of mental health counselors, nurses, occupational therapists, psychiatrists, psychologists, and social workers. Staff mix is diverse in terms of age, gender, sexual orientation, and educational level beyond undergraduate education, but most are white.

The unit has a long hallway with six semiprivate rooms and two single rooms. The nurses' station, a quiet room, and a sensory room, used to provide a calming space, are at one end of the hall, with a kitchen/dining area, the occupational therapy room, staff offices, a small conference room, and community living room at the other. The occupational therapy room has one long rectangular table, a small circular table, and workbenches and activity supply cabinets along the walls. The room is painted in soft green; patients' projects are scattered about; and there are many hanging plants by a Plexiglas window over a large work sink. A wide range of activities can be conducted in the occupational therapy room and unit kitchen/dining areas. However, the hospital design and the unit in particular are not large enough to accommodate group activities that require a lot of movement, physical sports equipment, or space.

The emotional climate on the unit varies according to the patient population. At times, the atmosphere appears calm and quiet, and at other times it is noisy, high-keyed, and energetic. There are occasional outbursts (yelling, crying, screaming, physical or verbal threats) by patients, which are addressed by staff trained in de-escalation techniques. Physically or verbally abusive behaviors are not tolerated. Patients who are unable to respect this requirement are provided with individualized schedules and one-to-one services as needed for their own safety or the safety of others.

The chief of psychiatric services, a psychiatrist, has ultimate authority over the goals and structure of any therapies conducted on the unit. In addition to this group, patients attend daily community meetings, group therapy, individual therapy, and individual occupational therapy sessions. The primary focus of treatment is problem identification and symptom management in preparation for discharge to home or the next level of care. Most members are also being treated with psychiatric medications or are being evaluated for such treatment. Each patient has his or her own case manager, and the patient's attending psychiatrist supervises all treatment. Patients who cannot (or refuse to) participate in their treatment program (as established by the individual patient, in conjunction with the treatment team, family members if applicable, and nursing staff) are often transitioned to long-term treatment at other facilities. Some patients' conditions require readmission to the hospital; therefore, they have attended treatment groups during prior admissions. Others have no group treatment experience or have participated in groups in other settings or contexts (i.e., AA, NA, clubhouse model recovery groups, outpatient therapy).

The occupational therapy department has direct responsibility for designing, implementing, and evaluating this group. This group is an open group, with the membership changing on a weekly, often daily, basis. Due to the high rate of patient turnover, the sessions must be planned and held daily. Leaders attend morning rounds or community meetings to get a sense of the unit and treatment plan issues that may be affecting members.

Because membership changes, the group is always, in a sense, in the formation stage. Therefore, the group needs leader direction and structure to facilitate the group process through phases of development and closure (termination) in each session. The group leaders consist of a licensed occupational therapist and mental health counselor. The minimum criteria for group membership are having unit-based privileges and being able to maintain personal safety in the presence of other group members and while using supplies (i.e., media such as pens, scissors, etc.), as evidenced by self-control of urges to harm self or others. In addition, prospective candidates for the group should at a minimum be able to communicate verbally in a simple manner, understand simple communications in written and verbal form, concentrate on a structured task in the presence of seven other patients and two therapists for a minimum of 30 minutes, and understand the goals and methods of the group.

After assessing the needs of the hospital's psychiatric inpatient population, the leaders, in consultation with the interdisciplinary team and unit nursing staff, determined that at any given time there would be eight patients who might benefit from a semistructured group. The group, generically considered parallel to a project-level activity-based group, is metaphorically named "Getting It Together." The group members are mixed in gender, and membership is voluntary in that patients can choose the group as part of their treatment program. However, once patients elect this service, during a pre-group interview they are asked to agree to a group contract that outlines that members are expected to:

Participate in the group project: at a minimum, getting or distributing materials to other group members or contributing ideas during group activities.

Express feelings about their individual participation, inclusive of interactions in the group, contributions to the project, and the group's final product, if applicable.

Assume positive group member roles by offering encouragement, agreeing to compromise at times, listening to others' ideas or opinions, asking for information, giving opinions, or expressing wishes in a socially acceptable manner.

Members are told that they are expected to attend sessions on a regular basis unless unusual circumstances prevail (i.e., safety issues, laboratory appointments). Should such circumstances arise, members, if possible, or their designee should notify leaders before the session. Members are required to remain in each group session for the 45 minutes or to negotiate with the group or leaders if a special contract or arrangement for reduced time is necessary. Information discussed by other group members is not to be shared outside of the group unless within the confines of a therapeutic relationship with unit staff or by group leaders in the context of maintaining safety or documenting and reporting member progress. If members are unable to fulfill the requirements of the group contract, they will be asked to leave or be removed from the group.

The group meets daily for 45 minutes. The group time is scheduled for 4:00–4:45 p.m., right before the dinner hour. Because of other treatments scheduled, the unit schedule for meetings, activities of daily living (ADL)/instrumental activities of daily living (IADL) times, the hospital meal schedule, and evening patient visiting hours, the group meeting time is on a fixed schedule and cannot be changed. Some group members return to the unit on readmissions and therefore have attended the group during prior hospitalizations. Other patients have no group treatment experience or have had psychosocial treatment in other settings.

Group size ranges from four to eight (maximum) members. The general purpose of the group is to increase member ability to engage in meaningful activity as well as to demonstrate pro-social participation. In past groups, members have been able to identify personal goals for the session when cued by the leaders. However, processing goal achievement at the close of group sessions has been problematic as members primarily seek leader (vs. peer) feedback about their performance. Currently, the group follows a cognitive-behavioral frame of reference (i.e., that thoughts, feelings, and behaviors are related), as has been integrated into the therapeutic milieu of the unit, under the direction of the chief of psychiatry. This frame of reference is integrated with a biopsychosocial frame of reference and a functional group approach in accordance with the functional group model.

Demographically, members are between 16 and 70 years of age and primarily live in the urban communities surrounding the hospital area. Culturally, many of the patients identify themselves ethnically as Chinese, Irish Catholic, African American, Vietnamese, Puerto Rican, or Russian. English is not the primary language for approximately half the patient population. Socioeconomic status ranges from middle-class and upper middle-class to destitute (homeless). Hospitalization costs are primarily covered by third-party payers (e.g., private insurance, Medicare). Diagnoses include mood disorders, schizophrenia and other thought disorders, personality disorders, substance use disorders, and eating disorders. Some patients have medical problems such as cardiac conditions, arthritis, diabetes, and multiple sclerosis, but these conditions are generally stabilized and secondary to their psychiatric disorder.

Group members' disposition plans range from returning to their homes to live alone or with family, being discharged to a more suitable living arrangement in the community, or awaiting transfer to longer-term inpatient treatment settings (i.e., private facility, state hospital, Veteran's Administration hospital). In the community contexts, members will be expected to resume roles as parents, workers, students, group home residents, or retirees. Of the current mix of group members, two are college students, one is a homemaker, one is retired, three are employed (an office manager, a chef, and a freelance writer), and one has a long-term history of unemployment. All are independent in basic ADLs (i.e., bathing, dressing). However, they have difficulty making decisions, especially when social interactions are involved, in managing more complex personal hygiene and grooming or with IADLs such as care of others/pets, and with fiscal, health, and home management (shopping, banking, bill paying, nutrition/ exercise, general personal item, and household maintenance). All members have expressed dissatisfaction with their use of leisure time. Some feel they have few to no interests; others are either overwhelmed by work obligations or do not have the motivation, energy, or resources (time, place, money, relationships, or interpersonal ability) to participate in leisure or volunteer activities. Some patients have identified that they tend to sleep during the day, take medications only when they remember or are reminded, spend their time predominantly watching television or on the Internet, and use smoking or drinking as a means to "relax."

Members identify estrangement or conflict in family or peer relationships and avoidance of structured community activities (clubs, church/synagogue, library membership, voting, etc.), which may for some be due to experiencing symptoms such as paranoia, delusions, flashbacks, or phobias, thus resulting in a high degree of isolation, even when around others. All members are ambulatory, and all have adequate gross- and fine-motor coordination and range of motion to perform routine ADLs. They are all able to maintain balance when performing activities seated, standing, walking, or moving about during simple gross motor activities (such as sweeping the floor, reaching for objects, and simple exercise routines). Many are unable to perform tasks with the strength and endurance required for the members' pre-hospitalization routines; for example, they may take frequent rests or complain of strain or fatigue. Some are experiencing medication side effects such as dry mouth, numbness or stiffness, tremulousness, or motor restlessness, some of which may or may not diminish.

Most members have intact memory skills for factual information, but some experience cognitive distortions in recalling verbal interactions and information involving affect. Members are generally oriented to time, place, and person. The majority of members have some insight into their current difficulties as being related to their mental illness. Some become anxious and have difficulty sequencing a plan of action when solving problems, whereas others are able to make abstract judgments but have difficulty with simple decisions involved in daily living. On admission, in addition to being at risk of harm to self or others, members presented problems such as poor self-esteem; preoccupation with internal stimuli; withdrawal from family, friends, or coworkers; loss of interest in vocational or avocational activities; indecisiveness and disorganization around daily routines, resulting in an inability to complete tasks required for daily functioning, such as food shopping, meal preparation, physical care of children, and attention to personal hygiene regarding care of hair, skin, teeth, cosmetics/shaving, etc.

Most members have difficulty recognizing and verbalizing their emotions. Although members are able to imitate behaviors, they have difficulty identifying when a change in action is needed. Some members rely totally on others to fulfill their needs, whereas others are unwilling to accept suggestions or help. Most are unable to identify their strengths and therefore focus their discussions on their limitations. Several members are unable to handle frustration with a task and show their anxiety by not completing the activity, moving about restlessly, being irritable, devaluing the task, and asking or demanding to leave. Some members attempt to interact with others in the group by always offering help (often to the exclusion of attending to their needs), others by demanding assistance and withdrawing if it is not immediately available. Some members vacillate between extreme expressions of affect or relatedness (anger or silliness; poor physical or interpersonal boundaries; tangential, paranoid, or distorted thought processes such as wishful, blaming, or "black white" thinking; neediness; or rejection).

The group needs to be advised on how to select relatively short-term activities with little complexity and minimal opportunity for error. The leaders need to assume an active role in adapting the activities so that members can hold a variety of group membership roles. Leaders also need to observe the group's process in order to make process comment, set limits, suggest alternative behaviors, and assume group membership roles when the members are unable to do so. A highly supportive, genuine, and consistent emotional climate in the group must be established and reinforced by the leaders.

CASE STUDY 2

CLOSED GROUP IN AN OUTPATIENT OCCUPATIONAL THERAPY CLINIC

• LEADERS: RUSSELL LEE, MS OTR/L, AND ALICIA WALL, COTA/L

The outpatient clinic has been offering a support and psychoeducational group for patients dealing with community re-entry for the past year under the direction of the director of rehabilitation, an occupational therapist, and chief physiatrist. This is a closed group, composed of eight members. Although membership is voluntary, the group contract outlines that once members agree to participate, they understand daily attendance is required. The group meets four times per week for 2 weeks. Program evaluation has found an outcome of the group to be that the patients require less follow-up care at home. The group is held in the occupational therapy clinic with plinths, mirrors, mats, weights, pulleys, a single bed, an adapted kitchen, a prevocational area with a Baltimore Therapeutic Equipment machine, computers with adaptive keyboards/mice, various tools, an indoor garden, an activity area with tables and chairs, and a reception desk and offices in the foyer of clinic space. Members are referred from the inpatient, subacute, and transitional care units of the rehabilitation hospital. Members must be age 17 years or older and in need of help with community re-entry issues such as energy conservation, time management, and adjustment to diagnosis or current disability status. Member diagnoses generally include hip fracture, total hip or knee replacements, mastectomy, traumatic brain injury, cerebrovascular accident (CVA), Guillain-Barré syndrome, and cardiac conditions. Members may have mild to moderate impairments in body structures and body functions that may be affecting motor, process, and communication skills such as balance, mobility, coordination, energy (pacing and endurance), and speech. Often, pain management and sleep disturbance are stated concerns of members. Members frequently express they find returning home very stressful, identifying strained family, friend, and coworker relationships; fatigue and difficulty completing routine tasks (activities of daily living, work, home maintenance); depression; anxiety; and feelings of uselessness as primary problem areas.

Group members are screened once a referral to the group is received. Members must be oriented to person, place, and time; be able to communicate verbally and understand oral instructions; be relatively stable emotionally (i.e., without presenting as highly labile), and be able to concentrate on group tasks for up to 60 minutes. The group is structured in a series of eight sessions sequenced to facilitate the group's phases of development. The group is intended to teach skills while providing a group-centered and cohesive support group. The leaders, an occupational therapist and an occupational therapy assistant, have the responsibility for planning and implementing the group. The group is developed according to the functional group model. However, person-environment-occupation and biomechanical frames of reference also inform leader reasoning.

Current group membership is seven adults, ranging from 31 to 66 years of age. There are four women (two are post CVA, one is post hip fracture, one is post bilateral total knee replacements secondary to arthritis) and three men (two have traumatic brain injury, one post motor vehicle accident that occurred when driving while intoxicated, one secondary to anoxia due to a myocardial infarction (heart attack) resulting in triple bypass surgery, and one has chronic pain secondary to spinal fusion for ruptured lumbar discs). Many members seem to become restless and irritable or slightly agitated when expected to perform an activity. The members demonstrate various amounts of gross and fine motor impairment resulting from their primary medical conditions or secondary to arthritis, neuromuscular disorder, chronic pain, general lethargy, or deconditioning. The range of problems includes poor dexterity and coordination in hand functions or gait, postural instability or problems with balance, limited active range of motion, and fatigue or strain when using muscular force required for certain activities. Additionally, many have poor sensory awareness and poor visual-spatial awareness. The range of member self-care skills includes complete independence in daily living skills (i.e., grooming/hygiene, feeding/eating, dressing, functional mobility, functional communication) to dependence in functional mobility (wheelchair mobility, transfers, ambulation), dressing, grooming/hygiene, and feeding/eating, requiring minimal to moderate assistance with these tasks or activities. Two currently require the services of a personal care attendant.

All group members report feeling depressed or anxious but are able to concentrate on a task or concept for 60 minutes and have immediate and recent memory. Range of insight varies from excellent to poor. Problem-solving ability ranges from being able to make decisions to reliance on concrete cues for evaluating decisions and plans. Most members seldom initiate conversation with individuals other than the staff or their own family. All express concern about how they appear to others, an inability to be productive, and feeling burdensome to friends, coworkers (if applicable), family, and loved ones.

Group members live in suburban areas and cities within a 90-minute drive and live at home, either alone, with spouses or significant other, or with other family members. Two members are retired, one active in retirement and one completely dependent on family with no outside interests; two are homemakers, one with high school–age children and one with an infant; one is currently unemployed with work potential (formerly employed full time as a lawyer, wanting to resume practicing part-time), one runs a small family business, and one is a music teacher.

Members' leisure skills range from active to quiet and sedentary pursuits. Identified interests include golf, exercise (walking, jogging, gym membership), volunteer work, cooking, music, computer, reading, and handicrafts such as sewing, knitting, and jewelry making. One member was unable to identify activities or social situations they perceived as enjoyable or fun. All express concern regarding their ability to adapt leisure activities, daily routine, or home environment to enable them to participate in what they want or need to do upon return home.

Members identified experiencing difficulty with transitioning back into social settings, including family routines, spiritual communities, work, and other community venues (grocery store, hairdresser, library, or settings such as health club or community service venues—rotary club, PTA, etc.). Members indicate that they are uncomfortable about or struggling with loss of traditional roles (driver of family car, head of household finances or maintenance, etc.). Most were unable to identify community resources available.

This group is one of the services offered through the occupational therapy department. The leadership responsibility rotates among the inpatient and outpatient occupational therapy staff of 18 occupational therapists and 2 occupational therapy assistants. The director of occupational therapy provides supervision as needed. Consultation is also available from the hospital physicians, nurses, speech language pathologists, social workers, physical therapists, and neuropsychologists.

The group is conducted in the occupational therapy outpatient clinic, which has an adapted kitchen, prevocational area, activity area with tables and chairs, reception desk, and offices. The clinic is wheelchair-accessible. Staff strives to promote a cheerful, warm, friendly, relaxed, and supportive environment in which therapists are open and direct in their communication with patients. Most therapists schedule patients in one-to-one therapies in the clinic. Therefore, coordination of use of supplies, equipment, and space with other staff and therapists is a necessity. The group is scheduled 10:00–11:30 a.m., so the leaders need to work with other staff to coordinate patient scheduling. Some members need transportation assistance to bring them to and from the occupational therapy clinic.

One of the aims of the group is to evaluate performance problems related to skills or behaviors necessary for functioning in life roles. Leaders can initiate referral to other outpatient or home-care services if additional areas of need are determined. The group is structured to help members identify task or role changes that may be necessary as a result of disability related to homemaker, work, or leisure roles. This includes helping group members to identify changes in living environment and relationships that may be necessary as part of adaptation to current disability. Discussing the use of orthotics, prosthetics, and assistive devices or adaptive equipment, as well as learning about the acquisition and maintenance of such equipment (which may require involvement of other individuals such as family members), may also be part of the group's agenda. Potential barriers to adjustment to community living (i.e., overindulgence by family members, architectural barriers, physical isolation, limited mobility, or emotional withdrawal of friends, family, lover, and coworkers) as well as strategies for intervening (i.e., asking for and accepting help, planning alternate routes and modifications of physical environment or use of mobility devices so that mobility is increased, giving feedback, suggesting compromises or alternatives) are common topics addressed. Additional strategies, such as focusing on abilities and strengths, seeking a peer support network in the community to aid adjustment to disability, and balancing activity participation through organizing a schedule to make optimal use of energy, are reviewed as part of the group's curriculum. During group sessions, members are taught joint protection and body mechanics principles to minimize stress on joints and maximize safety. To reinforce learning, members are cued during the group to position themselves physically for optimal performance and safety.

The group was established because, although expected to be functioning at a moderate level of independence at discharge, members need strategies and support to maintain themselves physically, emotionally, and socially in the community and to work toward their maximum potential. Similarly, patient education is necessary to prevent further debilitation or disability. Members referred are often highly dependent on staff or family members to fulfill needs. Family members have also often expressed concern over being able to cope with a disabled person at home.

▪▪▪▪▪
▪▪▪▪▪ ## CASE STUDY 3
▪▪▪▪▪

COMMUNITY-BASED GROUP

* LEADERS: MARY MUNROE, WELLNESS DIRECTOR; SAGE STILTON,
  VOLUNTEER; CONSULTANT: JACKI WRIGHT, OTD, OTR/L

This is a new group designed to be 10 weekly sessions. The group will meet at a community center for senior citizens in a suburban neighborhood. Members are local residents who come to the center from their homes. The director of the center has contracted with an occupational therapist to design, supervise the implementation of, and evaluate the group. The center's wellness director and a center volunteer will lead the group. Membership is voluntary and composed of members currently attending the center. This will be a closed group of seven to nine members in order to have a stable group of members with similar abilities. It will be designed for frail elders or those who need support to engage in center activities. The group will meet once a week for 90 minutes.

The members interviewed for this group currently visit the senior center 1 or 2 days a week and have ongoing medical difficulties, which include various levels of dementia, arthritis, diabetes, and history of stroke. One person has been receiving chemotherapy for cancer, and some members are showing signs of depression. Ages range from 70 to over 90 years of age. The group member composition will consist of five women and two men whose educational backgrounds range from elementary school to graduate education. Physically, members demonstrate various levels of ambulatory ability: three use walkers, one a cane; some have visual or hearing deficits; a few have difficulties in motor coordination and strength, with limited range of motion in their upper extremities, including their hands. All members are able to maintain sufficient balance to perform tabletop activities.

During the pre-group interviews, all members appeared to understand that the purpose of the interview was to seek membership for the new group. All presented as oriented to time, place, and person. Two members appeared withdrawn at the time of the interview, and an accompanying relative gave most of the information. One member was having trouble with her hearing aid. Others appeared reluctant to initiate conversation, although they politely answered all questions asked.

Some members live independently, others in the home of a relative. Roles include family members (grandparent, parent, sibling, aunt/uncle), friend, and community member. All are retired and on fixed incomes. Information regarding use of leisure time and interests was vague. Family members reported the need to instigate most leisure activities and outings. Most leisure pursuits are solitary and quiet/passive, including watching televsion; reading; doing crossword or word search puzzles (large print); handicrafts such as needlepoint, cross stitching, or crocheting; or card games (alone or with family members). Members are either at risk of or experience social isolation. Members manifest various levels of decreased role performance and social participation as well as decreased ability and competence in physical, cognitive, and social skill performance.

Members' self-care ability ranges from independent to partially dependent on assistance. Home health aides, relatives, and/or household help assist with bathing, dressing, or other personal needs (toileting, medication management) and home maintenance. Meals are delivered to some members, and others eat with their families. Transportation to the center is provided by friends, relatives, and occasionally by taxi or minibus.

Members arrive at the center between 9 and 10 a.m. Some have tea or coffee, which is provided for them by the center volunteers, but few participate in center activities. As part of agreeing to be members of the group, participants are expected to agree to do their best to attend the 10 sessions and to notify the leaders if they will not be able to attend. The group contract also asks that members keep group conversations confidential when outside the group.

A group structure that provides carefully selected activities as well as a safe emotional climate will be needed to encourage members to interact in the group. The leaders will have to assume an active role in adapting activities and attend to the task and social-functions of the group when members are unable to do so. A supportive, genuine, and consistent climate will need to be established and reinforced by the leaders.

The senior center is funded via grant money, city funding, and private funds. There is a board of directors that oversees center administration. The center director makes policy and administrative decisions in conjunction with the board and is directly responsible for the program and staff supervision. The center director negotiated with the board for the funds to engage the occupational therapist as a consultant. The center also has a dedicated group of volunteers who help the wellness director lead group activities as well as assist in the day-to-day functions of the center.

The senior center is a modern, two-story building with a large recreation room, kitchen and eating area, and meeting rooms on the first floor. Offices and additional meeting rooms are located on the second floor. There is a large parking lot in the back that provides direct ground-level entrance. The recreation room, where the group will meet, contains supply cupboards, a sink, and a large rectangular table. The room is well lighted with a row of windows on one wall. The room is easily accessible for walkers, wheelchairs, and so on, and it is possible for a wide range of activities to be performed while sitting around the table. Other rooms might be available should more private space be required. Materials are available in the cupboard, and special purchases can be made as needed.

The general climate at the center is friendly and warm. Members support one another. The center's objective is to help members to remain as independent as possible, living in their home environment if that is where they are happiest, and their quality of life is maximized. The structure of the senior center allows for the creation of a weekly closed group where the same participants will come for a session every Wednesday 10–11:30 a.m. The length of time has been selected to give participants ample opportunity to complete the short-term activities without feeling pressured. The occupational therapy consultant will review the group structure and provide weekly consultation for the group leaders (wellness director and volunteer, who has agreed to attend the group consistently for 10 weeks to assist). The wellness director and volunteer will meet for 20 minutes per week to plan and discuss the group sessions.

The leaders will seek suggestions and encourage input from members in planning activities and sessions. Leaders will be coached by the occupational therapy consultant regarding ways to seek member involvement by encouraging and modeling desired group norms including listening, participating verbally, being supportive, and giving feedback. Within the group structure, the leaders will need to adapt to the changing needs and dynamics of the group while maintaining a safe and caring environment that provides the right amount of challenge per the occupational therapist's suggestions or recommended modifications to the group, task, or environment.

Individual Learning Activities

CASE STUDIES

Choose a case study and complete the group history, group assessment and plan, and functional group protocol. Compare your write-up with those provided in Appendix C.

REFLECTIVE QUESTIONS

1. What is meant by a group plan? Why is it needed?

2. Why is the leader role in designing a group important to the group's ultimate success?

3. What is meant by a group contract, and how might one be designed?

4. What is meant by flow experience, and how may this be achieved?

5. Why might it be desirable to have an alternative group plan for the first sessions?

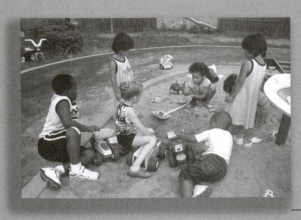

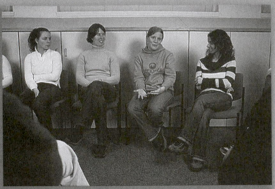

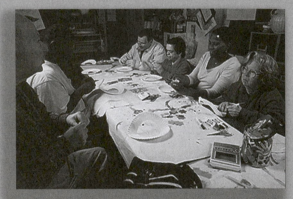

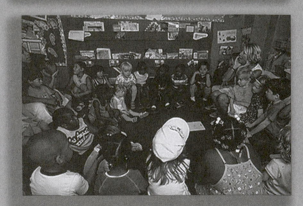

How Is a Functional Group Formed?

The design of a functional group requires care and attention to the individual and the group context. As the group forms, this concept continues in its dialectic application to both leader(s) and members as the group dynamics evolve. Admittedly, as a group begins, a combination of anticipation and apprehension is often felt, on the part of the leader(s) and the members. Therefore, the initial sessions of a group generally involve a process of orientation and deliberation, as the group's process needs to allow members to work through the anxiety and ambiguity to:

• Get acquainted
• Learn how the group functions
• Develop norms that will shape their behavior in the group

It is possible that the group will need to invest a considerable amount of time and energy in exploring hopes and fears about the group situation, trying to formulate goals, and dealing with issues related to feeling "in" (included) or "out" (excluded). Members may even struggle with deciding to stay in the group and get involved or to leave. The manner in which leaders deal with these issues, their own feelings, those of the group members, and resultant behaviors will, to a large extent, determine the amount of trust and cohesiveness that will be present at any time during the life of the group

The features of a group's process that develop with time are pertinent to the starting phase of individual group meetings. In the functional group model, each meeting may be considered a microcosm of the three developmental stages of a functional group: formation, development, and closure (termination). In looking at how a functional group is formed, there are specific characteristics that leaders need to address:

• Feelings of belonging and acceptance
• Dependence on the leader and testing the leadership
• Individual versus group goals
• Trust versus mistrust

These are listed here in the order in which they usually arise in many groups, but this may vary according to the membership and design of the group.

Forming and Group Actions

Each of the four types of action characteristic of the functional group model (purposeful, self-initiated, spontaneous, group-centered) can be used to address issues that may emerge in all stages of a functional group. Each action, in conjunction with leader skills, can serve to facilitate the group process as well as achievement of individual member and group goals (Table 6-1). This chapter outlines how each action can be applied during the formation stage of a

Table 6.1	**Group Issues and Membership Needs Related to Action: Formation Stage**

Formation stage issues: Concern over belonging and acceptance, formation of individual and group goals, dependence on leader; testing leader style.

Group member needs (related to action):

Purposeful action provides:	Self-initiated action allows:	Spontaneous action occurs via:	Group-centered action yields:
Structured activity that includes all members and can provide successful outcomes	Safety of polite social behavior	Encouragement of expression of ideas, feelings, and thoughts related to "here-and-now"	Building knowledge of group resources
Guidance regarding expectations of members	Expression of negative and positive feelings	Opportunity to interact with leader and test extent of freedom and control	Gradual sharing by members taking initiative
Clear options and alternatives in goal selection	Opportunity for safe behavior and risk taking		Examination of group goals and exploration of norms appropriate to achieving group goals
An accepting climate	Group support and encouragement for individual roles and goals	Member sharing of perceptions and reactions as to what is going on in the group	Group-centered decision making
Expression of respect for opinions and feelings of members		Overt support and acceptance of diversity or difference	Developing consensus and awareness of group's own process
			Establishing patterns of behavior/norms

Leader Actions and Skills Employed
Discussing confidentiality
Clarification of individual or group goals; use of group contract; establishing group rules
Strong involvement in task analysis, selection, and adaptation
Encouragement of member roles exploration
Structuring action and interactions for member comfort and growth
Modeling
Genuineness and empathy
Listening and responding
Tolerance of ambiguity and tentativeness in planning
Giving and receiving feedback
Sharing rationale for leader action
Using concrete language
Classifying themes
Setting climate for supportive interpersonal relationships
Providing input and support as needed

functional group and using the three case study forms, session narratives, and postgroup leader reflections to illustrate how these issues relate to the formation stage (see also Appendix D).

Purposeful Action

Purposeful action in the formation stage of a functional group can contribute directly to the development of feelings of acceptance and belonging in the group. All members need to feel included and invited to participate in the group action. Given the postulate, "The principle concern of every healthy group is to survive as long as possible, or at least until the task is done" (Berne, 1963, p. 77), then for a group to work together on a task, individuals must be drawn together as members in the group. Individuals are drawn to a group that promises to meet their needs and interests. Therefore, because the prospect of success also increases the attractiveness of the group for the members, the activity must be carefully matched with the skill level of the participants so members can expect a successful outcome. The leader(s) must seek opportunities to guide the action at the proper level of challenge for the group members (Fig. 6.1), thereby creating a "flow experience" (Csikszentmihalyi, 1990, p. 6).

Members' feelings of acceptance and belonging in the group are also increased when the purposeful action of the formation stage provides them with sufficient structure to allay

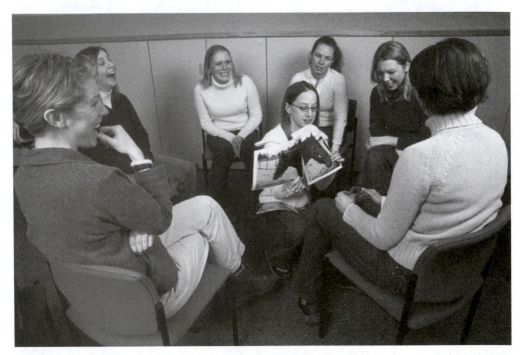

FIGURE 6.1 Flow as a successful outcome. (Photo by Mark Morelli)

some of their uncertainty about what will be happening. A clear structure helps new members recognize what behavior is desirable in the group, which, in turn, helps them to feel more comfortable. A structured task supplies members with a sense of predictability through clearly defined roles, goals, and limits, often reducing member anxiety. For example, a common activity in a new group is an exercise or game frequently referred as an "icebreaker." The purposeful action of this type of exercise is to help members interact, learn each other's names, and begin to establish interpersonal connections that facilitate communication with each other. The directions of an icebreaker activity need to be simple and clear. Members can then participate according to the structure of this type of activity, and member interaction is achieved.

Purposeful action in the group influences the extent of authority held by the leader. When the activity is highly structured, the leader holds an authoritative role. When the group activity is less structured, it allows the members more freedom in terms of choice or control over their actions. Members can potentially assume more authority in regard to group decision making within the group process. Purposeful action can thereby serve to regulate the amount of dependence or independence exhibited by members. The choice of task can influence the extent to which members will be able to function independently of the leader. Similarly, purposeful action aids the process of addressing individual member as well as group goals. The characteristics that are present in an activity can provide an initial structure for reaching specific goals. Through participating in carefully selected tasks, the group can formulate and clarify goals.

The manner in which purposeful action is carried out in the Formation stage can also be closely associated with the level of trust or mistrust in the group. When the comfort level in the group is high, trust is enhanced. When the comfort level is low, mistrust is common. A task successfully completed often enhances trust. Members can start to give each other feedback, both positive and negative, on aspects of their participation in the activity, thus purposeful action develops further in the group, which in turn, facilitates self-initiated, spontaneous, and group-centered actions. As the group begins to acknowledge feedback, from the leader and each other, and then act on it, group trust and cohesiveness develop. It is crucial as a group forms that members understand or be taught how to give and receive feedback constructively. Modeling the type of feedback given and the manner in which it is conveyed is one way this may be achieved.

Self-Initiated Action

A group characteristically begins with an initial introduction and a brief synopsis of the overall purpose or general goals of the group by the leader, after which a period of dramatic silence usually ensues. This silence is often characterized by members as stemming from their uncertainty about how to behave. Members may feel ambivalent about being in the group.

They may become increasingly anxious and not know how to address their own discomfort. They may look to the leader to make them feel comfortable and, perhaps in an effort to avoid dealing with their presenting problem and possible reason for being in the group, project that the source of their anxiety and discomfort is the leader. Resistance and hostility may therefore be directed toward leaders by some of the members. Other members might seek acceptance through polite social conversation. Those who feel awkward during moments of silence will seek to keep the conversation flowing on almost any topic. Members who feel most comfortable with action versus discussion will become impatient to get started on any kind of group task or activity, and will make comments in this regard.

Consequently, self-initiated action in the formation stage is usually directed toward the leaders. Members may feel highly dependent on the leaders for guidance around personal or therapeutic goals at the outset. They often consider the group leader as an all-knowing authority figure and themselves as persons who must comply with authority figures. It is common for members of new groups to direct their statements to the group leader rather than to their fellow members. As time goes on, leader dependence may shift to the opposite extreme of counterdependence. Members may display resistance to leadership, becoming highly suspicious of the leaders and afraid of being manipulated. This resistance may be manifested in statements of dissatisfaction with details about arrangements for the group. Members may complain about the time or place of group meetings or present as victimized or powerless in relation to decisions made in the group, format of group sessions, or types of activities chosen. Once leaders and members become more acquainted with each other, self-initiated action takes a different form. Gradually, questions about group goals emerge, and members begin to discuss, clarify, and develop goals. Through taking risks of verbalizing personal fears or perceptions about what is happening in the group, members gradually build a climate of trust. Carl Rogers (1969), a strong advocate for working through issues in the here and now, reflected, "If this self-initiated learning is to occur, it seems essential that the individual be in contact with, be faced by, a real problem. Success in facilitating such learning often seems directly related to this factor" (pp. 58–59).

Spontaneous (Here and Now) Action

Early in the formation stage, there may be little spontaneity, as members often seek acceptance through polite conversation about current or past events. Members' ability to listen may be affected by their anxiety or other issues. Thus, an exchange of ideas may be difficult. Suggestions are made, but there are few respondents to support or explore them. Again, Carl Rogers (1970) correctly observed, "the first expression of genuinely here and now feeling is apt to come out in negative attitudes towards other group members or towards the leader. Frequently the leader is attacked for failure to give proper guidance to the group" (p. 18). As time passes and a sense of group purpose is determined, safety and comfort in the group increases among the group members and in their relationships with the leader(s). Positive and negative opinions may be verbalized. As sharing of opinions is supported, a climate of respect for the feelings and opinions of individual group members develops.

The issue of dependence on and independence from the leader is highlighted via spontaneous (here and now) action. Through the process of the group experience, members realize that the leaders can neither answer all their needs nor make all decisions. If these tasks are carefully redirected back to the group, members can learn to be less reliant on the leader (Box 6.1). They begin to test the amount of freedom and control they can manage within the setting of the group. They also begin to feel more comfortable with group silences and learn to tolerate them with less anxiety.

The process of establishing norms and goals in a group helps the group members interact in the here-and-now context because, in the formation stage, group norms often deal with immediate concerns. Immediacy gives impetus to a genuine exploration of conflicts and problems as members share their reactions to what is happening in the group. Through interaction and sharing their perceptions of the group experience, members sort out individual concerns. They may state they feel pressured or perceive they are being forced by other group members or the group process to conform with group norms or plans against their will or inclination. Within this spontaneous action, group trust can grow if leaders facilitate a climate in which the members feel safe and experience support and acceptance around issues of difference (Box 6.2). These discussions can help members develop tolerance that can build understanding of matters pertaining to diversity within the group. The development of trust in the early stages of a group requires a climate of respect for the opinions and feelings of others (Corey & Corey, 1982).

Group-Centered Action

As the formation stage progresses, group-centered action develops. As members begin to feel a sense of belonging and acceptance, a climate of respect for the ideas, feelings, and perspectives of individual members emerges. Members become better at listening and commu-

Box 6.1   **Reducing Dependence on the Leader**

In a newly formed art group working with adults with MR, leaders notice that a male member is seeking attention via asking for assistance from the male leader. Additionally, a more capable female member often puts her head down on the table when not given individual attention. Leaders work with the members to establish and review group rules and expectations and alter their role in the opening phase of each group to allow more time for members to gather needed materials. They begin to direct the needy male member to seek assistance from the more capable female member.

Box 6.2   **Facilitating a Safe and Accepting Climate for the Group**

In an after-school program, leaders observe that preteens are subgrouping within the group according to familial (sibling), racial, and school district ties. As part of the groups' initial sessions, leaders use icebreaker activities that are structured to randomly assign pairs and subgroup teams. Group rules, established with member input, are frequently used to reinforce limits set on signs of resistance in the form of nonparticipation, whispering, or negative comments about the group activity or other members. Gradually, leaders see a shift in the group as subgroups more spontaneously merge to offer support or praise to a member attempting a difficult physical task (rock climbing wall, swimming), inquiring about the spelling of one another's names while doing art, or giving each other bracelets made during beading activity.

nicating their needs or point of view (Fig. 6.2). A positive and open climate encourages members to assume more leadership roles. In some instances, members may even vie for leadership by challenging the leader's statements or asserting their ideas or suggesting a course of action. As some of the leader responsibility is relinquished to group members, different relationships develop. Also, as a group forms and establishes norms and routines, it may spend the final minutes of a meeting planning for the next meeting and then spend the initial period of the subsequent meeting altering the previously made plans. Interdependence develops as the group works out new procedures, norms, and values to best use its resources to reach its goals. Interdependence in this context is defined as learning to accept dependence when it is truly needed and relying on leader and member expertise to help the group to function. Leaders can reduce the importance of their role by assuming the role of a consultant or troubleshooter as the group forms and members' dependence on the leader decreases (Box 6.3).

As a group begins to form, poor decision making can be characteristic of early group decisions (Gibb & Gibb, 1967). This can represent beginning attempts for group-centered action. Gradually, as the group forms and the emotional and social needs of the members are met, the group develops norms around providing individual support. At this point, members may begin to restate and reexamine the group's goals. The group's decision-making process alters to allow for taking the time to seek every member's opinion and establish a group consensus. This type of group-centered activity can contribute to an atmosphere of trust. Ironically, however, it is not uncommon to find members raising issues of confidentiality to test the extent of group trust as the group forms.

Ultimately, the goal of the formation stage is to achieve a "psychological group" (Bradford, 1978), which forms under the following specific conditions:

• Patterns of interaction are proved effective
• Differences in perceptions about task, communication, and procedures are clarified

- Relationships to other persons and groups are delineated
- Standards for participation are set
- Methods of work that elicit rather than inhibit member contributions are established
- A respected "place" for each person is secured
- Trust is established among members (p. 5)

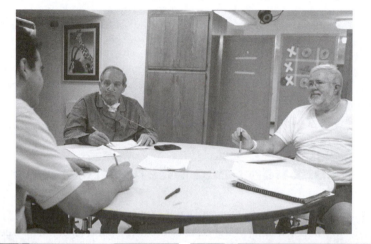

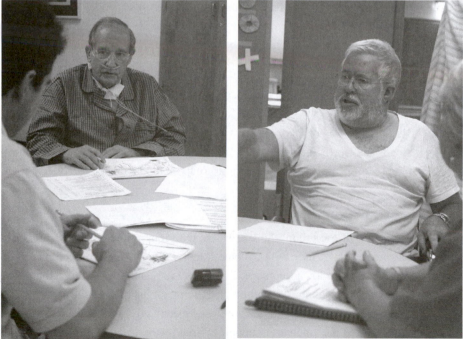

FIGURE 6.2 Listening and communicating needs and point of view. (Photos by Julia Ide)

Box 6.3   **Decreasing Importance of the Leader**

A wellness director requests assistance with wellness groups for seniors. During the first session, leaders arrive and find that members have arranged the seating in rows and are "saving" seats for peers who they are expecting to come to the session. Throughout the session, communication follows that pattern of members addressing leaders as the "experts," with little member-to-member sharing or interaction. In consultation with the wellness director, they ask that, for the next session, seating be set in a circle or horseshoe arrangement with a focal point (dry erase board or easel) on which to list member concerns or ideas that are brainstormed in regards to wellness topic to be addressed that session. As this norm develops, and leaders reinforce members' knowledge and experience with maintaining their own wellness, more group-centered communication through sharing of concerns and ideas occurs.

Leader Functions and Intervention Strategies

In the formation stage, the four group actions (purposeful, self-initiated, spontaneous, group-centered) are predominantly initiated and directed by the leader. This section considers the role of the group leader in the formation stage and presents specific leader tasks followed by self-assessment strategies for monitoring personal performance as a leader. Two primary issues of the formation stage that must be addressed are:

1. Members' need for acceptance
2. Development of relationships between leader(s) and members

By attending to selected elements of the group process and aspects of one's role as leader, members' need for acceptance can be addressed productively, and the process of developing relationships with and amongst group members can be facilitated.

Setting the Group Climate

As the organizer of the group, the leader sets the group climate. Apart from specific leader strategies, interpersonal style will, to some extent, influence the group climate. The ability to genuinely convey warmth, acceptance, and respect for each member contributes to a supportive group climate. A supportive and empathetic relationship with the leader has been positively correlated with group member progress. Specifically, a significant positive correlation was found between the amount of support offered by the leader and group member outcome

(Truax & Mitchell, 1971). The more support offered by the leader, the better the results achieved by the members.

During the early group sessions, while members search for what is acceptable behavior, they are dependent on the leader for guidance. Members look for direction and structure as well as approval both openly through their statements and covertly through their actions. It is the role of the leader to determine how much structure the group needs to have at this point. Leaders seek to achieve a therapeutic balance between too much and too little structure: "Although patients desire and require considerable structuring by the therapist, excessive structure may retard their therapeutic growth. If the leader does everything for patients, they will do little for themselves. Thus, in the early stages of therapy, structure provides reassurance to the frightened and confused patient; but persistent and rigid structure, over the long run, can infantilize the patient and delay assumption of autonomy" (Yalom, 1983, p. 123).

Thus, although it seems members like leaders who provide the greatest structure, they are less likely to achieve therapeutic changes in a highly structured group context. Monitoring one's own wish to be liked or the amount of discomfort experienced on shifting from what was conceived as the group plan is a crucial part of effective leadership.

Another role as the leader is to teach or empower members to assume responsibility for themselves and their group. This can be accomplished by sharing the rationale for leader actions with the members. Modeling certain behaviors that demonstrate a variety of group member task or maintenance roles can also be a means of teaching members to facilitate increased participation. Leaders can support members in a variety of ways:

• Treating the patient with respect and dignity
• Identifying and reinforcing the patient's strengths and virtues
• Refraining from undermining defenses but bolstering them
• Encouraging patients to employ defenses that are at least one step more effective than the one they are currently using (Yalom, 1983, p. 128).

It is a leader's job to create a climate that is experienced by members as constructive and supportive, one in which members can feel safe and can learn to trust the group.

Developing trust takes time and hard work. Members cannot trust each other until they know each other, respect one another, believe that they will be listened to, and feel that a sincere attempt will be made to understand them. Trust grows from working and learning together in a safe and supportive environment. A group may be successful in task functions but still not achieve trust among its members. Achieving a climate of safety and trust is crucial to the emotional maintenance functions required for a group's continued existence and effectiveness.

Clarifying Goals and Norms

The group leader should state the purposes and goals of the group at the first session and then help the group establish a method to review them, such as developing an opening ritual for every session. This is especially important if the group has an open group format or members need assistance with remembering the group's purpose and goals due to age (young children) or conditions that may impair memory (e.g., dementia). Leaders may also wish to express, in a manner appropriate to the context, personal feelings and hopes they have for the group. Key information that sets the parameters or ground rules and clarifies expectations of group members should be clearly stated. For instance, the leader or co-leader of a group may begin with the following statement: "This group is designed to be a safe place to help you learn to how to communicate and interact more comfortably and effectively with others in your work or social situations, or within your family. We will meet every Wednesday from 10:00 a.m. to noon in this room for the next 10 weeks. I (We) expect that you will attend all meetings, and ask that you let me (us) know if you will be absent. From time to time, new members will join the group. I (We) will plan what we will do as a group and then work together to put our plans into action. At times what we've set our sights on achieving may seem hard, but we hope we can support one another and also have some fun together. I am (We are) looking forward to being part of this group, getting to know you, and working together to achieve our goals." The leader may then pause and invite member reactions and comments. Although the purpose of the group as stated may be clear to the leader, it may not be clear to the members. Members should be encouraged to ask questions and make comments. The leader has established specific norms for group behavior:

1. Group members are expected to attend and communicate with the leaders and group if that will not be the case.
2. The group environment is to be one that is both safe and fun for members.
3. Group members will be asked and empowered to:
   a. Take an active role in planning how the time spent together is used.
   b. Talk about individual needs and goals.
   c. Discuss group tasks and goals.
   d. Share their perceptions of social interactions that occur within or outside the group.

The leader has conveyed participation in the planning process but that planning and learning will be a total group effort. Although it is made clear in the opening statement that regular group attendance will be expected, the fact that this is an open group where new members may join is also noted.

Leaders modeling established norms and redirecting unproductive ones will help create a safe climate in the group for learning. Norms that the leader can encourage include:

People should be listened to and recognized. The leader should acknowledge a questioning look or tentative statement (Fig. 6.3). The norm of personal respect and equal rights of membership in the group is established.

The group is a safe place. Members are reassured that what happens in the group stays within the group. A member will not be ridiculed or reprimanded for speaking out. The leader's behavior can be discussed just like any other point of discussion. The leader will encourage quiet members to speak more often and talkative members to speak less often.

Feelings are important. The leader encourages expression of feelings and establishes the norm that expression of feelings is vital if the group is to use its energy toward resolving problems and reaching its goals.

Objectivity is encouraged. The group learns that when the leader asks for information from members or asks if others have feelings similar to those expressed, those feelings will not be dismissed or smoothed over as nonexistent. The leader encourages observers to share their observations to demonstrate that members and leaders can help the group to look at what is happening in the group.

Members learn from doing things and analyzing them. Focusing on the "here and now" is a major learning method.

Planning is a joint effort. The leader is involved with the members in planning for group sessions. The leader does not have sole responsibility for the success of the group (Napier & Gershenfeld, 1983).

These norms, established through the leaders' verbal and nonverbal actions, provide examples that influence the behavior of the members and invite members to participate in various group roles.

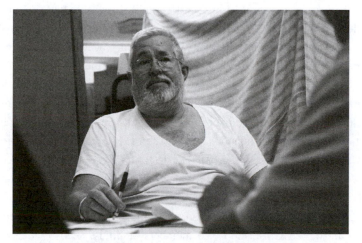

FIGURE 6.3 Questioning look. (Photo by Julia Ide)

Clarifying group and individual goals is essential in the early stages of a group. As the group develops, members become better able to formulate goals. Through helping others identify ways of learning from the group, members get a better idea of how they, too, can profit from the group experience. Thus, through the experience of setting goals in displacement, members can have opportunities that help them become more adept at identifying and sharing personal goals. The leader may be able to help members outline steps for reaching their personal goals and then demonstrate their commitment to this plan by asking members to make an individual contract with the group. A contract is a statement made by the member to the group regarding what he or she is willing to do or work on during a group session and possibly outside the group meeting. This contract states specific behaviors the member is willing to explore or change. The structure of the contract provides opportunities for self-assessment of performance as well as feedback from the group leader and members. By establishing or agreeing to the contract, the member assumes responsibility for his or her behavior and takes an active role in personal behavioral change.

Facilitating Purposeful Action

A primary purpose of the formation stage is to assist members with feeling accepted and included as valued members of the group. Therefore, the leader needs to carefully select and adapt the elements of purposeful action. It is particularly important in the early sessions of the group that the leader select tasks in which all members are assured of experiencing some success. The tasks should be appealing to all group members on a real and perhaps symbolic level. Purposeful action draws in or engages group members in a manner each individual perceives as meaningful.

In selecting purposeful action, the leader must determine the extent to which control needs to be exercised over the group's proceedings. To what extent should the leader be in control of the format or process? To what extent can the members be in control or assume responsibility? The relative importance of control will vary according to the characteristics of the members. For some individuals, maintaining control of themselves or situations may be problematic. For others, letting go of control, or recognizing what is or is not in their control, may be difficult. Tasks must be chosen with this broad spectrum in mind. External forms of regulation can be provided or diminished, often calibrated by the number of choices available, the amount of structure in the agenda and procedures, whether rules and norms are imposed and stated versus developed by the group, and so forth (Fig. 6.4). For instance, if a group of adolescents has trouble accepting adult leadership, the leader should select a task with limits and controls that are inherent in that particular task (i.e., games with rules). Through varied task selection and adaptation, the leader can adjust the amount of control exerted over the group's structure and process in response to members' abilities, needs, and goals. This titration of leader involvement enables the group to develop and facilitates goal achievement (Fig. 6.5).

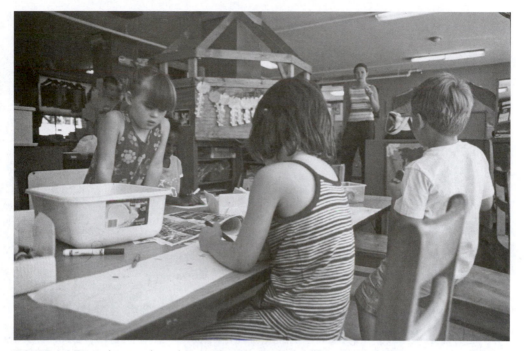

FIGURE 6.4 Titrated external regulation. (Photo by Mark Morelli)

Leader Emotional Response

Leader concerns in the formation stage may mirror members' emotional preoccupations. It is not uncommon for the leader to experience concerns similar to those of group members. Questions about the purpose or effectiveness of the group and concerns about safety or confidentiality are common. Fear of not being accepted or not belonging is often experienced by members joining a newly forming group or an existing one. Leaders, too, may fear lack of acceptance by the group and loss of members. If these feelings are unexamined or unacknowledged by leader, both the leader and members are in danger of unwittingly acting them out. For example, as strong reactions emerge in a group, the leader may not establish enough structure around group norms, such as being on time. Leaders and members may arrive late for the group as part of a wish to avoid dealing with feelings they are having or that are being expressed by others. Conversely, a leader might overregulate boundaries and be extremely rigid in rule enforcement. A member may also test a leader by violating group rules and norms or presenting as overly dependent on the leader. The motivations for these behaviors or reasons for these reactions may be unconscious or not yet understood by leaders or members.

There are many ways leaders can examine their emotional responses so as to identify patterns that emerge as the group works through issues in the formation stage. Processing feel-

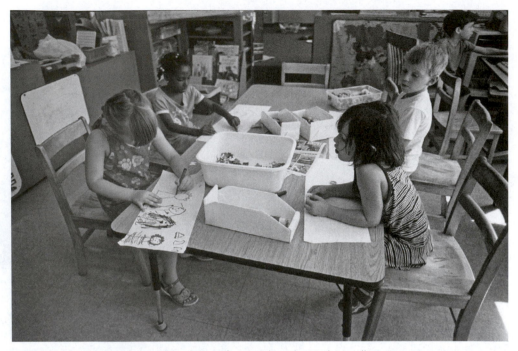

FIGURE 6.5 Outcome of titrated leader regulation. (Photo by Mark Morelli)

ings and group leadership experiences can occur in a supervisory or mentoring relationship or with a co-leader. Recording responses to semistructured self-reflective questions in a journal may help leaders understand their conscious or unconscious reactions to the feelings or issues that emerge as part of the formation stage of the group (Box 6.4). Using a structured approach to considering aspects of oneself that may influence therapeutic use of self (Display 6.1) or to self-assess one's skills in terms of leadership (Displays 6.2 and 6.3) may be a means to facilitate reflection. Using a consistent approach to assessing the group activity and leaders' facili-

Box 6.4   **Leader Emotional Response: Self-Reflective Questions**

- How do I react when excluded from a group?
- In what circumstances do I find that my behavior is overbearing or that I have difficulty asserting myself or, perhaps, find myself attempting to please?
- Do I find myself attracted to people who are overly dependent on me? When might this become problematic as a group leader?
- Am I comfortable with individuals who resist authority? When might this become problematic as a group leader?
- What resources are available to me for learning more about myself or developing skills such as being more assertive?

tation of maximal involvement (Display 6.4) may also provide useful insights as to what might be contributing to, or in some way affecting, the dynamics of the group in the Formation stage.

Session Evaluation

Completing a session evaluation is another means of reviewing and reflecting on the group's progress. The semistructured format of a session evaluation can help the process of reflecting as it allows one to gather thoughts about the group in a focused or coherent manner. Leaders are encouraged to consider whether the selected techniques and modalities seem appropriate for the group as well as the effect of their leadership. At each stage of group development, completion of a session evaluation can help monitor the group's process and members' progress in order to determine how effectively the group is addressing short- and long-term goals. The functional group protocol and session plans are then modified, as needed.

Display 6.1   **Self-Assessment of Aspects That Influence Therapeutic Use of Self**

Goal: The goal of this self-reflection exercise is to help you understand how these aspects of yourself may influence your engagement in culturally relevant and meaningful occupations and, in turn, potentially relate to your therapeutic use of self.

Note: This form is for personal use only and will not be viewed by others. Therefore, you control what and how much of this information is disclosed and to whom. Please save this document for future reflection and revision.

Directions: Describe yourself according to the following criteria.

Sex:

Sexual Orientation:

Race:

Nationality:

Ethnicity:

Language(s):

Age:

Socioeconomic class:

Religion/spiritual philosophy:

Disability status:

Health (describe):

Education level:

Occupational roles:

Physical size:

Mannerisms (tone and style of presenting toward and interacting with others):

Use of undesignated time:

Adapted from Wu J. (1998). Your Diversity/Cultural Competence Challenge: A Workshop on Engaging Diversity in Preparation for Practice. Tufts University, Department of Occupational Therapy, Medford, MA.

Display 6.2   **Initial Leader Self-Assessment**

Name:

Date:

Describe and rate your current level of leadership ability per the items below.

STYLE: Do you consider your leadership style to be DEMOCRATIC, AUTOCRATIC, or LAISSEZ-FAIRE? Why?

LEADER-MEMBER ROLE: LEADER-CENTERED/GROUP-CENTERED

Where does your emphasis lie? Please elaborate and give example(s).

SKILLS: Please rate your skills according to the following scale:

NO: No opportunity due to circumstances or setting

0: Poor, demonstrate behavior 0%–50% of the time

1: Fair, demonstrate behavior 50%–75% of the time

2: Good, demonstrate behavior 75%–95% of the time

3: Outstanding, demonstrate behavior more than 95% of the time

Note: Please include a comment for each item.

Item:	Score:	Comments:
Plan activities that:		
Are meaningful		
Offer choice		
Elicit adaptive response		
Can be graded to member's skill level		
Therapeutic relatedness:		
Genuine		
Demonstrates empathy		
Uses self as a model		
Reality-oriented		
Communication:		
Use active listening		
Demonstrate attentive physical posture		
Feedback:		
Nonthreatening manner		
Well timed		
Able to use concrete examples		
Able to confront member/sets limits		
Effective use of self disclosure		

Display 6.2   **Initial Leader Self-Assessment** (continued)

Summary/Goals:

Based on above ratings/comments:

a) What do you see as your strengths and growth needs in terms of your leadership skills? Why?

b) What do you see as potential barriers as well as resources available to assist you in this process?

c) What are your personal/professional goals in relation to leadership development? 1998 Tufts University-Department of Occupational Therapy, Medford, MA. Developed by Mary Alicia Barnes and Mike Miller.

Display 6.3   **Follow-Up Leader Self-Assessment Form**

Name:

Date:

Describe and rate your current level of leadership ability per the items below.

STYLE: Do you consider your leadership style to be DEMOCRATIC, AUTOCRATIC, or LAISSEZ-FAIRE? Why?

LEADER-MEMBER ROLE: LEADER-CENTERED/GROUP-CENTERED

Where does your emphasis lie? Please elaborate and give example(s).

SKILLS: Please rate your skills according to the following scale:

NO: No opportunity due to circumstances or setting

0: Poor, demonstrate behavior 0%–50% of the time

1: Fair, demonstrate behavior 50%–75% of the time

2: Good, demonstrate behavior 75%–95% of the time

3: Outstanding, demonstrate behavior more than 95% of the time

Note: Please include a comment for each item.

Item:	Score:	Comments:
Plan activities that:		
Are meaningful		
Offer choice		
Elicit adaptive response		
Can be graded to member's skill level		
Therapeutic relatedness:		
Genuine		
Demonstrates empathy		
Uses self as a model		
Reality-oriented		

(box continued on page 154)

Display 6.3   **Follow-Up Leader Self-Assessment Form** (continued)

Item:	Score:	Comments:
Communication:		
Uses active listening		
Demonstrates attentive physical posture		
Feedback:		
Nonthreatening manner		
Well timed		
Able to use concrete examples		
Able to confront member/sets limits		
Effective use of self-disclosure		

Summary/Goals:

1. Based on above ratings/comments:
   a) What do you see as your continued growth needs and goals for your leadership development?
   b) What do you see as potential barriers as well as resources available to assist you in this process?
2. Review your Self-Assessment of Aspects That Influence Therapeutic Use of Self. Identify at least one item that you feel may have influenced your level of comfort and degree of relatedness with clients and/or the system in which you are/were running your group.
   a) In what way was the situation challenging for you?
   b) What might be a personal/professional development activity you can do to address or overcome the challenge?

1998 Tufts University–Department of Occupational Therapy, Medford, MA. Developed by Mary Alicia Barnes and Mike Miller.

Display 6.4   **Assessment of Activity and Leadership: A Structured Observation Format**

Ask a peer, supervisor, or mentor to observe you leading a group activity (if possible) and to complete the structured observation worksheet below. After leading the group review feedback noted or if unable to obtain observers, conduct your own self-analysis to the best of your recollection.

Activity: Briefly comment on the activity in terms of:
   Applicability to population:
   Selection (level of interest/meaningfulness):
   Analysis (level of difficulty/skills needed):
   Structure (how much activity does/does not provide):

Display 6.4   **Assessment of Activity and Leadership: A Structured Observation Format** (continued)

Leadership/Facilitation of maximal involvement:
Orient Group: Did the leaders clearly indicate: (Yes/No)
_____Nature/Purpose of Group
_____Leader/member roles
_____Specific goals
Explain Procedures: Did the leaders explain or carry out to members' level of understanding: (Yes/No)
_____Agenda
_____Methodology
_____Specific tasks
_____Sequence of activities
Set up: Were members meaningfully involved in: (Yes/No)
_____Set up
_____Activity
_____Clean up
Follow Up: Did Leaders assists group in assessing group experience and connecting task experience to /individual member/group goals? (please give example)

Please comment on (using specific examples or suggestions):
Two things leaders did well:
Two areas in need of improvement:

2001. Developed by Mary Alicia Barnes, Tufts University–Department of Occupational Therapy, Medford, MA.

Conclusion

Being aware of the types of issues and member behaviors that may appear in the formation stage is vital to assisting group members as they go through the process of forming a group. Reflecting on one's practice as a group leader can help to analyze and interpret what may be contributing to the dynamics of the group or individual member's behavior. Additionally, reflection can aid the reasoning process and guide the selection of techniques and strategies available to facilitate the group's process and enhance members' ability to function. As leaders, it is essential to understand and accept that leaders cannot completely control the group's process or member behavior. It is important to anticipate or expect, and thus prepare for, certain behavior patterns frequently adopted by individuals who are confronted with an entirely new set of circumstances that may emerge as a group forms. Careful planning, thoughtful allocation of resources, and effective implementation of leadership skills and techniques can make possible the formation of a cohesive group capable of continued development.

A well-formed functional group can be ready to withstand the tests that will emerge as part of the group's development. As the relationships deepen, so do the complexities of the group process. The journey, or the group's life, has begun. The next chapter discusses facilitating the development of a functional group. As leaders, the reasoning process proceeds to incorporating awareness of potential issues in the development stage, assessing and reflecting on the group process as well as progress, and strategizing resultant leader actions.

CASE STUDY 1

OPEN GROUP ON AN INPATIENT PSYCHIATRY UNIT

Session Plan

Name of Group: "Getting It Together"

Date: Monday, June 6

Leaders: Lauri Levy, OTR/L; Jack Jones, MHC

Session Activity: "What's in a name?"—Introducing new members to the group

Specific goals for the group session: Given a task that is primarily leader-structured and -directed, members will:

- Learn other group members' names.
- Talk to another group member and address comments to the group as a whole.
- Take turns talking in a group.

Specific goals for group members:

Gary, Eric, Liz, and Pearl:

- To be able to state their names to new members and make one comment each to a new member re: "What I am working on in this group is (task or goal)."
- To express their feelings and reactions in a socially appropriate manner to leaders about being members of a group that has four new members (i.e., "It is hard for me to learn new members' names, have the group change," etc.).

New group members (Li, John, Betty, Lakisha):

- To verbalize feelings about being in the group and choose to participate in task and/or conversation with leaders and/or group members.

Description of methods and procedures:

Review and explain:

- Group's purpose, goals, and ground rules per written display board.
- Leader and member roles, group structure, and timeline.
- Describe icebreaker activity ("What's in a name?") in simple and clear fashion.

Rationale: Overall aim of activity is to facilitate introduction of new members into group, help previous members acknowledge change in membership, describe purpose of group, and instill feelings of safety and belonging for all group members.

Description of leadership role:

1. Provide task structure and support.

2. Limit set and redirect as needed.

Rationale: Reassure members that they are safe but not be so directive as to encourage overly dependent behavior.

Describe necessary preparations:

• Prepare new members for the group in individual pre-group interviews.
• Review session plan among co-leaders. Prepare flip chart with simple directions/pictographs.
• Gather supplies necessary for group activity.

List material and equipment needed:

Paper (lined and unlined)

Fine-tip, colored, nontoxic, erasable markers

Time and sequence outline for sessions (include what you will do and say as leader and what the group will do; consider both content and process):

• Explain group's purpose, leader and member roles; go over ground rules and expectations. (5 minutes)
• Explain that because so many new members are in the group today, the leaders have planned an activity to help group members get to know one another. Pass around paper, asking members to take a piece of either lined or plain paper and pass pile to person to the left. Place the remaining paper and packs of markers in the center of the table. Ask that everyone choose a marker and write down his or her first and last name across the top of the paper. Explain that each person is to write down two things they like and two things they might not like about his or her name. Tell group members that after they have completed the first part of the activity, each member will share some of what he or she has written with the person sitting to his or her right. Explain that, once everyone has finished talking, members will then take turns introducing that person by saying what he or she said about liking and not liking his or her name. (Co-leader will point out simple steps that are outlined on flip chart in both words and simple pictographs). (10 minutes)
• Ask if everyone understands how to proceed or if anyone has questions. Clarify as needed. Explain that group members will be encouraged to talk about the activity afterward and to say what they thought or felt about it at the end of the group. (5 minutes)
• Group will then do the described activities. Leaders will encourage member participation, keep group activity within time limits of session by prompting group to complete various aspects of task, and provide feedback or clarify directions as needed. (15 minutes)
• Leaders will facilitate member discussion re: task, summarize the purpose of today's session (getting to know one another), discuss potential plans for the following session with group members, and facilitate cleanup as necessary. (15 minutes)

Other information pertinent to this specific session: (i.e., will there be any new members, co-leaders, or guests? Is there an unusual tone in the unit or special event that is about to occur or just occurred for the individual member or group?)

In this session, half the group will be composed of new members. As one speaks only Mandarin Chinese, hospital translator will be present.

Session Narrative

Name of Group: "Getting It Together"
Date: Monday, June 6
Leaders: Lauri Levy, OTR/L; Jack Jones, MHC
Session Activity: "What's in a name?"—Introducing new members to the group

Prior to this session, as part of the admissions process, four individuals newly admitted to the unit over the weekend have chosen to participate in this group as part of their daily treatment regimen. To be most expedient and to share the work, each of us met with two members in individual pre-group interviews to give them a general overview of the group's purpose and expectations of members in the group contract. In the weekly co-leader meeting, the session plan was reviewed, and a flip chart with simple directions and pictographs was prepared. Immediately prior to the group, Lauri gathered supplies necessary for the group activity, an expressive task called "What's in a name?" placing on the table paper (lined and unlined) and fine-tip, colored, nontoxic, erasable markers. Lauri wrote out the group's purpose, goals, and ground rules on the dry erase board in the occupational therapy room.

During this session, the plan and task for us is to integrate the four new members into the group with the four members who have been in the group since the prior week. Members will be asked to participate in an activity to facilitate the introduction of new members to the group. The activity will initially be primarily leader-structured and -directed, as the stated group goals are to allow members to:

- Learn other group members' names
- Talk to another group member and address comments to the group as a whole
- Take turns talking in a group

Existing members of the group, Gary, Eric, Liz, and Pearl, are working on being able to state their names to new members and to make one comment each to a new member re: a task or goal they hope to work on during the group. Gary is displaying manic symptoms, so leaders are structuring the group to limit his participation to allow others to speak as a way to balance his participation in the group. Eric presents with some paranoia and needs frequent reassurances that he is safe. Liz remains quiet but has been able to state she is working on staying grounded when experiencing flashbacks. Pearl displays self-soothing behaviors of rocking and humming, but when asked directly she will state her goal is to "get the work done." In the weekend report, nursing staff had noted that Betty has displayed inability to attend any groups on the unit.

When the group began, Laurie took 5 minutes to explain our leader roles as helping members maintain safety, providing ideas for or assistance with tasks, and giving members feedback and emotional support as needed. Jack outlined member role expectations as: participation in tasks, sharing supplies, relaying information about oneself including thoughts or feelings, and providing feedback to others in a socially acceptable way. Jack reviewed the group purpose and goals, and ground rules written on the dry erase board were reviewed. Eric explained the ground rules to new members.

Laurie explained the basic group structure regarding opening the group, time for the activity, summarizing and closing the group, and general timelines for the session stating: "Because so many new members are in the group today, we have planned an activity to help group members get to know one another." Laurie distributed paper, asking members to take a piece of either lined or plain paper and pass the pile to person on their left. The remaining paper and packs of markers were placed in the center of the table. Jack asked everyone to choose a marker and write down his or her first and last name across the top of the paper. He then asked each person to write down two things he or she likes and does not like about his or her name. Laurie said that after people complete the first part of the activity, each member will be asked to share some of what he or she has written with the person sitting to his or her right. She explained that once everyone finished talking with the person on their right, members will then take turns introducing that person by saying what he or she learned from their neighbor in the group. (Jack pointed out simple steps outlined on flip chart in both words and simple pictographs). Laurie asked if everyone understood how to proceed or had any questions and clarified as needed. To redirect negative comments about the activity, she stated, "As we wrap up group today, we will talk about the activity afterward to give everyone a chance to say what you thought or felt about it'."

During the group, we tried not to be too directive in order to avoid encouraging behavior that seemed dependent on the leader. However, Gary had difficulty taking turns speaking in the group and interrupted several times while other group members were talking. Betty, a new group member who was sitting to Gary's right, remained in the group for 10 minutes and left, saying she was too "nervous" to sit any longer. We provided modeling and cues to the group as a whole to acknowledge Betty's departure and thanked her for coming as well as stating her reason for leaving. Laurie told Betty that the group understood being in a group was challenging for her and looked forward to her joining us for a little longer next session. Jack paired off with Gary for the remainder of the session and worked on providing feedback to Gary re: how he felt when Gary kept interrupting him and other members in the group. Gary acknowledged feeling too "revved up" to wait for others. However, members responded with imitation of Jack's behavior, beginning to encourage each other to listen and share. This was effective because it helped to model group norms and encouraged group-centered participation. Lauri's role shifted to that of primary group leader. After this point in the group, Lauri's feedback to members was met with offhand comments/jokes (i.e., "Yes, mother"; "You sound like my wife"; "Who are you, my mother?").

For most of the group members, the structure seemed to establish a nonthreatening climate. Jack (co-leader) wondered aloud if Gary realized he had interrupted others and shared with the group how he did not feel heard by Gary when Gary interrupted him, as a means of modeling feedback. Lakisha remained silent in the large group, but when Liz suggested another idea (acrostic of first name) for learning about others' names and how they would describe themselves, Lakisha completed an acrostic of her name and Pearl's name that she was willing to share with Pearl and show the group but not read aloud. John was able to share he was named after his father, but otherwise repeatedly asked Eric to remind him where we were (hospital) and what the date was (month, day, year). Li wrote his name using Chinese characters and predominantly addressed questions to his translator about when he could see his family. Leaders reassured and cued Li via the translator that he would see his family tonight during visiting hours. Liz quickly completed an acrostic of her name (Lonely Idiotic Zealot), completed one using Betty's name, and asked Li's translator about Li's family, writing out their names in English.

Gary, Eric, Liz, and Pearl were encouraged to share their goals for the group and express their feelings and reactions to the change in the group membership. We provided cues regarding how to do so in a socially appropriate manner (i.e., "It can be hard to learn new members' names, have the group change," etc.) to try to validate feelings as well as put it in a whole group context to avoid subgroups forming and to recognize that dealing effectively with changes is important for everyone to learn in order to manage stress. In this context, the new group members were also cued to verbalize their feelings about being in the group and asked to think about setting a goal for the next group, perhaps related to participating in tasks and/or conversation.

Generally, members seemed able to engage in the activity and able to converse or interact in a spontaneous manner to some extent when paired with another member. However, as leaders we needed to take a more directive role during group discussions, cuing members to share what was learned and to use strategies of referring to what was written down to help remember what was said. We asked group members to give feedback about what others had said about themselves or their names. During the discussion, we shared with the members that our overall aim of the activity was to introduce new members (Li, John, Betty, Lakisha) into the group, help previous members adjust to the change in membership, and to help all group members feel safe and a part of the group. Discussion regarding how members felt about the activity was more difficult for members and required more leader structure of dialogue.

Post Group Leader Reflections

Given the group's formation stage of development, the structure encouraged members to interact and enabled them to learn each other's names and something about one another. We feel the group structure encouraged a norm of doing one's best to adjust to changes, modeling our willingness to change our plan to incorporate Liz's idea, encouraging others to acknowledge how they feel about the change, and using the support of others in a group. Meeting new people and using strategies of verbal and written expression to identify feelings or assist with remembering information were also practiced. Except for Betty, the range of group processes enabled members to participate at a parallel through cooperative level. With our guidance, seven of the eight members completed the group task and participated in some aspect of large group processing that we facilitated. Members were encouraged to discuss their reactions to the session and ideas for future sessions.

During this session we felt we had ample opportunity to observe member behavior and their reactions to varying amounts of task structure. After the group ended, we noticed Eric and Liz informally chatting with Li via his translator. Liz also asked the unit staff if she could give Betty the acrostic of Betty's name that Liz prepared for Betty and overheard Betty thanking Liz for thinking of her. In future sessions we might provide Betty increased female leader support or avoid activities that require subgroup pairings to increase her sense of safety in the group. Also, extra time may be needed for Li's translations.

When Gary had difficulty taking turns and Betty said she was leaving the group, Jack had to assume more group task roles. Jack felt he was working too hard to model group maintenance roles through his interactions with Gary (risking rift in therapeutic rapport). However, members responded with imitation of Jack's behavior, beginning to encourage each other to listen and share. This was effective because it helped to model group norms and encouraged group-centered participation. However, it inadvertently created a sense of more authority in Lauri's role as "leader." Transferences about Lauri being a "good-enough wife/mother" seem to have emerged. Lauri remembers thinking about how to respond to members' perceptions of her as reflected in some of their offhand comments/jokes (i.e., "Yes, mother"; "You sound like my wife/mother"; "Who are you, my mother?").

We did not anticipate the effect that Betty's leaving would have on the group. The expectation that she remain in the group for 45 minutes was unrealistic and appeared to overwhelm her. In future we need to take time to make alternate agreements ("contracts") with patients who need to titrate the amount of time spent in the group. As this is a part of the group contract, making this explicit might decrease other members' sense of rejection. For example, Betty could have been told she could try contracting to stay in the group for 10 minutes the first time, 20 minutes the second, and so on, thereby encouraging success and establishing helpful limits.

We did not feel prepared to address the transferences and issues of rejection that emerged in conversation at that point as well as the now obvious symbolic connection of activity to parental figures. Accepting Liz's suggestion of using an acrostic (using the letters in one's name to describe oneself) as an alternate approach to task was very empowering to the group in a positive way and seemed to help shift member focus back to "getting to know one another." However, Liz's acrostic seemed laden with negative self-regard. We also need to consider more carefully the symbolic level of icebreaker activities as well as the effect of one co-leader assuming increased member role in keeping co-leader balance. Additionally, we need to attend to boundary maintenance as to the purpose of the group. We have found that co-ed co-leadership does afford opportunities to explore some of transferences in member reactions to our actions. However, the nature of acute inpatient psychiatric hospitalization is short-term, and focus is primarily problem identification with disposition recommendations for treatment upon discharge. Therefore, issues that lead to member regression need to be reframed as something to investigate in the future in an appropriate context and when a member feels ready and strong enough emotionally to do so. More frequent reminding members of the group name ("Getting It Together") as being linked to working together as a group to support one another in increasing one's ability to function (versus falling apart emotionally or in one's ability to manage from day to day) may be worthwhile. This may also serve as a helpful cognitive reframe for members.

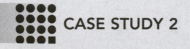

CASE STUDY 2

CLOSED GROUP IN AN OUTPATIENT OCCUPATIONAL THERAPY CLINIC

Session Plan

Name of Group: Community Re-entry: "Moving Forward"

Date: December 15, second of eight sessions

Leaders: Russell Lee, MS, OTR/L; Alicia Wright, COTA/L

Session Activity: "What I Value" collages (prioritizing valued roles/activities, examining time/energy use and personal concerns)

Specific goals for the group session: To identify priorities in life as a means to assist with setting goals related to time management, energy conservation, and adjustment to current disability status

Members will:

• Identify what they value and find meaningful in terms of time/energy use devoted to tasks via expressive art (collage) activity.

• Share what they value/find meaningful with group and discuss concerns related to being able to participate in valued tasks/roles/activities.

• Participate in group process to learn to prioritize and brainstorm ways to address concerns as method of problem solving and to receive group support.

Leader goal:

• Encourage development of group cohesiveness.

Specific goals for group members:

Jim (post MI): to identify priorities related to work and activities of daily living (ADLs) (including adding light exercise routine).

John (traumatic brain injury [BI] post motor vehicle accident [MVA]): to identify meaningful premorbid roles he can safely resume, such as home maintenance tasks (cleaning, sweeping, shoveling, laundry).

Steve (lumbar fusion): to identify realistic work (construction contractor–related), ADLs (related to exercise—stretching and strengthening—as well as pain management) and leisure activities.

Jeanette (post cardiovascular accident [CVA]): to identify ADLs (self-care) and homemaking/home maintenance tasks to support resuming these roles.

Wendy (post bilateral total knee replacement [TKR]): to identify work and ADL tasks safe to perform (to assist with adapted routine while recovering).

Brenda (post CVA): to identify tasks she can safely resume in role of mothering infant.

Juanita (post hip fracture): to identify tasks related to ADLs (exercise routine) and volunteering tasks (safe to resume while recovering).

Description of methods and procedures: Expressive art activity and group discussion

Rationale: To increase trust and member sharing of thoughts and feelings to facilitate sense of universality and to foster group support, cohesion, problem solving, and goal setting by establishing an environment that encourages free expression of common concerns paired with group support and problem solving re: how to address concerns

Description of leadership role:

1. Encourage expression of fears and perceptions in here and now through verbal and nonverbal means.

2. Clarify group goals and task.

Rationale: To enable group to establish a balance of individual and group goals and ensure that the group is a safe place to express concerns.

Describe necessary preparations: Gather art materials.

List material and equipment needed:

Magazines/newspapers (including a variety of precut magazine pictures/words representative of work, family members, leisure roles, etc.)

Alphabet stickers

Fine-tip markers

Glue sticks

Scissors

8" × 11" poster board

Time and sequence outline for session (include what you will do and say as leader and what the group will do; consider both content and process):

1. Introduce group to activity: state purpose, goals, and methods. (5 minutes)

2. Encourage group members to create individual collages as a means of identifying what is important to them in terms of time/energy use or describing feelings or concerns they have as they go through the process of community re-entry. Provide leader assistance/adaptation as necessary, but encourage members to help each other and ask for help when needed. (approximately 20 minutes)

3. Members show collages and/or share verbally what they identified. Process relationship to group's goals, and identify individual member goals related to any insights gained through activity or group discussion. Summarize common themes in regard to members' values, interests, goals, roles, and/or concerns. (10 minutes)

4. Close group with member feedback re: what was learned. Revise goals as needed, and review plans for next session. (10 minutes)

Other information pertinent to this specific session: (i.e., will there be any new members, co-leaders, or guests? Is there an unusual tone in the unit or special event that is about to occur or just occurred for the individual member or group?)

There may be possible impact due to time of year (weather, holiday season).

Session Narrative

Name of Group: Community Re-entry: "Moving Forward"
Date: December 15, second of eight sessions
Leaders: Russell Lee, MS, OTR/L; Alicia Wall, COTA/L
Activity: "What I Value" collages (prioritizing valued roles/activities, examining time/energy use and personal concerns)

During the group session, members were quiet and minimally involved in the collage activity. Russell posed to the group that they seemed subdued, and Juanita and John indicated that, for them, it was due to the time of year (weather, holiday season). Jim and Steve openly expressed their individual frustrations, fears of pain, and possible re-emergence of their physical conditions (myocardial infarction, ruptured discs). The general tone of the group seemed to be one of a pervading sense of loss. However, despite stating their feelings openly, only Brenda and Jeanette saw the value of the group as a means of support. Jim asked, "How will talking about this change anything?" Steve expressed dislike of the collage activity, declining to participate in that aspect of the group, and instead asked us to write out member concerns as a list on dry erase board. Wendy, although notably quiet, readily engaged in creating a very artistic collage, sharing that she enjoyed visual media, having studied graphic arts. However, most members did not appear comfortable with the expressive art activity format, seeming overwhelmed with its lack of structure. Jim questioned how doing a collage would help them with their issues related to community re-entry.

We decreased our emphasis on the collage task during this session, reverting to more verbal exchange. We related to the group that our reasoning as leaders comes from research study findings and our own experience that suggests support groups provide validation to participants and can empower them to bring about change in their lives. We openly acknowledged that the group seemed to need more time to get to know one another, build trust, and find activities that will support members with addressing the issues they face as part of community re-entry. We tried to reassure the group members that as this was only our second session together, needing more time to form as a group was to be expected. Alicia stated that as leaders our aim was to try to ensure that the group met their needs as members.

Through the process of introducing the activity option and subsequent discussion, all members openly stated feeling the loss of meaningful tasks and roles they had felt able to fulfill prior to illness or injury. Brenda stated she wanted more time to talk about her individual concerns and feelings of loss. With redirection, validation, support, and encouragement, all members were able to verbalize their individual concerns regarding managing life tasks and roles. By being encouraged to share these concerns, members began to talk about what they wanted to do as opposed to what their family and friends wanted to have happen or be done. Russell then summarized common themes that were raised in regard to members' values, interests, goals, roles, and concerns. Once Russell identified common themes, there was a group consensus in acknowledging commonalities such as feelings of fear and frustration as well as awkward or embarrassing experiences. We facilitated members brainstorming a list of possible options or strategies.

As the group came to a close, Jim and Steve identified they thought this group was the first time they openly discussed fears, frustrations, and concerns. However, they still questioned "What will being in this group do?" and seemed to need increased support around their feelings of loss of control of their bodies and in their lives. During this process, Alicia tried to probe members' thoughts to help members identify individual goals related to any insights gained through activity or group discussion.

Members were actively encouraged to give us feedback verbally and in writing via a session feedback form. Brenda identified that she would like to learn more about getting assistance in her home as getting a home health aide was mentioned as a possible way to address concerns. John and Steve identified that they wanted more time to talk about more choices in terms of activity (i.e., some can choose art, or some can use a worksheet to address topic of session). Jeannette was able to identify she hoped we would address getting around in the community in future sessions (i.e., community mobility).

As a group we decided that we will start each session with a check-in period with the specific aim of hearing member concerns to allow more opportunities for discussion and goal setting for each session. We agreed that as leaders we will offer some preset structure and topics but allow room for members' input and more group-centered visuals (dry erase posters/board, PowerPoint slides) as we want members to feel empowered to make choices as a means of moving forward.

Post Group Leader Reflections

As leaders, we were not prepared for the extent to which members wanted to talk about their feelings of loss and anger. The collage images and activity seemed to remind them of losses in roles, opportunities, body image, etc., more than was anticipated or intended. This tension suggests a need for individual member needs and goals, as well as group goals, to be further negotiated and tested in order for the group as a whole and individual members to see a connection between the two sets of goals in the group. The purpose of the group activity was not easily apparent to members. A more structured goal-setting activity might be preferable for these members at this early stage of the group's formation. Members seemed to need more structure and leader approval or input when making group decisions. As leaders, we expected more group-centered support and readiness to take action than was realistic this early in the group's formation. Members' personalities and circumstances suggest that they need more time and support to adjust and feel empowered to make changes necessary to improve their quality of life.

Although the value of the group as a means of intervention seemed apparent to us as leaders, members clearly need more time for discussion to learn what value it holds for them and how it will be helpful. In future we might consider devoting a session or part of a session to issues of loss and change. With this current group, we were able to address their need for a structure that allowed a balance of discussion and task (collage, writing on dry erase board). The task needs to be one that is readily adapted to individual members' comfort with and modes for expression to enable group members to feel more empowered to make choices and to assume group task and maintenance roles.

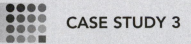

CASE STUDY 3

COMMUNITY-BASED GROUP

Session Plan

Name of Group: "Time Flies"

Date: September 21, 3rd of 10 sessions

Leaders: Mary Munroe, Wellness Director; Sage Stilton, Volunteer

Session Activity: Making scrapbook pages

Specific goals for the group session:

Members will:

• Share materials and meaningful verbal exchange through activity and reminiscence.

• Actively participate in group activity of creating scrapbook pages on verbal or nonverbal level (i.e., stating preferences/likes/dislikes in choice of materials, engaging in conversation re: memories about own or other members' life events).

• Express feelings (enjoyment, sadness, etc.) regarding activity and/or life events in a socially appropriate manner during the group.

Specific goals for group members:

Sophie (who is often anxious due to her mild dementia): To demonstrate increased comfort in the group setting via engaging in scrapbook task with familiar objects (personal picture or memorabilia) and/or in conversation with leaders or other members about personal memories.

Olga (who is easily fatigued secondary to chemotherapy for breast cancer): To attend and remain involved in the activity with short rest breaks, as needed.

Tom: To ask for assistance when needed vs. discontinuing the task.

Betty: To be more open to ideas of others and relate more positively to leaders and members (vs. presenting as negative or hopeless, i.e., "beyond needing or being worthy of support").

Irina: To communicate her needs more effectively with leaders and members.

Clara: To interact more with leaders and members.

Joe: To focus more on engaging in task and with members (vs. constant chatting and joking directed at leaders).

Agnes (who is frail and easily fatigues): To remain in the group the entire session and complete the activity with assistance.

Description of methods and procedures:

1. Provide members with an individual task that can facilitate group-centered sharing and discussion as well as leisure interest that can be pursued at home or in senior center outside of group sessions. Leaders will prepare and show scrapbook with pages made of the same materials being used as a model so that members can have an idea of how their finished product might appear.

2. Provide assistance with activity to adapt to the different skill levels of individual members. The methods for making the scrapbook pages range from applying stickers to gluing on foam, paper, and fabric cutouts/appliqués and/or small items such as photo corners. Members will be encouraged to ask for help and feedback about their scrapbook page from leaders and other group members should they need help.

3. Additional materials will be available to allow members opportunity to engage in making additional scrapbook pages to create their own scrapbook outside of group or senior center (i.e., at home, with family) should members (or their family/caretaker) identify this activity as a meaningful/enjoyable way to interact and reminisce.

Rationale: Decrease sense of isolation and building group cohesiveness through sharing of memories and materials.

Description of leadership role:

1. Help members understand the purpose of the group's activity.

2. Encourage and facilitate group members' participation in activity, sharing of materials/memories, and getting to know one another more through conversation.

3. Provide cuing/assistance as needed and promote group discussion and interaction.

Rationale: To instill feelings of safety and belonging in the group.

Describe necessary preparations:

• Review session plan with co-leader.
• Purchase scrapbook supplies necessary for group activity. Prepare four different sample scrapbook pages. Remind members, in person the afternoon prior and via follow-up phone call on morning of the group, of the activity plan made last group session and that they are to try to bring at least one photo or memorabilia item (postcard, newspaper clipping) for scrapbook activity.

List material and equipment needed:

Scrapbook pages of several colors so that group members can choose a color
Old issues of *Time/Life/Newsweek* or travel magazines; precut magazine pictures
Postcards of local attractions
Scrapbook appliqués, stickers, photo corners, etc.

Craft glue, glue sticks, markers, scissors, cropping tools (i.e., pinking shears to cut artful edges)

Sample completed scrapbook pages/scrapbook

Time and sequence outline for sessions (include what you will do and say as leader and what the group will do; consider both content and process):

1. Greetings and distribution of member name tags. (10 minutes)
2. Introduction to group activity, purpose, goals, and methods with visual cuing. Show model of scrapbook pages, and point out how different materials were used. (10 minutes)
3. Members choose scrapbook materials with assistance as needed from bins passed around, which are then placed around the table as space permits. (10 minutes)
4. Members assemble scrapbook page with assistance of leaders and adaptations in approach to task as per occupational therapy consultant's recommendations as necessary (i.e., magnifying lens, securing project to table with dycem, encouraging use of both hands, adapted scissors, etc.). Leaders assume group task and maintenance roles as needed to facilitate group members' participation in task and/or discussion about feelings, memorabilia, memories, or scrapbook supplies. Members are encouraged to help each other and to ask for help and feedback about page arrangement as needed. (40 minutes)
5. Bring closure to the activity. Reassure any members who have yet to complete their page that there will be opportunities to do so, either within or outside of the group. Ask members to rate their degree of satisfaction or dissatisfaction with the scrapbook activity or group session (rate on a scale of 1 = satisfied to 10 = dissatisfied), and discuss their ratings as member is able or time allows. Generate ideas for next session.

Other information pertinent to this specific session: Occupational therapy consultant will be observing as part of contractual arrangement for feedback and mentoring of group leaders. Leaders will introduce consultant and briefly address her role as observer at beginning of session.

Session Narrative

Name of Group: "Time Flies"

Date: September 21, 3rd of 10 sessions

Leaders: Mary Munroe, Wellness Director; Sage Stilton, Volunteer

Activity: Making scrapbook pages

On the day before the group, we reviewed our session plan during our consultation meeting. Sage, as agreed, had purchased scrapbook supplies necessary for the group activity and prepared four different sample scrapbook pages of varying levels of detail and media in our group scrapbook. We both reminded members, in person that afternoon and via follow-up phone call on morning of the group, to bring at least one photo or memorabilia item (postcard, newspaper clipping) for scrapbook activity per the plan agreed upon last group session.

Sage opened the group by greeting the members and asking them to distribute and put on their name-tags to help all of us remember each other's names. Mary announced that Olga would be absent due to side effects of her chemotherapy (fatigue and need to avoid crowds due to risk of illness). Joe expressed concern for her (saying cancer was an awful disease, frowning, closing eyes, slowly shaking head back and forth), and Clara stated she would pray for Olga. We thanked members for their concern on Olga's behalf and stated we would pass on their kind words.

We then asked members how they were and reviewed the group ground rules and purpose. Mary reintroduced the occupational therapy consultant who had been present during pre-group interview and stated that she will be observing to give us feedback as group leaders. Sage showed the sample scrapbook and pointed out how different materials were used (10 minutes). Mary outlined the session's agenda as:

1. Choose scrapbook materials from bins being passed around, with assistance as needed
2. Assemble scrapbook page (with our assistance and adaptations in approach to task as per occupational therapy consultant's recommendations as necessary—i.e., tabletop magnifying lens, securing project to table with dycem, use of both hands, adapted scissors, etc.).
3. Discuss feelings, memorabilia, memories, or scrapbook task; Sage encouraged members to help each other and to ask for help and feedback about page arrangement as needed.
4. Close session by rating amount of satisfaction or dissatisfaction with the scrapbook activity or group session (rate on a scale of 1 = satisfied to 10 = dissatisfied), and discuss ratings as able or as time allows.

Mary then explained that in today's session we would like members to:

• Actively participate in creating scrapbook pages.
• Share materials and reminiscences.
• Express feelings regarding activity and/or life events.

As the group began, some members needed cuing to get started, but all participated to the level of their ability. Irina showed enjoyment of this activity by smiling, and a few expressed feeling satisfied with their finished product. Sophie, who is often anxious due to her mild dementia, began to demonstrate increased comfort in the group setting via engaging in the scrapbook task with familiar objects (personal picture or memorabilia) and shared some personal memories. She often looked at the sample, which seemed to present a specific guide for her to follow as she decided how to assemble her page. Agnes, who is easily fatigued, was able to attend and remain involved in the activity with Joe's assistance. She stayed the entire session, with short rest breaks every 15 minutes. Tom asked for assistance and advice from Sage when needed instead of discontinuing the task. He needed repeated encouragement to ask for feedback from other group members when he seemed to be having difficulties in the creative process or with making a decision. Tom eventually was able to ask Betty to cut out a picture from a magazine for him and asked her for approval as to where to mount the picture on the page. Betty responded to Tom's request for help and gave him the reassurance that he seemed to need regarding the quality of his work. Irina was able to communicate with other members to procure and share materials. Clara remained withdrawn but sorted through materials, collecting items and images. She continues to smile and nod when others are speaking about subjects she appears to enjoy or to which she may relate. Joe presented as friendly and gregarious but also shared a number of somatic complaints that seem to be related to his diabetes. Mary redirected Joe to follow up with his primary physician as his physical symptoms were of concern. Sage indicated that, if helpful, we could arrange after the group for him to use the center phone in a private space to call his doctor. Joe also occasionally needed prompts to interact with peers (i.e., assist Agnes) rather than leaders. Topics members reminisced about while they were working were marriages, children, hobbies, world and political events (i.e., war, assassinations), and former career pursuits.

When members shared a memory, we would repeat to the whole group what they said to ask if others had similar life experiences or recollections of time periods. This was done to ensure all members could hear what was said and facilitate group-centered sharing and discussion. At times Irina would revert to speaking in Russian, so we would ask her to take her time when speaking and to please repeat what she had just said in English for us. As the group reminisced, many members commented on similarity in experiences or feelings about past events. Members displayed a number of responses in conversation (e.g., "How interesting," "What a tough job to be a...," etc.) and emotional reactions (surprise—"You don't say!"; sorrow/sympathy—"How terrible for you!," "What a shame!"; empathy—"I know how it feels to lose a loved one" or attentive body language such as frowning, sighing, nodding, clasping hands together, smiling, laughing).

These moments of interpersonal connection and sharing recollections of past events or experiences created a sense of group togetherness. Betty acknowledged feeling surprised to learn things about others and felt glad to be getting to know other people better. Clara remained quiet but task-focused and receptive to peers' feedback/comments (smiling, nodding, saying "Thank you"). We provided ongoing positive feedback to members regarding their efforts and productivity, making a conscious effort to direct the feedback to individuals as well as the group as a whole. Sage took the role of being primarily involved with the task of the group as members occasionally said they feel they do not have the energy to be creative or productive at this point in their lives. Mary focused more on the physical and emotional needs of members per the occupation therapist's recommendations regarding adapting task or interpersonal interactions to meet members' needs. Eventually all members became so involved in the activity that we had to cue them re: amount of time remaining in the session.

At the end of the group, Sage reminded members that materials were available should members want to make additional scrapbook pages to complete their scrapbook outside of group time (i.e., at senior center, at home, with family) if they found this activity to be enjoyable. We reassured any members who had yet to complete their page that there would be opportunities to do so, either within or outside of the group. Agnes expressed a desire to continue the activity in future group sessions or with a family member or volunteer outside of group sessions. A number of members addressed their feedback and comments to the group as a whole, and this led to an active discussion about what to do in future sessions.

Post Group Leader Reflections

Informally, we have noticed some members congregating during the morning coffee hour (while awaiting arrival of other center members and beginning of morning group). This suggests that the closed group format seems to be helping these members to get to know each other. Reminding members in person of the activity plan the afternoon prior framed as "confirming our decision made at the previous meeting" and in the morning as "calling to confirm our meeting time today to work on…" seemed to be helpful for members who are experiencing memory loss. Presenting the model of a scrapbook with completed pages using the same materials also seemed a specific way to help convey the concept of making scrapbooks together as a means to reminisce and get to know each other better, which also served to clarify the activity goal.

We did not anticipate members' concern about the absent member. This created a sense of group identity not previously manifested and suggests the group is becoming more cohesive and cooperative. We are wondering if, despite our own discomfort with the topic, we need to be willing to allow more open discussion around loss of friends and loved ones to support members with dealing with these ongoing issues and feelings of grief at this stage of life. However, with this group we also feel a strong need to keep the activities positive and the tone of the group hopeful. Some members have said they feel they do not have the energy to be creative or productive at this point in their lives. Therefore, we feel we need to provide structured opportunities for creative expression and feeling productive. We feel this can serve as a means for members to give and receive support as well as encouragement that in fact they are still capable of doing things, perhaps more than they think or believe.

Individual Learning Activities

CASE STUDIES

Choose a case study and complete a session evaluation. Compare your evaluation with that provided in Appendix D. Write a session plan that might be used to address issues that are part of the formation stage.

REFLECTIVE QUESTIONS

1. When does the formation stage begin in a group, and what are the characteristics of this stage?

2. What are two primary issues of the formation stage of a group?

3. What kinds of group-centered actions might be realistic to expect in the formation stage?

4. What does "setting the climate" mean?

5. How might a leader teach members to assume responsibility for themselves in the group?

6. What types of information might a leader include in his or her introductory statement to the group?

7. How does the structure of the group session influence the amount and type of member participation in the group?

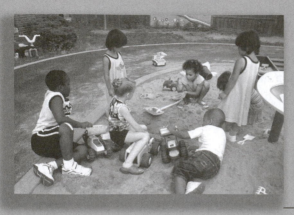

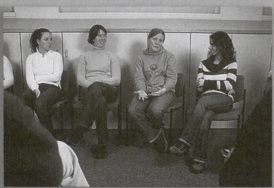

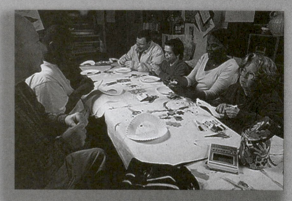

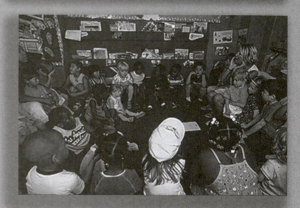

How Does a Functional Group Develop?

If we use the metaphor of group development as a journey or a life story, we can imagine the possible variations. Some travel or approach life with excited anticipation; others are consumed with worry about what may happen. When traveling, some pack lightly; others are burdened with their baggage. Therefore, one can expect that patterns in group when traveling, development will vary. Nevertheless, all groups demonstrate certain features. This principle has been explored in the formation stage of a functional group. In this chapter, the features characteristic of a group in the development stage (Table 7.1) are described. More specifically, this chapter emphasizes leadership issues in facilitating the group and individual and group expectations. It describes how to assess progress and identify and manage problems in the context of group action in the development stage.

This chapter also outlines dynamics that emerge as part of the group process and in the role of leader. It explores leader functions and strategies that may need to be employed in the development stage. Leader strategies include understanding and dealing with anger and aggression in the group, acknowledging the paradoxical elements of the group (strengths can be perceived as, or possibly become, limitations), and staying vigilant to promoting member interaction. If the destructive and regressive potential of the anti-group (Box 7.1) is not recognized and addressed by the leader, it is likely the group's development and member growth will not occur. Building one's skills and comfort with techniques for limit setting, managing anger and aggression in the group, and timing the use of interpretive reflections to the group are necessary to facilitating a group's development. Case studies demonstrate these concepts and describe leader functions such as involving members in setting goals, adapting the task to the stage of the group and individual members, and encouraging group members to assume task and maintenance roles (see Appendix E).

The life of a group is multidimensional. At a concrete, or manifest, level, a functional group is composed of individuals, an activity, and a physical environment. At a latent, or symbolic, level, the group has a purpose (both implicit and explicit), a set of dynamics and processes, and internal and external motivational forces. All these factors are interacting at any given moment. In a sense, these factors characterize the group's "meta-space," which is the experience of the moment. Neutral observers and group members could describe the group content and the process of the group's activity in similar ways, yet it is likely that each would also experience it a bit differently. Hence, the concrete and symbolic levels of a group are not readily distinguishable.

The main purpose of a functional group is the promotion of health and adaptation for its members. To accomplish this, the leader strives to create an environment conducive to purposeful, self-initiated, spontaneous, and group-centered action. As the literature has consistently shown, groups progress through developmental phases with unique characteristics (Agazarian & Gantt, 2003; Cohen & Smith, 1976; Corey & Corey, 1982; Garland & Frey, 1970; Garland, Jones, & Kolodny, 1973; Klein, 1972). Therefore, a leader must use a variety

Table 7.1	**Group Issues and Membership Needs Related to Action: Development Stage**		
Development Stage Issues: Concern over acceptance or rejection as result of change; testing the safety of the group; struggle between safety and involvement; control and power struggles (conflict) with leader and other members (Corey & Corey, 1977, 1982).			
Group Member Needs (related to action):			
Purposeful action provides: • Structured activity that includes all members and can provide successful outcomes • Guidance regarding expectations of members • Clear options and alternatives in goal selection • An accepting climate • Expression of respect for opinions and feelings of members	**Self-initiated action allows for:** • Support of exploratory behavior • Encouragement of task involvement and expression • Opportunity to express positive and negative reactions and feelings • Accepting environment	**Spontaneous (here and now) action occurs via:** • Encouragement of expression of ideas feelings, and thoughts related to here and now • Opportunity to interact with leader and test amount of freedom and control • Member sharing of perceptions and reactions as to what is going on in the group • Overt support and acceptance of diversity or difference	**Group-centered action yields:** • Leadership emerging from group membership • Sense of ownership as "our" group • Increased member-to-member interaction • Members looking less to leader for approval or needs to be met • Increased cohesiveness and support • Increased tolerance for limitations of group (time, materials, attention)

Leader Actions and Skills Employed
Reviewing confidentiality
Continued clarification of individual and group goals; use of group contract; redefining group rules
Continued leader involvement in task analysis, selection, and adaptation; activity demands must match member abilities for task and social interaction
Leader encouragement for members to assume group task and maintenance roles
Gradual increase in expectations for action to level of member tolerance and growth
Modeling
Genuineness and empathy
Active listening
Giving and receiving feedback
Assuring that conflict can be worked through if not acted out or avoided
Sharing process commentary as indicated

(table continued on page 180)

Table 7.1	**Group Issues and Membership Needs Related to Action: Development Stage** (continued)

Using concrete language; reframing potential hostility and anger as possibly related to disappointment with leader, frustration with limitations of group context, unmet needs, etc.
Connecting themes
Creating a climate or holding environment that allows for supportive interpersonal relationships
Leader input, support, and limit setting as needed

of strategies, depending on the needs of the group and individual members at each stage or phase of development. In the development stage of a functional group, the leadership functions may vary a great deal. The following is a general scheme for assessing the group's ongoing progress and identifying and managing problems. Certain issues are typical of this stage; whenever possible, leaders best serve the group by addressing these issues as they emerge. To facilitate a group's development, leader reasoning must balance individual needs with those of the group as a whole.

Assessing Progress

Evaluating the progress of the group, in addition to that of individual members, is an ongoing part of a leader's role. Structured and unstructured observation methods can be used. Structured methods provide the leader and members specific formats for systematically noting and recording behavior, events, and reactions. Some of the methods discussed earlier

Box 7.1   **Anti-Group*: A Process Rather Than a Fixed Entity**

- Varies in groups from hardly evident to taking over the group
- Has latent and manifest forms
- Occurs at levels of the individual, subgroup, and group as a whole
- Pertains to aggression, in particular toward the group
- Has a destructive and constructive developmental function
- Exists in relation to the creative and transformational potential of a group
- Exists in social organizations and institutions and wider culture of groups and is mirrored in sociocultural and political structures

*A concept developed by Nitsun (2000) that describes negative attitudes toward a group.

include a session evaluation, a sociogram, and a form designed for eliciting member feed-back. Leaders may choose to design observation formats specifically suited to a group member's goals or a group's stated outcomes. In contrast, unstructured observation methods require leaders or members to examine progress as part of the here-and-now action by spontaneously analyzing the group's process and dynamics.

Two techniques that are useful in elucidating process (as a means for assessing progress) involve reflecting observations as leaders back to the group via:

1. "Trainer process comments" (Miles, 1981, p. 115), which:
   a. "Illuminate the immediate problems facing the group"
   b. "Help build in the process-analysis function as a central feature of the group's work structure" (p. 115)
2. "Intermittent process analysis" (p. 117)

Once the group has some experience with trainer process comments, the group may establish as a norm members spontaneously commenting on what is happening. "In effect, group members are continually asking, 'What is happening? What is making these things happen? How can we change our behavior for the better?'" (Miles, 1981, p. 117).

A leader needs to gauge whether there is sufficient trust before making "process commentary" (Brown, 2003) (Box 7.2). It is advised that leaders be "somewhat tentative" (p. 238) in the early stages of a group and save process commentary for the conflict and working stages. Brown suggests that leaders make statements rather than pose questions so as to not push members to accept comments or to avoid being seen as critical or blaming. This technique is useful in moving a group forward when it seems stuck or loses energy or when discussions are circular. Brown cautions that leaders need to be prepared for members to resist process commentary because often the group is keeping material hidden for a reason. Brown suggests that the group will get back to the issues when it is ready. Behaviors such as withdrawal, dependency, and subgrouping serve the group and members' sense of safety. Until trust and cohesiveness are felt, aggressive feelings, such as jealousy and competition, or loving feelings, such as admiration or interpersonal intimacy, may be unconscious or experienced as too threatening if they emerge openly in the group.

Projective identification may be a possible variable in unconscious interpersonal transactions that may be occurring and contributing to group member behaviors. Projective identi-

Box 7.2   **Process Commentary**

"Process commentary makes visible what and how the group and its members are acting in the here and now....The leader speaks of what is hidden or not understood and the effect of these on the group and its members" (Brown, 2003, p. 238).

fication is the process "in which one person or subgroup finds a willing container for unwanted projections; the recipient then identifies with these projections, that is, the disowned parts of the projector" (Weber & Gans, 2003, p. 408). Leaders may also observe certain members experiencing role lock. Role lock is the process in which a member and the group confine that member's participation in the group "to a restricted aspect of the individual" (Weber & Gans, 2003, p. 408), such as always being the first to speak, role of group historian, or perhaps even that of group scapegoat. In scapegoating a group member, other group members place their "disavowed feelings and undesired aspects of themselves onto another group member" (Weber & Gans, 2003, p. 408). As group leaders, having an awareness of these processes is paramount so as to not inadvertently collude with the group in these behaviors.

If members are encouraged to be evaluators and observers of the group process to help determine the validity of the leader's assessment, the methods should yield feedback pertaining to the group's outcomes and operation at both the symbolic and concrete levels. The information used in this process of assessing progress focuses on members' actual functioning in the group environment and reports of behavior outside the group. Three questions guide the assessment:

1. As a result of the group's interaction, are members learning the adaptive skills and behaviors necessary for occupational performance?
2. Are members better able to fulfill their health needs?
3. Are the group's structure, process, and content conducive to facilitating the group goals and appropriate action (purposeful, self-initiated, spontaneous [here and now], group-centered) in the development stage?

Identifying and Managing Problems

The leader and, whenever possible, the group should attempt to identify problems at the concrete and symbolic levels. Such a review might occur at the beginning of a meeting, at the end of a session, at the completion of a task, or intermittently during the session. Some leaders prefer to designate a period for evaluating the session, such as the final 10 minutes. Others believe this sort of strict scheduling breaks the flow of action or activity. The timing will depend ultimately on the immediacy of the problem, an individual leader's style, and the group members' attention span, ability to delay gratification, and need for closure.

In the development stage of a functional group, one may expect problems that are characteristic of group members learning to work on a mutual task. Problems may originate from the group as a whole or from needs of individual members. In attempting to identify the group's needs, leaders must ask themselves: "What is inhibiting the group's movement toward purposeful, self-initiated, spontaneous, or group-centered action?" Every aspect of a functional group may need to be examined.

Nitsun's (1996; 2000) concept of the anti-group provides a framework for expecting and understanding the negative processes within and toward a therapeutic group. Attending to the anti-group phenomenon allows the leader to facilitate the inherent potential for creative process and positive progress to emerge out of destructive impulses and fantasies. By recognizing and effectively containing negative attitudes of hostility, anger, and aggression, the leader can facilitate a group achieving its purpose. Recognition of aggression as a natural phenomenon is central to a group's survival and growth. Nitsun (2000) also emphasizes the impact of powerful countertransference responses. Leaders are not immune to these processes and the effects of the anti-group. In leader countertransference, certain aspects of the leader's personality become strongly activated by group members. This can elicit either overly positive or negative reactions or responses to either individual members or the group as a whole. Without awareness of these processes and support to achieve clarity, leaders are left vulnerable to feelings of anger, incompetence, failure, and helplessness (Nitsun, 2000).

Some common group problems in the development stage include:

• "Conflict or fight"
• "Apathy and nonparticipation"
• "Inadequate decision making" (Bradford, Stock, & Horwitz, 1978, p. 63)

There may be specific origins for these group problems. Members who demonstrate fight behavior may feel "frustrated because they feel unable to meet the demands made of them" (p. 63). Their main goal may be "to find status in the group" (p. 64) rather than follow the goals or task set by the leader or other members. These members may feel a greater loyalty to "outside groups of conflicting interests" (p. 64). Members who demonstrate conflict behavior may feel they are "involved and are working hard on a problem" (p. 64) and therefore resent disruption or conflict from others.

Members may respond with apathy if the problem being worked on:

• "Does not seem important to the members"
• "[Seems] less important than some other problem on which they would prefer to be working"
• "May seem important to members, but there are reasons which lead them to avoid attempting to solve the problem" (p. 67)

Members also respond with apathy when a group has "inadequate procedures for solving the problem" (p. 68) or members feel "powerless about influencing final decisions" (p. 68). Another reason for apathy may involve a "prolonged and deep fight among a few members" (p. 68) that is dominating, and therefore undermining, the group. Inadequate decision making may also result from unsatisfactory group interactions such as:

• Premature calling for a decision
• Decision being too difficult
• The group being low in cohesiveness and lacking faith in itself
• The decision area being threatening to the group, because of unclear consequences, fear of reaction of other groups, or fear of failure for the individuals (p. 72)

In addition to a group's difficulties with task and maintenance functions, individual members may lack the skills or experience necessary to function in the group or to accomplish his or her role. A group member may also have unrealistic notions regarding his or her skills or ability to complete the task. In facilitating members' self-initiated action, it is important to remember that "perhaps the most salient element of the flow state is a sense of control over the environment. A person has to feel that his ability to act is adequate to meet the opportunities for action available. 'Inner' skills and 'outer' challenges must be in balance before the flow state can be experienced" (Csikszentmihalyi, 1975, p. 191).

The problems presented by individual members vary, and leaders should consider the following when trying to identify possible causes:

• Lack of opportunity for skill practice and modeling
• Inadequate positive reinforcement
• Secret or conflicting goals
• Insufficient information
• Poorly formed defense mechanisms
• Low self-esteem
• Process, communication, or interaction skill deficits
• Motor skill deficits
• Over- or underappraisal of skills
• Over- or underappraisal of activity demands

Problems in the group's structure and processes can inhibit group development. Inattention to group needs and lack of leadership skills can also foster group problems, such as the following:

• Activity is not matched to the group's abilities, processes, goals, or environment.
• Activities fail to meet members' interests or basic needs (safety, approval, self-esteem).
• Group goals are unclear, unrealistic, or not understood.
• Emotional environment does not support the group's efforts or those of individual members.
• Group members lack the necessary skills to perform a specific task.

- Insufficient mechanisms for receiving feedback or communication result in hidden conflict.
- Physical environment is not conducive to achieving the group's purpose (i.e., the room is too hot or too small or too big for everyone to be heard or understood).
- Group composition is too varied (age range, ability range, group readiness, etc.) or group size too big to allow for cohesiveness.
- Members are not encouraged to contribute to the goals or procedures of the group or to help each other directly.
- Group procedures, process, and effectiveness are not evaluated adequately. Leader may be summarizing group themes and actions prematurely or questioning verbal and nonverbal communication in a manner that group members perceive as judgmental.
- Distribution of leadership and membership roles is inadequate.
- Group members are not given the opportunity to test ideas and possible courses of action.
- Clear limits and expectations are not established or the leader is passive in dealing with disruptive behavior in the group (or interference from outside the group).
- Favoritism to particular group members or to subgroups is shown by the leader through nonverbal or verbal communication.

Problems can also arise on the symbolic level. Even the savviest of leaders, using sound clinical reasoning and principles of evidence-based practice, may find themselves viewing a group member as a "difficult patient" (Gans & Alonso, 1998, p. 312). However, if one looks more closely at the powerful dynamics at play, "the difficult patient" is, to an extent, a coconstruction of interactions among the leader, the group members, and the group as a whole (p. 312) (Box 7.3). Leaders are human and make mistakes (Box 7.4). By reflecting on their practices, however, leaders can learn from their mistakes and build their skills and competency, thereby increasing their effectiveness.

Mistakes, such as the ones outlined above, can serve as a guide for self-examination, supervision, mentoring, and identification of leadership problems. In some instances, solving a seemingly minor problem of the physical environment can eliminate apparent leadership problems. For example, if members feel they are not heard adequately, a change from a noisy room may create an environment in which leader and members are more relaxed and there-

Box 7.3 Factors Contributing to the Creation of the Difficult Patient

- Patient dynamics and characteristics of those dynamics
- Leadership competency and mistakes in leadership
- The role of intersubjectivity in the group construction of the difficult patient
- Dynamics of group as a whole (Gans & Alonso, 1998, p. 312)

Box 7.4   **Leadership Competency and Mistakes in Leadership**

- Faulty patient selection
- Inept or harmful handling of boundary violations, scapegoating, and group norms
- Inability or unwillingness to acknowledge mistakes
- Refusal to be a lightning rod for negative feelings
- Failure to set limits on members' expression of sadomasochism
- Failure to accept one's own limits as they affect clinical practice during the inevitable, painful vicissitudes that punctuate one's professional career and personal life (Gans & Alonso, 1998, pp. 317–318)

fore listen to each other more easily. An advantage of co-leadership is that leaders can share the task of identifying problems. One leader might more naturally address leadership problems at the concrete level, and another may attend to problems at the symbolic level.

Leader Intervention Strategies

Many strategies can be used to intervene and address the numerous problems described. To address issues at the symbolic level or those involving transferences and anti-group, leaders must work to address their own attitudes toward and acceptance of "the importance of aggression in the group" (Nitsun, 1996, p. 175). This requires that leaders express members' potential frustrations or disappointments that may exist by virtue of being in a group. Examples of this might be acknowledging limited time for task completion, having to take turns when talking, or sharing materials or leader attention. Leaders need to gain comfort with members' expression of affect, whether it be disappointment, sadness, hostility, anger, or aggression (Fig. 7.1). In group self-initiated action, expressions of dissatisfaction are often the first signs of a group's formation. Additionally, expressions of anger and hostility should be expected as part of a group's development. Leaders must be able to recognize the "defensive function" (Rosenthal, 1987); this may serve as members resist the difficult work being a group member will require of them. Leaders also need to work to develop their ability to face conflict as well as to allow members to express their anger and disappointment by redirecting it toward the leaders. This can serve to reduce scapegoating of members as well as provide an opportunity to examine unmet needs. If leaders can remain open to member criticism and feedback, this can serve as a means to model this process for members. Certainly this process of dealing with hostility, anger, and aggressive or competitive forces in the group still requires that leaders maintain safety by providing limits and containment in the group. It is vital that group rules and norms be upheld during the group. Additionally, to influence the group's process

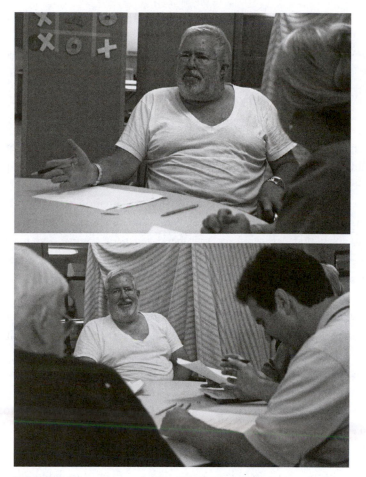

FIGURE 7.1 Expressions of affect. (Photo by Julie Ide)

and outcome, leaders can consciously and actively work to alter the group's structure through three strategies:

1. Involving members in setting goals.
2. Adapting the task more closely to the group and individual members.
3. Encouraging group member roles.

Involving Members in Setting Goals

A client-centered approach has always been a cornerstone of the functional group model (Box 7.5). Therefore, a key leadership function is to enable the group members to become involved in establishing goals. The strategy employed varies according to the individual's readiness and abilities as well as the group's maturity or social/emotional cohesiveness.

Box 7.5   **Choice Is Fundamental to Occupational Therapy**

"Occupational therapy has been unique, historically, because of the client's participation in his own treatment. Choice has been so fundamental to our thinking that we have questioned whether procedures which are done to the person, over which he has no control, should be called occupational therapy" (Yerxa, 1967, p. 3).

The value of group member involvement in goal setting should not be underestimated. In a study on making choices, it was found that "subjects who were not permitted choices in completing the activity perceived themselves as less powerful only when they participated in the activity in the presence of others in the same situation" (Henry, Nelson, & Duncombe, 1984, p. 249). Encouraging group members to make choices about the group's goals establishes a norm that can reinforce members' sense of control and mastery. The aim is to empower members by teaching, through experience or action, the value of achieving a personally selected goal. It appears likely that, having a sense of choice is particularly important to individuals when an activity is conducted in a group setting.

Even if explicitly stated, group goals often seem ambiguous to the members in the initial phase of a group's development. In the case of a short-term group with limited time or an open group, leaders must rapidly focus members' attention and energy on goal setting. The many factors that influence the selection of goals by the group make member involvement in goal setting an ongoing leadership task.

To understand the intervention strategy for involving members in goal selection, factors that can influence formation of group goals need to be examined. Three factors have been identified:

1. Motives of members: these can be of a personal interest to individual members or solely in the best interests of the group.
2. Superordinate group goals: these focus on long-term purposes and group objectives.
3. The group and its social surroundings: this includes other groups that exert influence on the group's goals (Cartwright & Zander, 1968).

Early research demonstrated that members were willing to take greater risks and were more willing to work together toward the group's purpose if they were involved in making a group decision or specifying a group goal (Cartwright & Zander, 1968).

How can leaders instill hope and facilitate member involvement in goal setting? If a functional group is conducted within an institution or with some outside directives, leaders should first and foremost keep members informed of the group's general purpose and resources. After giving general information on these factors, the leader should ask members what they see as their needs. Leaders can also give members feedback and encourage members to give each other feedback about behaviors displayed in the group. Members may also find it useful to hear about the procedures and formats used in similar groups or in past groups to address member needs and goal setting. Through these various strategies, the leader helps members, and the group as a whole, define problems, needs, and goals.

Functional group members may be severely impaired in their ability to cognitively, emotionally, or socially impart information or formulate goals. Insecurity about performance skills can also contribute to difficulty in goal setting. Therefore, leaders, in the course of a group's development, must at times actively establish formats for goal setting by:

- Structuring various activities to help members clarify their goals
- Actively listening to members and reflecting back what is being said, or not said, in concrete terms
- Observing members and reporting what is being done or not done
- Encouraging group members to report back to the group their experiences outside the group when pertinent to the spontaneous (here-and-now) action in the group

Through their verbal and nonverbal behavior, leaders must demonstrate that every member's opinion is important to the group's functioning. Similarly, leaders must be aware of members' changing needs and the necessity for involving members in goal setting throughout the course of the group's development.

Task Adaptation

In the functional group model, the development stage builds on the formation stage of the group. In the formation stage a group climate is established, group goals and roles are clarified, and the basis for trusting relationships is formed. The development stage includes a "transitional phase of a group's development" (Corey & Corey, 1982, p. 194), also known as a "transition stage" (p. 194). Group member behavior is characterized as "marked by feelings of anxiety and defenses in the form of various resistances" (p. 194). In a functional group, the transition stage would occur as part of the development stage. Certain member behaviors, anxieties, or possible "resistances" (p. 194) might appear as:

- Concern over group acceptance or rejection if members change
- Testing the safety of the group
- A struggle between safety and involvement
- Control and power struggles or conflicts with the leader or with the other group members (p. 194)

After the group has worked out these issues, it proceeds to a "working stage" (Corey & Corey, 1982, p. 194). At this point, there is a shift in the group process wherein members are more able to function as a cohesive unit. Communication is more open, and leadership functions become shared. In this working phase, members often feel there is hope for change. Interestingly, novice group leaders commonly feel that they have done something wrong when developmental problems arise in a group. These problems are characteristic of groups learning to work together; for a group to progress, it must work through these issues, which are common in the development stage.

Group leaders can use specific strategies to adapt the group's task structure and process in the development stage. First, the dominant characteristic being displayed by group members should be identified. Second, the leader structures the activity in graded increments to allow the group to learn how to work through the issue. For example, a leader might notice that members are late for a group meeting and do not bring the agreed-upon materials necessary to complete a planned activity. By confronting the group with empathy, the leader can begin to clarify if a power struggle exists. Perhaps some members feel the leader or a subgroup of members is imposing the activity choice on the group. In this instance, the group can be supportively encouraged to examine alternative ways to approach the decision-making process. The leader might suggest the group discuss how it feels to confront an authority figure or to role-play and practice ways to address a difference of opinion or offer information. Ultimately, through use of such strategies and being accepting of member actions and feedback, the leader allows a safe rebellion. Opportunity is provided for members to learn new behaviors or adaptive skills, and the safety of the group is protected.

If the group is an open group, one can expect that issues will recur as the membership of the group changes. Similarly, if the membership is heavily weighted with individuals who are experiencing difficulty with a particular problem—such as separation problems of childhood and adolescence—one could expect the problem to be reflected in the type of group development issues that arise (Fig. 7.2). For example, power and control struggles relative to the leadership or task might become problems. Leaders must be able to process the group's actions, limit-set certain behaviors, and plan strategies on the basis of the developmental needs of the group and its members.

Encouraging Group Member Roles

For group members to be encouraged to fulfill member roles and develop leadership, they must be involved in planning the group. This planning process must provide opportunities that will allow members to assume responsibility for action in accordance with the group members' abilities and the group's stage of development. Therefore, members need to be taught process skills (at the level of their cognitive ability) such as:

• Active listening
• Giving and receiving feedback
• Using "I" statements

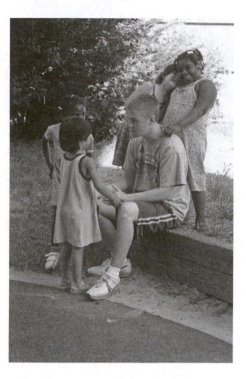

FIGURE 7.2 Processing separation and attachment issues. (Photo by Mark Morelli)

- Reality testing their perceptions in the here and now
- Speaking in the present tense
- Decision making
- Assessing progress

These skills should be modeled by the group leader and practiced by the members. To enable group members to gain these skills, leaders can encourage members to more actively assume the task and maintenance functions of the group. This can be facilitated through the use of the following techniques:

- Involve all group members in defining the group's name, purpose, procedures, rules, and norms as well as in observing the group's behavior.
- Positively reinforce members' strengths, compensate for members' deficits through structuring the group's task at levels members can manage, and avoid focusing exclusively on members' limitations.
- Allocate the resources necessary for task completion, such as an appropriate room and access to needed materials.
- Act as a resource person and facilitator rather than an authority or rescuer, as members should feel the leaders are present to enable the group to achieve positive action.

- Use a co-leader, if possible, to model ways to collaborate, share responsibility, and give support.
- Provide some structure, but do not overwhelm the group with structure, as members may feel useless or not understood. Too much structure fosters dependency and stifles self-initiated action; too little may result in chaos or apathy.
- Sanction members testing a variety of behaviors within the limit of the group's safety. This may involve helping members to realistically assess or reality-test the consequences of their actions and the possible relationship between behavior in the group and behavior outside the group.

Leader Emotional Response

The development stage of a group presents special challenges to leaders, especially those with a high need for control or being seen as an authority figure. As the group becomes more cohesive, members will have less need to perceive the leader as all-knowing. As stronger interpersonal bonds are developed, members will struggle with each other and the leaders for power and control. Acting out behaviors such as lateness and unexplained absences test the group's limits and stability. Although these reactions are to be expected, they can still cause strong emotional reactions in leaders as well as members.

Countertransference difficulties arise in a group because powerful emotions naturally emerge within the group format. Challenges emerge within the process of countertransference that can lead to leader role difficulties and elicit "therapist shame" (Weber & Gans, 2003) (Box 7.6). Therapist shame can be viewed as a natural occurrence when working with groups. Although often overlooked, therapist shame nonetheless has a potent effect on group leadership. Weber and Gans (2003) explain how leader aspirations can be grandiose and contribute

Box 7.6   **Common Challenges Evoking Countertransference and Therapist Shame**

- Collusion with role lock or scapegoating
- Containing and detoxifying noxious projective identifications
- Negative transferences in which aspects of a group member's personality strongly activated by group leader
- Idealization of the therapist (Weber & Gans, 2003, p. 407)

to group therapist shame, describing Brightman's narcissistic triad in the grandiose professional ego ideal:

- Omnipotence (the wish to be all-powerful)
- Omniscience (the wish to be all-knowing)
- Total benevolence (the wish to be all-loving) (Brightman as cited in Weber & Gans, 2003, p. 399).

To mitigate being overwhelmed by the experience of therapist shame, Weber and Gans (2003) offer their conclusions of the "good-enough" group therapist to provide a framework to help leaders replace the "grandiose professional ego-ideal" with a "realistic professional ego-ideal":

- Mistakes will happen when leading groups.
- Learning about oneself from mistakes and sharing the learning in a positive way can be empowering to a group.
- Trust times when beliefs run counter to group outlook, and speak up against the attitude.
- Enjoy knowing the fact that group members often get more from each other than from the leader.
- Leaders are important to group members because of the functions leaders perform, such as being steady, fair, empathic, and dependable.
- The leader being with group members as they experience disappointment in uncontrollable aspects of the group experience, such as lateness and absenteeism, is of value to the members.
- Peer supervision with respected colleagues nurtures leaders to enable them to sustain group members and identify with their experiences as group members.
- It is a privilege to do the work of a therapist. Keeping this in mind can help to neutralize the criticism received when serving in the role of emotionally containing others (Weber & Gans, 2003, pp. 412–413).

Peer supervision or mentoring in dyadic or small groups can help leaders monitor reactions counterproductive to the workings of their groups. Co-leaders may find disruptions in their working relationship that mirror struggles in the group, such as vying for control, favoritism, and so on. Monitoring these co-leadership relationship disruptions, to prevent these types of acting out behaviors on the leaders' part, is paramount to the group's survival in the development stage. Self-reflective questions (Box 7.7) can help leaders examine their emotional responses and identify patterns in their own reactions that emerge as part of the process of working through issues in the development stage of the group.

Box 7.7   **Leader Self-Reflective Questions for Development Stage**

- In the past, how have I dealt with conflict in a group situation?
- What is my reaction to the group becoming more cohesive and members assuming more authority over their own process and procedures?
- Have there been unusual behaviors in the group, such as premature loss of members, absences, or lateness? If so, what is my reaction?
- What strategies have I used to manage boundary violations?
- Are there conflicts in the group that may be contributing to such behaviors?
- How can I support and guide the group at this point in its development?
- Have I (or my co-leader) been acting differently in or outside of the group?
- Are there feelings that have not been discussed or unresolved conflicts at the root of the turmoil? For example, do I feel competitive with my co-leader? Does this resonate with unresolved sibling rivalry from my own primary family relationships or from an adult partnership?

Conclusion

Just as in the formation stage, the development stage of a functional group has particular issues and problems requiring carefully considered responses from leaders. The issues that arise are part of the growth essential to the well-being of the group and its success in reaching certain goals. Understanding the potential impact of dynamics, such as those of the anti-group, projective identification, and transferences, is the underpinning to realizing the group's growth needs. Additionally, having an appreciation for the power of these processes supports using leader strategies effectively. Strategies such as allowing choice, limit setting, process commentary or analysis, and facilitating group members' abilities to assume group task and maintenance roles become instrumental to the transitional group processes. It is vital that leaders incorporate their own reflective practices to identify and manage problems in the group. As a group develops, leaders need to stay vigilant to the processes of the group. The development stage of a functional group requires that leaders use their understanding of these processes to involve members in setting realistic goals for themselves and the group to meet the changing group and member needs.

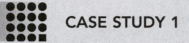

CASE STUDY 1

OPEN GROUP ON AN INPATIENT PSYCHIATRY UNIT

Session Plan

Name of group: "Getting It Together"
Date: Wednesday, June 8
Leaders: Lauri Levy, OTR/L; Jack Jones, MHC
Session Activity: Arts and crafts for hospital flea market fundraiser
Specific goals for the group session: Members will:

- Express feelings and thoughts in the present tense.
- Express positive and negative reactions and feelings.
- Complete at least one item per member for annual hospital flea market fundraiser.

Specific goals for group members:

- Maggie (new member): Integrate into group.
- Lakisha and Pearl: Increase comfort within group to decrease tendency to subgroup.
- Eric, Li, Liz: Express feelings about having a new group member; identify one project to complete; state personal goals for group session.
- Gary: Self-monitor pressured speech with cues; decrease number of verbal outbursts (interrupting others).
- Betty: Remain for 30 minutes and engage in activity.

Description of methods and procedures:

- Summarize previous session to reinforce learning for existing members and to integrate new member.
- Review goal of supporting hospital fundraiser to raise funds to purchase books for patient library and stuffed animals for children's unit.
- Offer choice of activity: beading, small wood crafts (i.e., birdhouses, bookends), and decorating keepsake boxes.

Rationale: To provide an opportunity for expressing and processing feelings regarding having a new member in the group; activity is familiar to existing members and provides choice within a larger group project and member levels of ability—hence, little opportunity for failure.

Description of leadership role: Encourage members to talk about their feelings in the group and possible anxieties experienced as new member enters group; encourage members to support and assist one another with elements of chosen activities (providing feedback, advice, physical assistance with task as needed).

Rationale: Provides group an opportunity to reality-test expectations of leaders and group; recognizes stage issue of dependence versus independence and reinforces that it is safe to express feelings in the group while allowing self-directed, spontaneous, purposeful, and group-centered action; provides opportunities to explore how individual choices and group dynamics can affect action.

Describe necessary preparations:

• Lauri will gather necessary supplies.

• Jack will prepare new member for group in a pre-group interview. Discuss with her recent activities of group, its goals and norms. Reinforce notion that new members are encouraged to participate at their own pace until they have some experience with the group's procedures and processes.

List material and equipment needed:

Beading supply cart
Nontoxic paints/stains/clear coat
Birdhouse/bookend kits
Prefabricated keepsake boxes
Decorative items (self-sticking gems, magazine pictures, etc.)
Nontoxic craft glue

Time and sequence outline for sessions (include what you will say and do as the leader and what the group will do; consider both content and process):

• Introduction of new member; review of group's purpose and procedures. (approximately 5 minutes)

• Review plan to work on creating items for hospital fundraiser. (approximately 5 minutes)

• Outline project options, encouraging members to make choices. (approximately 5 minutes)

• Members work on projects. (approximately 25 minutes)

• Process and plan next session. (approximately 5 minutes)

Other information pertinent to this specific session: There is a new female member (Maggie) joining the group; a group member (John) was discharged yesterday. Maggie had a pre-group interview with Jack, who discussed recent activities of the group, its goals, and norms. She appeared highly anxious even in the 1:1 context of the pre-group meeting.

Session Narrative

Name of group: "Getting It Together"

Date: Wednesday, June 8

Leaders: Lauri Levy, OTR/L; Jack Jones, MHC

Session Activity: Arts and crafts for hospital flea market fundraiser

Prior to the group, Lauri made sure that there was an adequate supply of beading materials, birdhouses, bookends, and boxes. She arranged the materials to facilitate members making choices and accessing needed supplies quickly and easily. During the session we bridged from previous sessions this week by summarizing what was done and highlighting what was learned to reinforce learning for existing members and integrate new member (Maggie). We reviewed accomplishments of members and announced that Betty was hoping to stay for 30 minutes today. We reinforced that new members are encouraged to participate at their own pace. Laurie stated that, as leaders, our expectations were that the group would:

• Discuss feelings and thoughts about the group or activity in a constructive way
• Share positive and negative feelings in a safe way
• Express feelings about adding a new group member (Maggie), as related to the ongoing theme of change
• Work as a group and take responsibility to support each member in completing at least one item for the fundraiser

Laurie explained to the group that we believed arts and crafts provide an opportunity for personal expression through the creative process. Jack provided support and feedback when Liz was able to talk about her fear and anger regarding perceived loss of attention and Maggie expressed her own anxieties she was experiencing entering a new group. When Gary stated leaders were not helping the group enough, Laurie chose to reality-test what reasonable expectations there might be of us as leaders and of the group members in terms of making decisions and engaging in project work more independently of us. Laurie asked group members to try to see their own resources, identifying what we saw as each member's strengths and abilities. Jack explained that we considered the project as representative of how when individuals work together toward a common goal or interest, something "greater" can be achieved (raising funds for books for library, toys for children's unit). We reinforced that it is safe to express feelings of disappointment in our lack of participation as leaders in the projects and our decision making regarding limiting members' choice of project.

When needed, we made process commentaries regarding member behaviors and wondered aloud what might be contributing to individuals' actions (i.e., is Liz holding back perhaps due to fear of suggestions not being accepted? Gary looking to us as leaders to approve of his work?) and how these group dynamics were possibly affecting group member interactions. Lakisha made several bead bracelets and shared that she felt ready to make decisions, stating she would have to in order to return to her job as office manager. Pearl told Gary she would help him "get the job done" and was able to pass along to him needed items and assist with cleanup at close of the group. Eric shared with the new member that he had both positive and negative feelings about the group. He worked cooperatively with Li, who worked silently (the hospital translator was not present) painting the bookends and the birdhouse Eric built. It was at this point that Maggie was able to state that she did not feel very creative or artistic and wished she could team up with someone or just provide assistance to someone. The group members responded with validating comments regarding how some of them found being creative hard at first due to their depression or low self-image and identified ways in which she could be of assistance to them (finding certain colored beads or decorative gems, gluing things together, holding birdhouse while member painted/nailed, etc.).

Laurie summed up the group as being one in which it seemed that rather than heightening a sense of deprivation and isolation, members expressing their thoughts and emotions, both verbally and artistically, enabled them to acknowledge feelings of hopelessness and hope. Liz identified that she developed bonds with members in the group in a relatively short time and felt gratified by the group's efforts to work together to support a good cause.

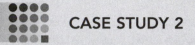

CASE STUDY 2

CLOSED GROUP IN AN OUTPATIENT OCCUPATIONAL THERAPY CLINIC

Session Plan

Name of Group: Community Re-entry: "Moving Forward"
Date: December 17; fourth of eight sessions
Leaders: Russell Lee, MS OTR/L; Alicia Wall, COTA/L
Session Activity: Energy Conservation, Adapting Activities or Environment, Pain Management
Specific goals for the group session: Members will:

• Learn energy-saving procedures.
• Practice work simplification techniques.
• Discuss potential plans for organization of home/work environments to minimize energy output.
• Address apparent ambivalence in regard to dependency on leaders, outpatient providers/insurance, and significant others as a potential barrier to "moving forward."

Specific goals for group members:

Jim (BI post MI): To identify strategies for planning routines to incorporate energy conservation into activities of daily living and work-related tasks such as e-mail.

John (traumatic BI post MVA): To incorporate work simplification and safety awareness into home maintenance tasks (cleaning, sweeping, shoveling, laundry).

Steve (lumbar fusion): To learn to incorporate strategies for pain prevention and management into work tasks (construction contractor–related).

Jeanette (post CVA): To incorporate pacing into homemaking and home maintenance tasks to support success in resuming these roles.

Wendy (post bilateral TKR): To practice use of adaptive devices and identify environmental adaptations necessary to enable return to work.

Brenda (post CVA): To pace child care tasks and identify modifications to task or environment needed to support her to fully resume tasks performed in mothering role.

Juanita (post hip fixation): To reinforce need to follow current precautions and identify interim strategies to remain active (exercise routine, volunteering tasks safe to resume) while recovering.

Description of methods and procedures: Lecture, PowerPoint slide show, demonstration, practice, and discussion.

Rationale: Audiovisuals will make procedures more specific; discussion gives members an opportunity to vent feelings and get group support; practice allows for some skill development.

Description of leadership role: Teacher, encourager, supporter, and confronter.

Rationale: To model techniques, assess member performance, reality-test leader and member perceptions, and support members' emotional needs.

Describe necessary preparations: Prepare audiovisuals, lecture, handouts, and work simulations.

List material and equipment needed: Laptop, screen, LCD projector, and items for work simulation stations.

Time and sequence outline for session:

PowerPoint slide show and lecture
Group discussion
Practice techniques at work/task simulation stations

Other information pertinent to this specific session: Holiday season and weather concerns persist.

Session Narrative

Name of Group: Community Re-entry: "Moving Forward"

Date: December 17; fourth of eight sessions

Leaders: Russell Lee, MS, OTR/L; Alicia Wright, COTA/L

Activity: Energy Conservation, Adapting Activities or Environment, Pain Management

Russell opened the group by outlining our aim as: "Today we will be focusing on energy conservation techniques that can assist you with pain management and adapting to your current condition or disability. We have prepared a PowerPoint lecture to introduce the topic and show some of the recommended techniques. We are also providing you with handouts to help you use the concepts at home. We have set up work simulation stations for us to try out what will be reviewed in the lecture, which includes:

• Energy-saving procedures
• Work simplification techniques
• Potential plans for organization of the home/work environment to minimize energy output

During the lecture, we would like you to feel comfortable to ask questions or express feelings or concerns related to using the suggested tips and techniques presented and practiced in today's session."

After reviewing the concepts via the lecture format, Alicia asked members if they had any questions about the material and were met with silence. The simulations (meal preparation, yard work, housekeeping, sustained reading, keyboarding tasks) prompted some discussion in subgroups. The work simulation gave us a chance to observe members' skills and performance and gave members an opportunity to practice and give each other feedback. Members were able to demonstrate some energy conservation techniques, and many began to identify specific activities of daily living and independent daily living tasks with which they are currently struggling, requiring significant others or family members to do for them. Jim expressed his frustration with how slowly he seems to be recovering, stating that desktop activities such as e-mail and reviewing lengthy documents were taking longer than he felt he had time to devote to these tasks. Brenda identified that she is also frustrated by her inability to perform diaper changes for her baby due to her decreased strength and limited motion in her "bad" (affected) arm. Jeanette stated her fatigue and difficulty with balance were making cooking "near to impossible." Steve declined to participate in certain simulations, complaining of pain. Juanita and Wendy identified that they need to work directly on tasks they currently find difficult to do due to decreased range of motion and being wheelchair-bound. John willingly participated in all simulations but appeared to grow restless, especially when members were discussing how and why they felt the procedures would or would not work at home. Russell facilitated discussion by classifying common themes and issues and highlighting members' suggestions regarding alternative approaches to tasks.

In closing, Alicia acknowledged to the group that perhaps we should have intentionally divided the group into subgroups for practice simulations to increase member time for sharing and decrease time required for each work simulation as it was clear members wanted more opportunity for problem solving and practice. Russell reflected to the group that as leaders we may have unwittingly responded to what we would term "dependency" issues in our structuring of today's session. We openly shared our observations that members have seemed dependent on us as leaders of late, passive in terms of recommended follow-up with outpatient providers/insurance, and acquiescent to the wishes of significant others versus their own stated plans and goals in the group. Russell wondered aloud if members might be feeling ambivalence in regard to facing the issues of community re-entry. We asked members for feedback regarding our perceptions, stating we shared our observations to raise awareness as a precaution, as such behaviors might become potential barriers to "moving forward" in terms of increasing independence as part of community reintegration.

Members were able to express concerns about feeling dependent on their families and their anger toward leaders for not allowing the group to continue beyond the eight scheduled sessions to help them progress more. The group members were more irritable and angrier than expected, which Alicia reflected back to the group as perhaps due to additional stress of the holiday season and weather conditions (ice/snow). As members articulated their feelings, they were able to acknowledge fears of falling on ice, getting their wheelchair stuck in snow, experiencing anxiety when riding in cars (fearing car accidents), and feeling abandonment and isolation in losing the support of leaders and each other. Once feelings were validated, we were able to incorporate addressing these feelings as part of setting realistic goals for remaining sessions.

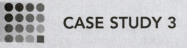

CASE STUDY 3

COMMUNITY-BASED GROUP

Session Plan

Name of Group: "Time Flies"
Date: October 12, 6th of 10 sessions
Leaders: Mary Munroe, Wellness Director; Sage Stilton, Volunteer
Session Activity: Greeting Cards: Part II: Collaborative Verse
Specific goals for the group session: Members will:

• Increase initiative in planning group activities.
• Express feelings and thoughts in present tense (here and now).
• Verbalize positive and negative reactions to group activities.
• Interact socially.
• Experience enjoyment in self-expression.

Specific goals for group members:

Betty and Irina (who were late for the group last week): To be able to discuss this issue in
   the group if they are late again.
Sophie (who is often anxious due to her mild dementia): To demonstrate increased comfort
   in the group via engaging in familiar tasks and/or in conversation with other members
   about personal memories.
Agnes: To remain involved in the activity and discussion for the entire session with two to
   three short (5-minute) rest breaks as needed.
Tom: To continue to ask for assistance when needed instead of discontinuing the task.
Betty: To be more open to sharing ideas or giving feedback to others (instead of avoiding
   topic, subgrouping, arriving late, or complaining).
Irina: To communicate more openly and effectively with leaders and other members besides
   Betty.
Clara: To take more leadership with peers.
Joe: To continue to focus on engaging in task and discussion with peers.

Description of methods and procedures:

Summarize activity of previous session in which members decorated greeting cards.
Clara had observed that they had written no verses on the cards. A plan was made for
group to write a verse in this session. With a collective verse, group members each contribute

at least one word, idea, or line about a selected topic (i.e., birthdays, holidays, get well, sympathy).

Rationale: Writing in a group will allow participants to channel reminiscences and synthesize them into the verse, if desired. Writing also encourages a deeper level of social interaction than previous group activities. The process of creating a collective verse validates everyone's experience and contribution.

Description of leadership role:

• Assist members in reminiscing process and in the selection of a topic for verse.
• Provide support for and acknowledgement of member contributions.
• Provide visual and verbal structure for writing and repeating lines or phrases for those members who have auditory or visual deficits by writing in large letters on newsprint and reading each contribution aloud.

Rationale: Structure will support and encourage group discussion of positive and negative feelings about reminiscences.

Describe necessary preparations:

• Review and discuss session plan with co-leader.
• Select examples of verses to read to the group.
• Describe in detail the procedure for collaborative writing, reassuring members that a contribution can be just a word, a phrase, or a line.

List material and equipment needed:

Large newsprint paper, an easel stand, and markers

Center laptop and mini LCD (networked to printer) to type out and display verse as agreed upon and to print out final copies to be distributed to all members to cut and paste into cards

Glue sticks

Scissors

Time and sequence outline for sessions (include what you will say and do as the leader and what the group will do; consider both content and process):

• Greetings, distribution of name tags. Review group purpose and procedures. (approximately 5 minutes)
• Review of last session and group planning for today. (approximately 5 minutes)
• Introduce the activity of collaborative writing. Describe how a topic for the verse will be chosen from member suggestions. Read selected examples of verses. Describe that the process of writing will involve each member in turn, contributing a line, word, or phrase. (approximately 10 minutes)

- If needed, leaders can start by reminiscing about a meaningful occasion on which they received greeting cards, and then ask group members to do likewise. As members come up with topics, co-leader will record them on the newsprint and repeat them aloud. After approximately 10 minutes, the leader will read the list of topics, and members will choose a topic for the verse.
- As each group member makes a contribution to the verse, the co-leader will type it on the laptop and read aloud what is displayed via LCD projector for all to hear. The members will be given a chance to change any wording. Gentle prompting by the leader will help to ensure that members have satisfactorily expressed themselves before the next member will have his or her turn. The group will continue to go around so that all group members have the opportunity to participate and contribute to the collective verse. (approximately 10 minutes)
- The completed verse will be read aloud in its entirety and copies printed.
- Members will cut and paste into cards as desired. (10 minutes)
- Ask members to share how they felt about today's activity and group experience. (approximately 10 minutes)

Session Narrative

Name of Group: "Time Flies"
Date: October 12, 6th of 10 sessions
Leaders: Mary Munroe, Wellness Director; Sage Stilton, Volunteer
Session Activity: Greeting Cards: Part II: Collaborative Verse

As we began the session with our opening ritual of greetings, Sophie spontaneously gave each person, including leaders, a name tag. We then asked how people were doing since last meeting when Olga told us she would be leaving to go to a hospice. John replied that he felt bad for her and that he hoped to create some card message to send to her in today's session. We reviewed our group purpose and procedures, including that in our last session members had designed greeting cards and agreed with Clara's suggestion that this session be devoted to writing verses that could go inside some of the cards.

Mary introduced the idea of collaborative writing and our belief that it could be a more personal way for members to reminiscence and share thoughts and feelings about specific life events (birthdays, wedding, losses, accomplishments). Sage read selected examples of verses (congratulations, get well, thinking of you, and sympathy cards). Sage suggested that the collaborative process of writing involve each member contributing a line, a word, or a phrase (approximately 10 minutes).

At this point, Sage contributed a memory of a difficult time in her life when she received cards and how special and loved she felt to get all those cards. She asked group members if anyone had ever had a similar experience. As members remembered occasions, she recorded them on the large pieces of newsprint we had posted on the wall and repeated them aloud. After approximately 5 minutes of sharing, she read the list and members chose the theme "Thinking of You" as the topic for which they would write the first verse.

As each group member made a contribution to the verse, Sage repeated what was said aloud as she typed. When Mary noticed subgroupings of members asking each other what was written or said, she suggested that perhaps Joe could give Sage a break and repeat what was said aloud for all to hear. Mary also asked that members hold off on critiquing or editing until all members had an opportunity to share their thoughts. She repeated this redirection when she noticed that disruptive talking was continuing between Irina and Betty. Gentle prompting was needed to ensure that members satisfactorily expressed themselves before the next member had his or her turn. The group format became a sort of round robin of members going around in the seating formation of the table circle. The members were then given a chance to change, omit, or select from what was brainstormed any wording they liked for their verse. Completed verse(s) were read aloud for members to give final approval. Copies were printed via the center's networked printer. Members then cut and pasted verses into cards as desired (10 minutes).

In closing Mary asked members to share how they felt about today's activity and group experience (approximately 10 minutes). We reflected to the group that we noticed that the writing component of the activity dragged on somewhat and that we were surprised that they required so much direction from us as leaders. Tom said that he did not really understand the activity but liked the poems the group came up with, as he pasted one of each in his cards from last session. Sophie asked Tom if the group could sign one of his completed cards to send to Olga. Joe said he was just happy to listen to others' ideas and that a card would be sent to Olga. He indicated he enjoys the group more when conversation occurs in addition to activity, versus the pressure of having to come up with ideas of what to talk about. Betty and Irina said that they did not enjoy the writing as it felt like too much work. Clara, Sophie, and Agnes agreed that they just liked reminiscing about special occasions and found it difficult to stop this part of the activity and proceed to writing. Clara stated that if she knew how much work it was she would never have suggested they put verses in the cards. Members were praised for their honesty and encouraged to take a more active role in the planning. Mary suggested that in the future, the group could consider changing or modifying session plans when they feel it is not working out rather than sit in silence, complain to a neighbor, or carrying on despite not enjoying what they were doing. Members agreed to try to speak out in future. Sage reassured the members that their contributions to the selection of or changes to group tasks are welcome and supported. Mary emphasized that if we care enough about each other, we have to feel comfortable to be honest with each other about how we are feeling. She clarified that not liking someone's idea does not mean an absence of care for that person or a desire to hurt their feelings, just that the idea does not appeal. Sage encouraged members to become more involved in future discussions of activity selection. We acknowledged that everyone has likes and dislikes and strengths and challenges and that we want members to feel safe to talk about these things with the group. As the group dispersed, we heard Joe saying to the group "We should eat lunch together so we can talk some more about the good old days."

Individual Learning Activities

CASE STUDIES

Choose a case study and compose some post-group reflections. Next, complete a session evaluation. Compare your evaluation with that in Appendix E. Write a session plan that might be used to address issues that are part of the development stage.

REFLECTIVE QUESTIONS

1. Are the leadership functions of the development stage the same as those the formation stage? Why or why not? What types of control and power issues are characteristic of this stage? What is the role of the leader in addressing these issues?

2. What are some of the "metaspace" elements in a group at the concrete and symbolic levels?

3. How might a leader encourage group members to assume various group membership roles?

4. Why is testing the safety of the group an issue for members in the development stage? What group actions can address this need?

5. How might a leader alter the group's structure to influence the group's process? How can the activity be useful in influencing the group's process?

6. Recall a dinner with family or friends when you felt tense. Describe how you were feeling and concerns that you left unexpressed. How might the unspoken influence the group dynamics? What was being discussed overtly, and what was covert in the group? Recall shifts in the mood and what was said or done to elicit the change.

7. Describe how the wish to be "omnipotent" and "benevolent" can aversively affect group leadership. Identify how these wishes may be acted on in interactions as well as expectations held of yourself, within the group as a whole, with individual members, within subgroups, and with your co-leader.

8. Members of a group are all angry with one member. They blame her for other members having a negative attitude toward the group. Their anger toward her escalates week after week. How might this member be "coconstructed" as the difficult patient by the group and leader(s)? How might she be "coconstructed" as the scapegoat in the group? How can you intervene to shift the dynamics? Describe ways of limit setting and what you might say to encourage group members to direct their anger and perhaps disappointment with the group or the activities toward you as the group leader.

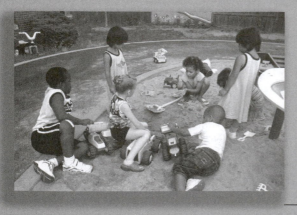

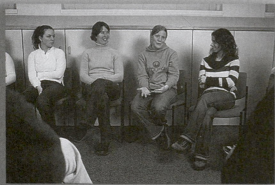

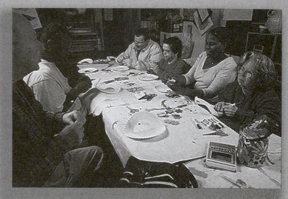

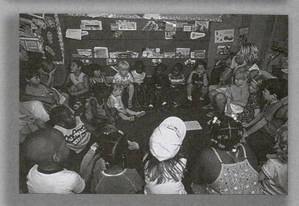

How Is a Functional Group Concluded?

The process of concluding a group can be viewed from a number of different vantage points: the termination of one member in an open group or the termination of an ongoing open or closed group. The issues and expectations are often similar in scope, although varied in intensity. The primary tasks of the closure stage are:

• Reviewing the group experience to consolidate what has been learned
• Dealing with members' concerns and feelings about separation and loss

The final meetings of a group are important because they give members the opportunity to clarify the meaning of their experiences in the group. This process makes members aware of what they have learned, what behaviors have changed, and what skills they may have acquired. In addition, members can decide which of these changes in behavior they can or want to bring to new situations. However, termination also often brings up a plethora of emotions, conscious or unconscious in both leaders and members. "Termination of a group, as in most human relationships, and especially where the participants have gone through a lot together and have developed a sense of closeness and mutuality, is fraught with sadness. It is akin to losing someone dear and feeling grief, or to feeling that one is being abandoned. It leaves one with the dread of loneliness and of having to 'go it alone.' It reactivates the fear of risk and the anticipation of inadequacy and hence failure. Mingled with these anxieties, if the group has been a help, are feelings of hope, of power to succeed, and of the adventure of facing a new day" (Klein, 1972, p. 283).

This chapter describes the issues a leader can expect to face during the closure stage of a functional group. Leader functions and intervention strategies for facilitating closure are also discussed. The needs of group members with regard to the four types of action in a functional group are outlined. The case study narratives present three scenarios related to the closure stage (see also Appendix F).

Issues and Expectations

As a group or a member's participation comes to a close, the leader should expect certain reactions to the termination by the individual, from other members, or the group as a whole. Although the term "termination" describes what occurs as part of the closure stage, it can also include the reactions in terms of members' ability to handle transitions. Termination is a transition to another stage in the life of the individuals involved. Therefore, whenever possible, the leader must support and guide the members as they face and begin the transition. A group may end prematurely because of a leader's personal situation, such as illness, moving, retirement, or death (Fieldsteel, 1996). Thus, the termination process is shaped by several factors: the extent to which earlier issues were resolved, the sociocultural background of members, and the group structure and culture (Wardi, 1989). The following four questions are central to address in considering approaches to termination (Klein, 1996):

1. What are the criteria for termination? Therefore, when should a member or group intervention end or not end?
2. What are the leader tasks of termination, and how do they differ from the ongoing work of a group?
3. What is the process of the group during termination? This encompasses:
   a. The role of the member and group in making a decision about ending
   b. How this differs from other phases in a group
4. What unique techniques does the leader use in the process of termination (Klein, 1996)?

When a member chooses or needs to leave a group, regardless of theoretical perspective, the following leader tasks are essential to the process of termination:

• Encouraging the member to explore the decision to terminate in the group
• Assessing the member's progress in the group in terms of what has and has not been achieved (Fig. 8.1)
• Examining the member's group experience and identifying options for the leaving process

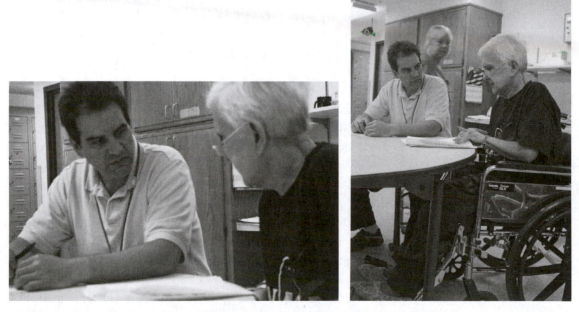

FIGURE 8.1 Left, Exploring decision. Right, Assessing progress. (Photos by Julia Ide)

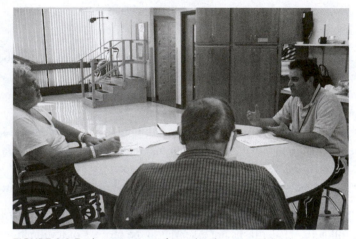

FIGURE 8.2 Exploring impact of member leaving. (Photo by Julia Ide)

• Encouraging both the member and group as a whole to say goodbye
• Helping the member plan for the future and, if needed, other intervention services
• Assisting members remaining in the group as they deal with the meaning and impact of the member's departure (Fig. 8.2)
• Discussing the possibility of adding a new member to the group (Klein, 1996)

As the chapter proceeds, it examines the issues that can emerge as part of the closure stage to build an understanding of what to expect and possible leader actions and reactions when working through termination with a group. Dealing with the following issues and reactions to termination will enable members to move beyond the group.

Denial and Avoidance

Group members may deny the reality of termination (Cohen & Smith, 1976; Klein, 1972) by not talking about it or by putting off dealing with their feelings until the last few minutes when it is too late to discuss them thoroughly. Groups may also deny the reality of termination by making elaborate plans for the group to meet again in a reunion. In such a case, the end of the group sessions is acknowledged, but the end of the group relationship is denied.

Premature Termination

Typically, some members withdraw from the group before issues of termination are discussed. Withdrawal is manifest through lack of participation (Cohen & Smith, 1976; Corey & Corey, 1982), lateness, or absenteeism. It is important as leaders to maintain realistic expectations regarding termination: "there can be no complete resolutions or perfect terminations, but to borrow from the wisdom of Winnicott, group members may seek and experience 'good-enough' terminations. A good-enough termination is one that fulfills the treatment contract, including its refinements during therapy" (Rice, 1996, p. 8).

In a premature termination, the contract is not fulfilled. Premature termination can include:

• Dropping out early
• Being unable to make a commitment to the group
• Ending the session early
• Having made a commitment to the group but leaving before the work is complete

The reasons for dropouts and early leaving are complex and can be harmful to the group. If circumvented by helping the member understand the wish for premature termination and having the member agree to stay, the attempted premature termination can become a turning point in continuing therapy. Ironically, late endings (session running over time), postponing the ending, and members' not leaving unless the group is terminated are also forms of premature termination in that the group contract is not fulfilled in a manner that effectively addresses the need for a group or member's participation to end.

Anxiety and Fear

It is quite common for group members to experience anxiety over the impending termination (Cohen & Smith, 1976; Corey & Corey, 1982; Klein, 1972). Fears usually concern members' doubting their ability to transfer what they have learned in the group to situations outside of the group. Such anxiety may manifest itself in regressed behavior, moving apart from the group to gain closure, or a return to behavior more typical of the formation and development stages of the group.

Anger, Depression, and Sadness

Feelings of anger may surface around the time of termination. At times, this anger is not expressed, and the grief is internalized; hence, members feel depressed and abandoned (Klein, 1972). The anger may also be directed toward the group in general for not having fulfilled the fantasies or goals of the member. Similarly, the anger may be directed toward the leader or the institution under whose mission the group was a service. Members may view the group experience as worthless and become depressed or express irritation with one another. As the group members seek closure, members may experience intense sadness (Cohen & Smith, 1976; Klein, 1972). As a result, members may reduce the intensity of their involvement.

Raising New Issues for Discussion

Some members, under the pressure of termination, may bring up new issues for the group to consider (when there is no longer time to discuss these issues adequately) in hopes of furthering the life of the group. Leaders should be aware of this possibility and acknowledge the importance of the issue raised in the context of validating the members' concerns and feelings about the group coming to a close. Identifying other resources for addressing their concerns may be necessary. In addition, leaders need to avoid the temptation of being drawn into members' wishes for the group to continue. The role of the leader in the closure stage is to help the group be realistic. Redirecting and limit setting the group at the level of the individual and group as a whole may necessitate re-enforcing the reality of the plan for closure. The group may need feedback that dealing with new agendas at the time of closure is unrealistic and a potential means of avoiding the process of saying goodbye.

Leader Functions and Intervention Strategies

The most important response of the leader to member reactions is to continue to acknowledge feelings as done throughout the group meetings. In attempting to classify the ways in which termination may come about, four types of termination have been identified:

1. Standard and planned
2. Standard and unplanned
3. Tapering and planned
4. Tapering and unplanned (Rose, 1989, p. 527)

As a gauge to guiding the planning, "groups composed of many members who are highly dependent upon the group require a longer period of time to reduce their dependence. These groups should be informed earlier about termination than groups of members who are not as dependent" (Rose, 1989, p. 530). Generally, the leader's role in assisting termination is to:

• Give members as much notice as possible
• Include members as much as possible in decisions related to its ending
• Be aware of the members' and one's own feelings
• Help members make transitional plans for after the group ends

Time-limited groups present unique circumstances in ending a group. When working with time-limited groups, it is useful to incorporate a reminder regarding the group's time frame as part of the group's opening and/or closing ritual. As termination of the group approaches, it will likely become necessary to structure the last session to address members' feelings and behaviors. Commonly emerging themes in regard to the myriad of emotions members may be struggling with include; "deprivation, resentment and anger, rejection, grief and loss, [and having to take] responsibility for self" (Mackenzie, 1996, p. 41).

As with time-limited groups, there are unique issues to address with termination of inpatient groups. Inpatient units are typically chaotic with quick turnover, unpredictable departures, and other services impinging on regular group attendance (e.g., blood tests). Some specific strategies (Brabender & Fallon, 1996) include:

- Addressing "the importance of the termination process at all levels of the system" (p. 84). This may include in-services, incorporating unit goodbye rituals inluding staff or interns
- Making other members of the staff or interdisciplinary team "aware of the importance of the group-termination process" (p. 85) to enlist their assistance with supporting member's participation in the group
- Discussing member's "discharge issues within groups" (p. 85)
- Providing leader "input into treatment planning" (p. 86) to maintain awareness of member needs, concerns, and progress as related to disposition issues
- Planning in advance with member and staff as to whether "group attendance on discharge day" (p. 87) seems feasible or realistic for member
- Recognizing, and addressing if possible, member's "attempts to avoid group attendance just prior to discharge as resistance to dealing with termination" (p. 87)
- Making "use of a single-session group" (p. 88); designing the group so that each session can be self-contained in terms of addressing closure at the end of each group

Leaders must explore, examine, and monitor their countertransference responses, both conscious and unconscious, working to make the unconscious known through supervision and reflection. These may arise in reaction to the reality of the group member's situation or that person's perceived needs and transferences, as well as in responses to the system (health care or administrative) and its potential inability to meet the patient's needs. Three common kinds of countertransference responses that may present in leader (or member) are: "disappointment over progress attained, anxiety resulting from frequent patient discharges, and powerlessness with regard to the lack of control over the discharge process" (Brabender & Fallon, 1996, p. 89).

Thus, when working with group members in acute inpatient settings, addressing closure must always be a part of the group process. Leaders need to work with members on countering feelings of loss to:

- Diminish demoralization
- Limit regression
- Help terminating members contain, organize, and understand feelings about loss
- Encourage the probability of member's continuing treatment (pre and post discharge (Brabender & Fallon, 1996).

Encouraging Members to Express Concerns

As in the early phases of the group, the leader needs to encourage expression of fears and expectations as members reach the final sessions of the group. These feelings may be as troubling to the members as were their initial feelings upon entering the group. The task of the leader is to draw attention to the cohesiveness and support the members feel in the group now and help the member identify how such a change is the result of their growth and participation in the group process. The leader should reminisce with the group to remind the members how each member contributed to creating the atmosphere they now experience.

Discussing Feelings of Loss, Anger, and Sadness

If leaders avoid dealing with feelings of loss and anger at the end of the group, members probably will avoid doing so as well. If the feelings of loss (and associated past experiences of loss that members may be reliving) are not discussed, members will most likely react with feelings of anxiety, depression, and anger. Withdrawal, absenteeism, silence, or tearfulness may result. Therefore, the leader must structure and facilitate an open discussion of the feelings of loss that may accompany the end of any meaningful experience or relationship.

Dealing With Unfinished Business

The leader must also allot time for reviewing and discussing unfinished business relating to transactions between members or to the group process or goals (Corey & Corey, 1982). Members may need to bring up unresolved conflicts with other members or with the leader. It is not always possible to resolve the issues that are raised, but an exploration of their current state can be helpful before the group terminates. Member needs, goals, and resources should also be assessed so that appropriate referrals can be made when necessary.

Review of Members' Participation in the Group

Members have been giving and receiving feedback throughout the life of the group, which has helped them assess their impact on the group. During the last sessions, more specific feedback may be helpful as part of a review of each member's participation. Asking members to report briefly how they saw themselves in the group in terms of their role or participation and what the group has meant to them might preface this process. This activity can be followed by feedback from the group concerning how they have perceived each other's participation in the group.

Transfer of Learning to New Situations

The closure stage can be a time for members to prepare for the new experiences that they will encounter in new situations or groups. The knowledge or skills they have gained from this group experience may help them cope with new situations. In the final sessions, members need to focus on how their experiences and actions in the group may relate to situations outside the group. To help generalize and integrate their experiences, activities such as role playing and behavioral rehearsal may be beneficial (Corey & Corey, 1982). Although the use of celebrations or parties as a final group activity may serve as a defense against experiencing feelings surrounding endings, such group rituals can aid termination when created by the whole group with the leader's attention to the interpersonal and intrapersonal meaning of the ritual (Shapiro & Ginzberg, 2002).

Reinforcing Confidentiality

At the time of termination, the leader should repeat the principle of confidentiality and remind members to respect confidences shared in the group after the group has ended.

Members' Action Responses

The issues raised as a functional group comes to a close lead to member needs, which require action. To support purposeful action, the leader should provide structure and encourage members to assume group maintenance roles. This is especially important because closure can activate withdrawal or strong emotions in people. These feelings may prompt members to return to self-initiated action in the form of behaviors displayed in the formation and development stages of the group. Hence, action may become centered on individual members' needs rather than on the group's needs. Spontaneous action may diminish somewhat, and group-centered action may focus on conflicts with the leader or with one another. Such responses require the leader to use the full range of skills in limit setting, process commentary, confrontation, and self-disclosure (Table 8.1).

Leader Emotional Response

As in other periods of growth, the closure stage raises many feelings and reactions. There is a parallel process between the therapist's and members' feelings of ambivalence with separation from the group (Wardi, 1989). Regression at termination may bring the group and the inexperienced therapist alike to a state of heightened anxiety and actual dependence. This may cause great difficulties in efficiently and constructively completing this phase of separation for both the group and the therapist (p. 97).

Group members and the leader may feel a sense of accomplishment coupled with anxiety, as well as sadness, over the loss of the group. The leader may experience feelings similar to those at the group's formation or when a member joined the group. If leaders have a positive experience with a group or an individual terminating, they will likely feel some sadness and happiness for gains made by the member(s). The leader (and members) may also experience a sense of relief if the group process or aspects of that member's participation in the group did not go well. When possible, these feelings need to be discussed openly and genuinely to validate group members' experience (Fig. 8.3).

Table 8.1	**Group Issues and Membership Needs Related to Action: Closure Stage**

Closure Stage issues: Denial and avoidance, premature termination, anxiety and fear, depression and anger, sadness, raising new issues for discussion.

Group members' needs or behaviors related to action:

Purposeful Action	Self-Initiated Action	Spontancous Action (Here and Now)	Group-Centered Action
• More focus on maintenance roles, less on task • Trust versus mistrust re-emerges as theme • Participation declines • More structure is needed	• Power struggles emerge or re-emerge • Withdrawal from group • Regressive behavior(s) may be revisited or re-expressed as means to demonstrate uncertainty about future or ability to function without group (i.e., question if "ready" for group to end)	• Becoming more concerned about individual needs • Wish or appeal for group to continue may be expressed • May devalue importance of group and learning or growth that occurred (viewing work done as worthless) • Anger toward leader and/or other members (possibly to avoid sadness about loss or anxiety about separation) • Feedback to other members provided with less intensity	• Review of group's history and process over course of sessions • Reminiscing about member participation • Recognizing and/or celebrating individual and group accomplishments • Group conflicts may predominate • Silences and inactivity may prevail • Unresolved issues may be raised

Leader Actions and Skills Employed
Review terms of group contract regarding number of sessions and confidentiality
Re-enforce group rules
Structure process to facilitate members addressing feelings about termination issues
Genuineness and empathy
Listening and responding
Modeling acceptance and tolerance of ambiguity
Giving and receiving feedback
Classifying themes
Use of metaphor or narrative in reviewing group stories and reminiscing about member participation
Structuring activity to allow for "transitional object"
Confrontation
Reality testing
Self-disclosure

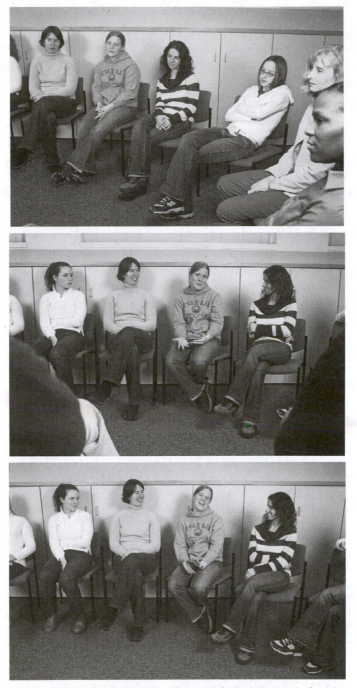

FIGURE 8.3 Leader facilitates undiscussed feelings in need of exploration. (Photo by Mark Morelli)

Sometimes, a member or group must end before being ready. Reasons for ending may be because a person moves, a schedule changes, or reimbursement is insufficient or time-limited. There are also situations in which a leader must ask a member to leave a group. The person may be unable to handle the expectations of the group, or an alternative modality may be more appropriate or beneficial. Leaders will react variously, of course, in relation to the particular group and member but also in relation to their own history and experience with loss and change. Furthermore, people react differently to success as well as to not meeting a challenge or goal. These reactions will get stirred in both the leader and the member as the leader helps the individual, as well as the group, come to a sense of closure.

Group collusion and complicity may also operate in the hasty departure of a peer member for reasons that are unconscious to the group (Billow & Gans, 2005). In such cases, group-as-a-whole interpretations can address the primitive projective identifications commonly found in a group that is not fully stable. An example of such unconscious projective identification is labeling one individual as the "sick" or "difficult" member. Billow and Gans advise the leader to examine countertransference difficulties. Lack of awareness can lead to acting out unconscious anger by turning a member into the group scapegoat, failing to find ways to protect a group member, and through reaction formation turning anger into ineffective caring.

It is vital that leaders or co-leaders be aware of their experience and monitor their personal reactions so as not to interfere with the growth of members. Self-reflective questions (Box 8.1) can help with examining emotional responses and identifying patterns in the leader's own reactions to the termination issues that arise in the closure stage. The extent to which the leader shares reactions will vary according to the type of group and the theoretical frames of reference. Settings may also have cultural norms of established methods they deem as supportive ways to bring a group to ending. Schools, for example, have many ceremonial structures in which people share their feelings about ending, such as graduation exercises and yearbooks. Camps may create scrapbooks of photos; art groups may create portfolios of

Box 8.1   **Leader Self-Reflective Questions**

- Do I feel the group or individual is ready to terminate? Is my appraisal consistent with the group member's perceptions or that of others significant to the member, such as family?
- If our appraisals are inconsistent, where is my reaction coming from? Is my satisfaction, disappointment, or relief relevant and appropriate from the member's perspective?
- How much of my response is useful to share? Am I assisting the member in a productive way to make a transition from the group to functioning without the group support or with other types of help?
- What have I learned from working with this group or individuals in the group?

artists' work; and so on. The length of time the group has been meeting as well as the intensity of the relationships may be a factor in deciding how best to address termination. Members' needs and the leader's own amount of comfort are equally important measures for calibrating the media used and the degree of self-disclosure appropriate to the context.

Conclusion

The termination of any role or relationship is difficult, and the leader must carefully guide members in effectively dealing with this event in the closure stage. At this point, members need support to make the final effort to absorb and consolidate their experiences. With the help of the leader, members may view the closure stage as a means to move forward and continue with their progress and gains made in the group. Closure can be viewed as an opportunity for members to realize the benefits of their work in the group via applications of what was learned to life outside the group.

In short-term groups, the issues surrounding the group's ending need to be addressed on a regular basis. For groups that are ongoing, such as those found in long-term care residential and day settings, members also face the loss of members, leaders, and programs. Further, attrition occurs for several reasons, including a mismatch between member and group format as well as lack of member readiness for the group experience. Closing interventions may include customs and activities to symbolize closure and exploratory discussion about future plans and opportunities outside of the group for members. In every case the leader needs to monitor both subjective reactions to the loss as well as objective circumstances such as the need for referrals.

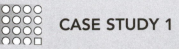

CASE STUDY 1

OPEN GROUP ON AN INPATIENT PSYCHIATRY UNIT

Session Plan

Name of group: "Getting It Together"
Date: June 10
Leaders: Lauri Levy, OTR/L; Jack Jones, MHC
Session Activity: Mural painting
Specific goals for the group session: Members will:

• Experience success in an interdependent task.
• Express feelings and thoughts in the present tense.
• Express positive and negative reactions and feelings.

Specific goals for group members:

• Liz, Lakisha: Express feelings about upcoming discharge.
• Betty, Maggie, and Pearl: Remain for the entire session, and engage in task and discussion without evidencing extreme anxiety (somatic complaints, ruminations).
• Gary, Li, and Eric: Take leadership role in activity, and engage in termination discussion with Liz and Lakisha (Li will require presence of hospital translator to facilitate verbal participation).

Description of methods and procedures:

• Summarize previous session to reinforce learning for existing members and to integrate new member.
• Decide on theme and group procedures for painting group mural.

Rationale: To provide an opportunity for expressing and processing feelings regarding having two members leave the group; activity is familiar to existing members and provides a role for all members; there is no one correct way to paint a mural; hence, little opportunity for failure.
Description of leadership role: Encourage members to talk about their fears and anxieties about leaving. Support members' addressing transition and disposition issues in the group.
Rationale: Provides an opportunity to reality-test readiness for discharge and reinforces safety in expressing feelings in the group; review individual gains and effect on group dynamics and action.
Describe necessary preparations:

• Lauri will gather necessary supplies.

List material and equipment needed:

Nontoxic acrylic paints in the primary colors

Paint texturizers and mixing palettes

Paint brushes of various sizes

Paper cups, water, and tape

Large piece of canvas for mural

Time and sequence outline for session (include what you will say and do as the leader and what the group will do; consider both content and process):

• Review group's purpose and procedures. (approximately 5 minutes)

• Review previous group session with group input. (approximately 5 minutes)

• Plan group mural, encouraging group member roles. (approximately 5 minutes)

• Members paint mural. (approximately 20 minutes)

• Clean up, process session, termination discussion, and planning next session. (approximately 10 minutes)

Other information pertinent to this specific session: This session will take place on a Friday, and the group will not meet again until Monday.

Session Narrative

Name of group: "Getting It Together"

Date: June 10

Leaders: Lauri Levy, OTR/L; Jack Jones, MHC

Session Activity: Mural painting

During this session Laurie bridged from previous sessions this week by summarizing what was done and highlighting what was learned to reinforce learning for existing members and continue to integrate new member (Maggie). We reviewed accomplishments of members and announced Betty was planning to stay for the entire session again today and that this would be Liz's and Lakisha's last group due to their upcoming discharge plans. Laurie reviewed that, as leaders, our expectations were that the group would:

• Discuss feelings and thoughts about the group or activity in a constructive way

• Share positive and negative feelings in a safe way

• Express feelings related to theme of change in light of members leaving

• Work as a group and take responsibility to decide on a theme and how member would like to go about creating a group mural

Jack explained to the group that we chose mural painting to provide an opportunity for expressing and processing feelings and to provide a role for all members in the creative process. He stated there is no one correct way to paint a mural; hence, we believed there was little opportunity for failure. The group provided support when Liz was able to talk about her fear that she will decompensate once she leaves the hospital. Gary reiterated his stance from an earlier group this week that he felt we were not helping the group enough in regard to the mural task. Laurie chose to reality test what members need from us as leaders in terms of making decisions more independently of us. We explored possible cognitive distortions that may be part of the relationship between member thoughts and feelings and behavior.

We reminded the group members of their personal strengths as potential resources to balance each other's limitations in regard to abilities. Jack explained that we saw the mural as also being representative of how, when a group works together, something symbolic of their time together can be created. Laurie questioned whether members were displacing their fears about having support after discharge to our participation as leaders. When needed, we would make process commentaries regarding our observations of member behaviors and query aloud what might be contributing to individual's actions (e.g., is Liz being critical perhaps due to fear of not being successful in her transition to supportive housing; is Gary still looking to us as leaders to approve of him?) and how these group dynamics were possibly affecting group decision making and member interactions.

Pearl suggested the mural be about New Beginnings. It was at this point that Li shared with the group (via his translator) that he was born in the Year of the Dog and hence must form new friendships to counter the hard times that will lie ahead for him this year. Maggie was able to state that she felt painting images was too much pressure and that she wished the mural could include pieces of fabric and other materials used in yesterday's group (i.e., buttons, beads). The group members welcomed her contribution to the mural in that format, and Jack assisted Maggie with locating needed items.

Existing members were able to acknowledge Maggie's work as adding nice dimensions to the mural and praise Li for his contributions to the group and the mural (Mandarin Chinese characters for friend). Liz joked about "out with the old and in with the new" and discussed her upcoming discharge next week. Betty became tearful as she reminded Liz to be nicer to herself as Liz had been to Betty by making an anagram of Betty's name in an earlier group. Eric stated he would miss Liz's creative ideas. Pearl told Lakisha to make sure she "gets the job done" in response to Lakisha talking about returning to work part time.

Laurie summed up the group as being one in which it seemed that members' expressing their thoughts and emotions, in words and artistically, enabled them to acknowledge opportunities that may arise via change and feelings of loss or sadness. Eric and Liz identified that they felt they would benefit from a similar group outside the hospital setting. Leaders discussed options members could explore in the community to find peer support and project-oriented groups such as clubs, consumer-run programs that offer support services, adult education classes, and so on.

■■■■■
■■■■■   **CASE STUDY 2**
■■■■■

Closed Group in an Outpatient Occupational Therapy Clinic

Session Plan

Name of Group: Community Re-entry: "Moving Forward"

Session activity: Group closure: conduct review of topics (revisit one or two topics in more depth per members' selection), evaluation of group series, party

Date: December 20, last of eight sessions

Specific goals for the group session:

- To prepare refreshments together (fruit salad, coffee/tea, baking cookies using commercially prepared cookie dough).
- To express feelings regarding group's termination.
- To review topics to emphasize progress and consolidate members' feelings about what was learned/accomplished.
- To conduct evaluation of group series to obtain specific feedback from members.
- To symbolize group's gains and termination by having a party.

Specific goals for group members:

Jim (BI post MI): to outline for group ADL and IADL tasks he is now able to complete; including; e-mail, exercise, and relaxation.

John (TBI post MVA): to verbalize safety awareness strategies he has learned and give an example of activity in which he applies them at home.

Steve (lumbar fusion): to update group on status of work hardening assessment and outline how he incorporates strategies for pain prevention/management in daily routine.

Jeanette (post CVA): to take leadership role in fruit salad preparation and kitchen cleanup to demonstrate gains in adaptive device use and resumption of valued role/activity.

Wendy (post bilateral TKR): to report on readiness for return to work.

Brenda (post CVA): to outline child care tasks and strategies she is finding useful as she resumes tasks in mothering role.

Juanita (post hip fixation): to review current precautions and employ them without cueing for entire session.

Description of and rationale for methods and procedures:

Review session topics listed on group evaluation, and ask members to rate each session topic via Likert scale and provide verbal/written feedback.

Have members bake cookies, prepare fruit salad, and facilitate discussion/progress reporting by asking members to provide each other with feedback; leader cues and input as needed.

Leaders will share personal perspectives and memories re group process and progress and mixed feelings regarding ending.

Rationale: To reinforce gains and ability to be independent; to provide concrete resources.

Description and rationale for leadership role:

Role-model feedback exchange and ways to cope with or address ambivalence about group ending.

Reality-test; clarify feelings and reinforce that although members may be able to or attempt to keep in touch/reunite, important to acknowledge that will be in different context (i.e., without leaders, in social settings, via e-mail, as subgroups, etc.). Therefore, need to acknowledge face-to-face in this final session that the group is ending and what time spent together has meant.

Rationale: To bring closure to group in a supportive manner.

List material and equipment needed:

Ingredients for cookies and salad
Schedule use of kitchen
Evaluation forms, pens

Time and sequence outline for session:

Food preparation and discussion. (30 minutes)
Complete evaluation forms with discusssion/sharing and cleanup. (15 minutes)
Final goodbyes. (5 minutes)

Other information pertinent to this specific session:

Holiday season, weather, potential for regression or avoidance in light of termination

Session Narrative

Group began 5 minutes late because members arrived late (congregating in lobby talking, therefore needed to be cued that group was due to start and reminded that it was being held in kitchen area). Initially, Jeanette was reluctant to take a leadership role in food preparation and stated that her kitchen was not like this one and that she was not sure what needed to be done. The other members reassured her that they would help find needed items; with Jim's cajoling and Juanita's supportive comments, Jeanette was able to demonstrate her skills in using rocking knife and dycem and managing oven.

This created a natural opportunity to transition conversation to safety and begin group discussion concerning progress made by asking John to be first to report to the group what he feels he has achieved (i.e., "Speaking of safety…). John had difficulty making the connection in terms of the activity (stating he does not do the cooking at home) but was then able to report that he finds going to AA meetings a way to stay safe as it has kept him from resisting the temptation to join his friends for a beer.

Wendy, Brenda, Steve, and Juanita continued with fruit salad preparation while simultaneously following John's lead and reporting to the group progress they felt they had made as well as goals they still have in regard to their own continued recovery. Jeanette reported that she has agreed to have various adaptive devices installed (grab bars, kitchen devices) and has rearranged some of her kitchen to make access of items easier. Brenda reported that, although awkward having someone in her home, having a home health aide has facilitated her interactions with her baby as she is less fatigued and stressed by knowing she is not alone if something were to happen. Wendy reported that she has worked a half day and will need to continue to adjust her expectations around how long it will take to get ready for work, get into her office, use the ladies' room, and so on, as well as needing to decide whether it is worth asking someone to get needed files or to attempt to do such tasks herself. Steve reported that he has a work hardening assessment scheduled but that he continues to struggle with resentment about residual pain and mobility restrictions. Juanita added at this point saying she also felt that she thought her hip should feel better by now and that she feels "stir crazy" and worries that once she can move around again, she might fall.

Russell took the lead in acknowledging each member's contributions, and Alicia provided suggestions by asking "what might you do about that or who should you talk to about that?" She often redirected members to follow up with their personal care attendant, their physician, or certain specialists. Russell role-modeled his goodbyes by stating how impressed he was with how the group came together, reminiscing about moments of group "rebellion" or anger as well as those moments he found touching or humorous. Russell verbalized his wish that the group could work together longer and acknowledged the reality of the capitations of insurance and the upcoming holidays.

Members followed suit with reminisces. Jim openly expressed a wish for the group to continue meeting outside of the hospital, suggesting at a coffee shop. Alicia reflected that the wish to continue meeting may not only be an artifact of enjoying one another's company but also that members have come to realize and value the support. Russell reported that the literature supports that recovery can often be facilitated by people working on their goals via meaningful activity in their natural environment, using Jeanette's graciously taking leadership in today's cooking activity as an example. Russell cautioned that continuing to meet may become more difficult than group members anticipate and pointed out some of the subtle differences that will exist (i.e., questionable handicap accessibility of a coffee shop, absence of himself and Alicia as leaders and sounding boards to process member reflections, concerns related to confidentiality and privacy). Jeanette responded by suggesting that the group try a reunion after the holidays at her home. Members agreed, and as the group came to a close they had prepared a contact list of phone numbers, home addresses, and e-mail addresses, which Jim took stating he would e-mail the list to everyone in the group. Member feedback on the evaluation forms turned out to be overwhelmingly positive, with main qualitative comments being related to having "more time." Members identified that the handouts would be most useful if provided as a complete resource notebook that was bound and easily identifiable.

CASE STUDY 3

COMMUNITY-BASED GROUP

Session Plan

Name of Group: "Time Flies"
Date: October 27, last of 10 sessions.
Session Activity: Group collages
Specific goals for the group session:

• Address group and individual members regarding feelings about termination.
• Evaluate the group experience and members' increased initiative and interest in avocational activities.
• Continue to support socialization between members.

Specific goals for group members:

For Sophie: to continue to engage in tasks and/or conversation with leaders and members about personal memories.

For Agnes: to attend and remain involved in the activity for the entire session with short rest breaks as needed.

For Tom: to offer assistance when needed by others.

For Betty: to continue to relate more positively with leaders and members (versus appearing negative or engaging in subgrouping).

For Irina: to communicate more openly with leaders and members.

For Clara: to continue to interact on own initiative with leaders and members.

For Joe: to assume leadership roles, balancing focus on engaging in task and discussion with members.

Description of methods and procedures:

- Remind members that this is the last group meeting.
- Decorate frames for photo collages.
- Engage in a group-centered activity creating photo collages from photos taken each session (per signed photo releases obtained with members' agreement in first session) to frame to hang in senior center as a means to symbolize their group experience and allow them to discuss their feelings about termination and memorable events in the group's history.
- Create digital images of completed collages so that each member can have smaller copies to frame.

Rationale: Members will use their own initiative to decide how to decorate frames as well as work collaboratively to choose which events will be portrayed in the collages.

Description of leadership role:

Encourage members to review the group's progress and concretize these memories via the collages.

To reinforce what has been learned and enjoyed in the group and provide an opportunity to listen to members about group coming to a close.

Material and equipment needed:

Collages: foam core backing for collages, photos printed via center laptop and printer on photo paper, glue, and scissors; center's digital camera to photograph final product(s)

Frames: buttons, silk/dried flowers, acorns/small pine cones, fabric/ribbon scraps to decorate frames

Time and sequence outline for sessions:

1. Greetings and distribution of name tags; review of the group plan for the session and reminder that this is the last session. (approximately 10 minutes)
2. Review of previous meeting and group discussion. (approximately 5 minutes)
3. Introduction of the activity, a collage representing memories of the group sessions. The group is to choose the desired photos for the collage and the process for completing it. (approximately 10 minutes)
4. Planning the collage; members select materials and complete the collage. (approximately 20 minutes)
5. Decoration of individual frames. (10 minutes)

6. Viewing the finished collage and discussion among members about what they chose to represent in their section of the collage. (approximately 20 minutes)
7. Processing the session and reviewing what members have experienced in the group. Leaders also allow time for the expression of feelings regarding the termination of the group. (approximately 20 minutes)

Other information pertinent to this specific session:

Leaders need to be prepared for members reminiscing about other losses in life (friends, loved ones, homes, abilities, etc.,) and support/redirect as needed.

Session Narrative

Joe had not arrived at the center yet when the session began. This proved difficult as no one had heard from him, and members were clearly distressed by his absence. Mary outlined our plan to have members work on subsections of a group collage and then reproduce the final product for individual members. Sage stated that once the group collages were assembled, members could decorate individual frames for their copy of the collages. Tom took initiative to suggest that the members work in subgroups of three, and Betty asked if either Mary or Sage could go call Joe to check to see if he was coming or was okay.

Clara began spontaneously to reminisce about lost friends/loved ones, relaying a story about losing a family member in a bus accident. Sophie became tearful and appeared anxious and confused, forgetting to pass out name tags and asking repeatedly where her son was (perhaps in reference to Joe's absence). With leader encouragement, Irina worked to soothe her, showing her pictures and asking her to choose which ones she liked best. Clara followed suit, offering favorite ones to Irina to cut and past on their section of the three-part collage. Tom, Betty, and Agnes had completed their collage and began to create a second one for the group frame when Sage returned to inform the group that Joe's family said he had a doctor's appointment and would likely be late to the center today.

The group became quiet. Tom offered to decorate a frame for Joe if he did not arrive in time. Betty began to reminisce about how quiet Tom was when the group first began meeting, saying something about his being a "doubting Thomas," seeming to want to complement his increased confidence and initiative. Irina rebutted by stating she felt Betty used to be the one who doubted she was worthy of love and attention. Mary reframed Irina's insight by reflecting how the friendships formed in the group seemed to have made a difference in members and even in their day-to-day lives at the center. Sage then asked Agnes and Sophie to point out their favorite photos in their group collage and placed them in the first section of the group frame, then did the same with Clara and Betty for the second collage.

Joe arrived as Tom and Betty were working to complete the final group photo collage. As the group greeted him, Joe stated: "Didn't think I would make it today," which led to Betty reprimanding him for not calling. Mary reflected to Joe that perhaps he was avoiding the group because it was the last session. Joe denied this, stating irritably, "You're the ones who told me to follow up with my doctor." Agnes stated, "I wish we would't fight." Irina began to console Agnes by saying she felt people were upset because the group would not meet again. At this point, Tom suggested that they "finish what they started," asking Joe to assist him with completing the final collage. Mary acknowledged that endings were hard for her personally but that she felt the group meetings have helped her immensely in her role as wellness director as she has realized that people getting to know each other has helped with finding meaningful activities to do together. Sage indicated that because time was running out, the frame-decorating activity would have to be done another time, perhaps as an activity offered during the center's open arts and crafts group.

Sage took photos of the completed collage, transferred the images to the center laptop, and began printing them. Sophie agreed to pass out the copies of each image to the group members. Each member thanked her as she gave out the copies. As the group came to a close, Joe apologized for being late, suggesting once again that they all have lunch together and thanked Sage and Mary for their hard work in offering the sessions.

Individual Learning Activities

CASE STUDIES

Choose a case study, and compose some post-group reflections. Next, complete a session evaluation. Compare your write-up with that in Appendix F. Write a session plan that might be used to address issues that are part of the closure stage.

REFLECTIVE QUESTIONS

1. How may issues of termination differ for an open group versus a closed group?

2. What are some of the ways group members deal with the termination experience?

3. What is the role of the leader in helping members deal with their feelings? What may happen if there is no discussion of these feelings?

4. What is the primary task of the closure stage? What leader skills are useful in this process?

5. What are activity goals for the closure stage? How can these activities help members review their participation and experiences in the group?

Occupational Therapy Practice Framework: Domain and Process (American Journal of Occupational Therapy, 2002)

DOMAIN

Occupational Therapy Practice Framework: Domain and Process

Engagement in Occupation to Support Participation in Context(s)

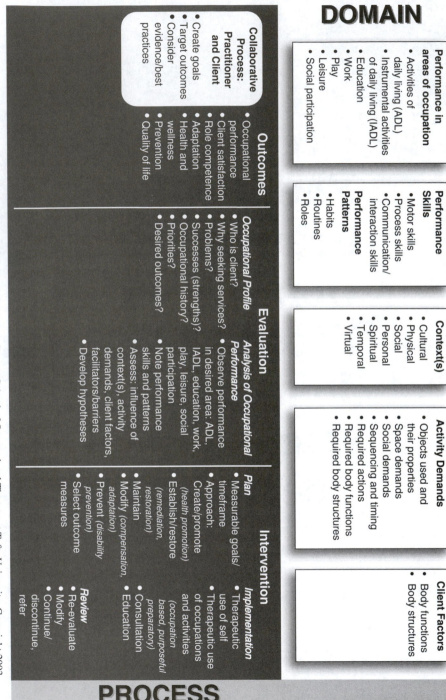

Performance in areas of occupation
- Activities of daily living (ADL)
- Instrumental activities of daily living (IADL)
- Education
- Work
- Play
- Leisure
- Social participation

Performance Skills
- Motor skills
- Process skills
- Communication/ interaction skills

Performance Patterns
- Habits
- Routines
- Roles

Context(s)
- Cultural
- Physical
- Social
- Personal
- Spiritual
- Temporal
- Virtual

Activity Demands
- Objects used and their properties
- Space demands
- Social demands
- Sequencing and timing
- Required actions
- Required body functions
- Required body structures

Client Factors
- Body functions
- Body structures

Collaborative Process: Practitioner and Client
- Create goals
- Target outcomes
- Consider evidence/best practices

Outcomes
- Occupational performance
- Client satisfaction
- Role competence
- Adaptation
- Health and wellness
- Prevention
- Quality of life

Evaluation

Occupational Profile
- Who is client?
- Why seeking services?
- Problems?
- Successes (strengths)?
- Occupational history?
- Priorities?
- Desired outcomes?

Analysis of Occupational Performance
- Observe performance in desired area: ADL, IADL, education, work, play, leisure, social participation
- Note performance skills and patterns
- Assess: influence of context(s), activity demands, client factors, facilitators/barriers
- Develop hypotheses

Intervention

Plan
- Measurable goals/ timeframe
- Approach: Create/promote (health promotion) Establish/restore (remediation, restoration) Maintain Modify (compensation, adaptation) Prevent (disability prevention)
- Select outcome measures

Implementation
- Therapeutic use of self
- Therapeutic use of occupations and activities (occupation based, purposeful, preparatory)
- Consultation
- Education

Review
- Re-evaluate
- Modify
- Continue/ discontinue, refer

PROCESS

Occupational Therapy Practice Framework illustration by Mary Alicia Barnes: Boston School of Occupational Therapy at Tufts University, Copyright 2003. Occupational Therapy Practice Framework: Domain and Process. American Journal of Occupational Therapy, 56, 609–639.

234

History of Occupational Therapy Group Intervention*

Historical Trends

Occupational therapists have been using groups as an intervention method since the 1920s. Today, groups can be found as an intervention tool in most areas of occupational therapy. As the use of group intervention increased, the role of the occupational therapist and the nature of the group as an intervention approach changed. We present the history of group work in occupational therapy based on our process of historical research, examining the trends and forces leading to the development of occupational therapy group intervention as it is known today.

Our synthesis encapsulates the history of group work in occupational therapy into six periods, or eras of focus: (1) the project era, (2) the socialization era, (3) the group dynamics–process era, (4) the ego building–psychodynamic era, (5) the adaptation era, and (6) the wellness era. Group work as an acknowledged tool of occupational therapists did not officially begin until 1922, when Adolph Meyer (1922/1977) described the use of individual craft projects in a group setting. Using group work as a tool for healing already had a long, if unappreciated, history in Western civilization. Kielhofner and Burke (1977) noted that "the use of occupation as a form of treatment for the physically or mentally ill is documented throughout recorded history" (p. 678).

*Originally published & adapted from Home, M.C., & Schwartzberg, S.L. (2001). A Functional Approach to Group Work in Occupational Therapy, ed. 3. Philadelphia: Lippincott Williams & Wilkins.

The moral treatment movement of the 19th century is cited most often as the immediate historical origin of occupational therapy (Bing, 1981; Bockoven, 1971; Gillette & Kielhofner, 1979; Kielhofner & Burke, 1977). The moral treatment movement emerged from the humanitarian trends of the 18th and 19th centuries (Gillette & Kielhofner, 1979; Kielhofner & Burke, 1977). The objective of this movement was described as follows: "The physical, temporal, and social environment was engineered so as to correct faulty habits of living and regenerate new ones. . . . It employed the moral remedies of education, daily habits, work, and play as therapeutic processes for normalizing disorganized behavior in the mentally ill" (Kielhofner & Burke, 1977, p. 678).

The patients' programs apparently included individual and collective activities. Group activities were developed solely by the therapist. Leuret, in describing an aspect of his program in Paris in 1840, presented group activity as it might have appeared to the casual observer: "To some I assign reading out loud, reading verses or singing. Reading is usually performed by several patients who recite alternate passages or sentences from a story according to a plan which I have devised. . . . Some do not enter into this exercise with much cooperation, but pray or grumble instead" (1840/1948, p. 64).

As his description continues, he discusses effects of group process that are still sought by therapists today: "Once they overcome their initial distaste, stimulated by the example of others and by the presence of an audience, they begin to apply themselves to the work which they eventually accept with pleasure. Those who read well, drill others and soon their self-esteem improves and they become better teachers than I could ever be" (Leuret, 1840/1948, p. 64).

Leuret's ultimate goal of engaging group members in meaningful activities and occupations within the structure of a group format is remarkably similar to the desired outcomes of occupational therapy group intervention today. Apparently, he structured the activity and group processes according to what would now be considered a developmental continuum. The proponents of the 19th century moral treatment movement thus strongly influenced the practice of early 20th century pioneers in occupational therapy by serving as models.

Identifying when and by whom the first occupational therapy groups were conducted is a difficult task. Perhaps the confusion stems from the numerous definitions of group treatment or from the failure of therapists to identify their practice as group treatment. Most likely, the first occupational therapy groups were groups of patients working on individual projects in a clinic or on a ward. They were probably an organized unit or, more accurately, a collective, not necessarily a group with a unified goal or interdependent tasks. During the early years of the 20th century, there was enough interest in this sort of activity to lead therapists to found a professional organization. In 1917, the National Society for the Promotion of Occupational Therapy was founded (Reed & Sanderson, 1980).

Project Era: 1922–1936

The project-oriented nature of the collective unit dominated the years between 1922 and 1936, giving rise to the name of this period. During these early years, there was little or no emphasis on the process of interaction among the members while they worked on their projects in the open setting of the collective. In the first issue of the *Archives of Occupational Therapy,* Adolph Meyer (1922/1977) and Eleanor Clarke Slagle (1922) described occupational therapy collectives. Meyer observed the following: "It had long been interesting to see how groups of a few excited patients can be seated in a corner in a small circle of two or three settees and kept wonderfully contented picking the hair of mattresses, or doing simple tasks not too readily arousing the desire for big movements and uncontrollable excitement and yet not too taxing to their patience. Groups of patients with raffia and basket work, or with various kinds of handwork and weaving and bookbinding and metal and leather work, took the place of the bored wall flowers and of mischief-makers" (p. 640).

Similarly, Slagle suggested a program that included collectives. Slagle advised moving the patient through a series of four steps. The steps progressed from individual habit training, to the "kindergarten group" for "stimulating the special senses," to occupational therapy ward classes focusing on the individual, and finally to the "occupational center," or "curative workshop," for helping the patient adapt to other members of the group (pp. 15–16). In the final phase, the patient was moved from supervised activity to a collective focusing on vocational goals. Slagle called this the "preindustrial group" (p. 16). Both Meyer and Slagle viewed the activities in collectives as a means for patients to develop socially acceptable habits to replace their pathological reactions. Thus, the Project Era begins with a formalization of the philosophy of 19th century moral treatment. This formalization, however, was only one thread from the previous century influencing 20th century professionals.

During the last decades of the 19th century, known as the Progressive Era, America was becoming a scientific and industrialized society (Wiebe, 1967). There were increases in scientific concerns, developments in technology, booming industrialism, increased urbanization and immigration, and a shift in industry from shop to factory (Wiebe, 1967). Women were fighting for the right to work in an occupation of their choice (Smuts, 1959). According to Wiebe, these changes called for a new set of values and a new kind of social order.

Like many other institutions, hospitals changed during the late 1800s, and these changes had a crucial impact on the developing health professions. Rosner (1979) points out that because of the economic and social forces of the depression of the 1890s, hospitals changed from charity institutions to organizations requiring payment for services: "The move away from charity to pay services was rationalized as part of the larger Progressive Era movements toward order, efficiency and bureaucracy" (pp. 118–119). By 1922, when Meyer and

Box B.1   **Cheap Labor**

> According to Rothman (1980), activities necessary for the daily operation of the hospital, such as farming, laundry, and sewing, were called occupational therapy. The occupational therapy collective thus became an economic unit in which the patient was also a worker.

Slagle described occupational therapy, these forces had already had an effect. Patients now did part of the labor of the institution (Box B.1).

Canton (1923) surmised that there was an economic rationale for prescribing work as occupational therapy, stating: "It is interesting to note that work originally was given only to state patients, planned to relieve employees rather than to effect cures, and managed from the viewpoint of utility. It was found that other patients wished to share in these employments and since the relatives who were paying for their care sanctioned the arrangement, they too were permitted to putter around so that now the proper use of time in some helpful and gratifying activity has become a fundamental issue in the treatment of all neuro-psychiatric patients" (p. 348). The recognition of a connection between activity and health led to several results for the collectives in which members worked on projects and performed minor jobs for the institution in which they lived.

When the National Society for the Promotion of Occupational Therapy was formed in 1917, its membership included medical doctors, social workers, teachers, nurses, and artists (Hopkins, 1978). Most of the members were women, and this was in character with what became the employment trend of the times. In fact, as Chafe (1972) reports, "The proportion of all women workers who were professionals grew from 11.9 per cent in 1920 to 14.2 per cent in 1930" (pp. 89–90). The role of women in founding and defining occupational therapy is sometimes neglected in historical analyses, leading to the erroneous conclusion that occupational therapy is similar to the male-dominated professions in health care. In fact, women in occupational therapy shaped the direction the field took in this early era, choosing collective work because of their backgrounds (Box B.2).

There was no mention of groups in the occupational therapy literature from 1923 to 1936. In 1936, 14 years after Meyer's and Slagle's papers were first published, an interest in

Box B.2   **Founding Women**

> Occupational therapy began as a female-dominated profession. These founding women were likely to be from upper-class families and to be familiar with handicrafts and family or group living. They were also probably quite comfortable directing groups of people in a collective milieu.

groups reappeared. Three papers on occupational therapy group treatment were published in 1936. These articles present evidence that occupational therapists were beginning to conceive of the gathering of patients as a group versus a collective. Further, occupational therapists were now dividing responsibility for a single project among several patients and viewing opportunities for involvement in a project as a device for restoring health.

Although the role of occupational therapy was not specified, L. Cody Marsh (1936) advocated that relatives of psychotic patients be given group treatment. In 1936, Davis and Dunton, as mentioned by Gleave (1947), described a form of large group occupational therapy in which patients had the opportunity to associate with a group project and to increase their self-respect through the group's accomplishment. Anderson (1936) suggested "project work" or "individualized group therapy" to improve the use of group activity. In project work, the therapist structures an activity to meet the group member's individual needs while still requiring each member to contribute to a larger group project. Anderson emphasized that project work should not be confused with the utilitarian worked-related activity usually offered by occupational therapy departments: "Project work, with its designated therapeutic aims and offered for its therapeutic values, must not be confused with that type of group activity often provided in many institutions as a part of 'hospital economy,' 'doing odd jobs,' time-filling activity, or furnishing labor needs of the institution with no reference to the value of the work for the individual concerned. Nor is project work the same as occupational therapy where the guest usually works in a group or alone on an individual project but not with the responsibility of contributing a part to a project which is the divided responsibility of an entire group" (p. 265).

This is the first clear indication that group work should be defined according to the patient and not according to the hospital and its economic needs or according to the physician's or therapist's interests.

Anderson clearly departed from the norm when he suggested occupational therapy should focus on the patients' therapeutic needs rather than fulfilling the institution's labor needs. Nevertheless, he emphasized that the occupational therapist was responsible for carrying out the physicians' "therapeutic aims" (Anderson, 1936, p. 265), which he identified as:

- An outlet for aggressions
- Propitiation of guilt
- Freedom for fantasy expression
- Opportunities to create (p. 265) (Box B.3)

In her historical analysis of the development of occupational therapy, Woodside (1971) pointed out that, between 1910 and 1929, occupational therapy developed into an active and organized profession. In the 1920s occupational therapy schools started to become

Box B.3   **Project Work**

"Therapeutic aims…designated by the psychiatrist in charge of the guest are followed for each individual and this permits and makes necessary individualization of the work within the larger group. In addition to the therapeutic values determined upon a psychiatric basis, this out-of-door activity has the additional advantage of being physical exercise performed in the open air and sunshine" (Anderson, 1936, p. 265).

affiliated with colleges and universities. In 1923, the first set of minimal educational standards were published. In 1929, occupational therapy became the first profession to require its membership to be registered with a specific set of credentials. According to Rerek (1971), the profession defined its direction in the mid-1930s by asking the American Medical Association to establish standards for occupational therapy education and to accredit each new school. This, Rerek assumed, was when the profession formally assumed a medical ancillary role.

The climate of the mid-1930s stimulated professionals to reconsider the form of occupational therapy group intervention. During the Depression, many occupational therapy departments closed, decreased their personnel, or struggled with limited supplies (Reed & Sanderson, 1980; Rerek, 1971). By this time, the field of medicine had become more established as a profession and had increased its interest in scientific pursuits (Markowitz & Rosner, 1979). In addition, the realities of the Depression meant fewer women could enter male-dominated careers (Chafe, 1972). The few jobs that did exist were given to men, as they were the primary wage earners in households. More and more women turned to those areas of the economy that were traditionally open to them for employment. This led to an increase in the number of aspiring professional women in fields such as occupational therapy, as it related to their professional interest in medicine.

It should not be surprising, then, that Rothman (1980) found in the 1930s that "the most popular and prevalent form of hospital 'treatment' throughout these years remained occupational therapy" (p. 344). According to Rothman, however, "occupational therapy involved daily assignments to endless chores, chores as meaningless to their lives as they were important to the survival of the institution" (p. 346). Patients were not yet free from an economic role. Jobs were selected because they were necessary for the maintenance of the institution, not because of any specific interests or treatment goals for the patients. Rothman emphasized that "occupational therapy…affected the very existence of the mental hospital, for inmate labor was essential to day-to-day maintenance of the facility" (p. 346).

Occupational therapy group treatment was clearly representative of the times. Hospitals established to treat patients needed patient labor. The strong interest of women in the profession shaped the content and structure of that labor. Because women were taught many crafts as part of their upbringing, they were perhaps most able to teach inexpensive craft activities to groups of dependents as well as to supervise group tasks involving daily hospital maintenance. Canton (1923) noted that early occupational therapists needed to function as both a teacher and a nurse: "She will be the kind of person who needs the little touches which would make even the most barren place a bit homelike, and a certain amount of buzzing activity which is part of every normal environment....In addition she must bring to the work the ability to teach certain projects now accepted as valuable occupations" (p. 355).

The willingness of female therapists to conduct group treatment under male supervision gave the physician, who was usually male, more time to pursue his new scientific and professional interests. As these elements combined to shape the outer form of the profession, researchers in the field were laying the groundwork for internal changes that would affect how occupational therapists provided treatment.

Anderson (1936) was probably the first to identify a therapy group structure that could change behavior. In his view, the group was seen as a curative tool rather than as a way to keep patients occupied. In Anderson's project group, the elements of activity and group process claimed to foster personality change. Anderson stated that group activities could fulfill ordinary health needs as well as therapeutic aims. His new vision of group therapy brought to an end the formative phase of the Project Era that had emphasized the economic and the therapeutic value of treating patients in groups.

Socialization Era: 1937–1953

During this period, the purpose of groups evolved, changing from individual activities to an environment providing opportunities for socialization among psychiatric patients. Occupational therapy groups afforded patients an outlet for social needs and a vehicle for experiencing gratification from positive social contact. Quilt making was described as a group activity that aided socialization (Dunton, 1937). A literary club was later supported for group treatment of schizophrenics to work out "social cravings" (Blackman, 1940). Lockerbie and Stevenson (1947) noted that group activities and clubs were valuable for socialization problems found in psychiatric hospitals. G. Margaret Gleave (1947), an occupational therapist, suggested using group therapy with children to provide a permissive, socializing atmosphere, basing her work on Slavson's group therapy approach.

Slavson, who has been called the father of group psychotherapy (Schiffer, 1979), had a major influence on group treatment in occupational therapy. His ideas were especially influential during the Socialization Era. In 1934, Slavson designed his first group treatment method for children (Schiffer). This method was based on the group work he conducted from

1911 to 1930, which was "concerned primarily with the personal enrichment of individuals through active participation in creative pursuits" (Schiffer, p. xiii). Around 1934, Slavson drew important conclusions about the curative effects of creative activities in a peer group environment. Schiffer reported what Slavson told him in an interview at the time: "...it was the element of *compresence,* the actuality of being and interacting one with the other in the peer group, the sense of self-worth gained from newly acquired skills, the self-selected, completed craft and art projects, fortified by the spontaneous praise of fellow members, and the improved social status that were responsible for the corrective effects on personality and character" (pp. xvi–xvii).

Games were also viewed as an effective means for improving the socialization of psychiatric patients in a mental hospital (Hyde, York, & Wood, 1948). White (1953) discussed the use of simplified, repetitive activities that could involve large groups of patients and could be structured for maximum involvement. Guided group activity, such as gardening, painting, and museum trips, were found by Koven and Shuff (1953) to promote cooperation, social awareness, and a sense of gratification through group achievement.

Taking a somewhat different approach, Halle and Landy (1948) recommended the integration of craft and art activities used in occupational therapy groups with group psychotherapy. They found that the subject matter in the art activities groups often correlated with the subjects being discussed by the psychiatrist in psychotherapy groups. These group techniques were developed and implemented during the Depression of the 1930s and during World War II and its aftermath (Rerek, 1971; Jantzen, 1972). The severe budget cuts of the 1930s were followed by an increased demand for occupational therapists during World War II. During World War II, thirteen occupational therapy education programs were founded in association with established colleges or universities (Jantzen, 1972). Before the war, there were only five educational programs: three in independent proprietary schools, one in a hospital, and one in an undergraduate liberal arts college (Jantzen, 1972). The 1940s brought the need for new educational programs in the field of occupational therapy to the forefront of educational growth.

The 1940s saw tremendous growth in occupational therapy services despite budget cuts. Groups enabled therapists to treat a greater number of patients within a limited time. Because there was still relatively little theoretical orientation, occupational therapists remained in need of supervision and continued to serve an ancillary role. As an extension of the physician, the therapist could treat many patients at a lower cost while continuing to provide necessary medical treatment. The close relationship between medicine and occupational therapy no doubt explains why physicians dominated as authors of the articles in occupational therapy. Of nine occupational therapy journal articles published on occupational therapy group treatment during 1937–1953, four were by male physicians, three were coauthored by a male physician and a female occupational therapist, and only two were authored by female occupational therapists.

Group Dynamics–Process Era: 1954–1961

The 1950s brought a shift in occupational therapy group intervention. Professionals now recognized the group's curative powers and sought to use these effects to achieve therapeutic goals. As group leaders, occupational therapists were also structuring their role (Box B.4), the groups' membership, and the activities to meet various patients' needs.

These changes resulted from two factors. First, occupational therapists were now exposed to the concept of group dynamics. Therapists learned how to manipulate a group to achieve specific therapeutic aims. They learned that the group could be used as an environment to produce change in or to support specific kinds of behavior through an understanding of group dynamics and process. Second, the introduction of somatic therapies, particularly medications, enabled patients to function more easily in social settings, thereby freeing the therapist of the earlier concern for socialization and social skill maintenance (Feuss & Maltby, 1959). Therapists could now concentrate on treating individual patients' specific problems and developing new forms of the group to meet those needs.

In 1954, Fidler and Fidler proposed ways that groups could facilitate treatment goals. They suggested a new concept of occupational therapy as a laboratory for experimentation of behavior. This concept and its model differed from previous models because Fidler and Fidler recognized the curative effects of the learning, practicing, and modeling of healthy interpersonal behaviors that occurred naturally in an occupational therapy group. Recognizing the limitations of verbal groups for helping patients who were chronically psychotic, Bobis, Harrison, and Traub (1955) observed the role of the occupational therapist in helping these patients make continued progress in an occupational therapy activity group. They commented: "Group projects were emphasized with patients working together or doing different parts of a project. Suggestion was used a great deal by the occupational therapist—steady, gentle urging to participate in the group or group project" (p. 20). Patients showed a higher adjustment level in the activity group setting, and thus the authors concluded that the group played an important role in the patients' improvement.

Nelson and colleagues (1956) developed groups for differing types of patients, diagnoses, goals, and objectives. They structured "group occupational therapy" for, among others,

Box B.4   **Grading by Ability**

The occupational therapist's role ranged from that of a leader-member (when facilitating groups with members with higher levels of functional abilities) to one of active encourager who meets members' needs and structures the activity (when leading groups with members who are less capable in the areas of activity and social participation).

male geriatric patients, patients on insulin, and patients post lobotomy. A graded group program in which patients were selected for one of three groups according to their level of adjustment was also designed especially for women. These group members were homogeneous in their level of ability rather than in their diagnoses, which enabled them to benefit from socialization opportunities in a particular group structure. Combs (1959) designed a group for elderly men in a chronic disease hospital receiving custodial care. Activities were structured so that the patients moved from being primarily concerned with individual performance to being concerned with group performance.

In 1958, Lakin and Dray implemented an experimental sheltered workshop program in a home for the aged. Because the authors believed that "for the group as a whole, work for which one is paid is worthwhile activity" (Lakin & Dray, p. 173), wage-earning activity was structured into a group situation as a therapeutic modality. There were several positive effects for the group, including maintenance of adequate self-image and increased social contact.

A pilot study to determine a method for resocializing patients who had been chronically ill was conducted by Springfield and Tullis (1958). The average period of continuous hospitalization for these patients was 31 years. All subjects were characteristically apathetic as a result of being institutionalized and socialized in a passive and dependent patient role. The researchers found improvement in socialization was more noticeable in the activity group than during times when a project was not being conducted. They noted, "We were fully aware that if our program was to succeed, the emphasis must be placed on interpersonal relations rather than on any special activity" (p. 248).

Moss and Stewart (1959) developed a program for geriatric patients to facilitate movement from hospital to community. They developed groups for particular patient needs, assigning patients to groups "according to their specific disabilities or needs" (Moss & Stewart, p. 268). For example, one group of patients was given training in self-care activities. A group of confused and withdrawn patients was given simple individual tasks that they could complete successfully because they needed motivation and reassurance. After several months in generalized activities, the therapist suggested that these patients work on different elements relating to one group product. In a similar group program, the therapists chose eight men who could benefit from intensive group activity. This group worked on one large project related to a common goal rather than on smaller individual projects.

During the 1950s, there was increased theoretical research and publishing. The American Occupational Therapy Association conducted an institute on the theme of "interpersonal relationships" (AOTA, 1955) (Box B.5). Similarly, Gibb (1958) wrote on general group process principles for occupational therapists. He described how to make groups more by effective using concepts of group dynamics as guiding principles. The 1956 Allenberry Workshop held a conference on the function and preparation of the psychiatric occupational

Box B.5   **Defining Theory**

The theme of the American Occupational Therapy Association's institute in 1955 was "interpersonal relationships." Topics such as "Diagnosing Factors in Interpersonal Relationships," "Developing Effective Patterns of Leadership," and "Understanding the Complexities of Staff Relationships" were discussed. Types of leadership, functions of leadership, group dynamics and factors, and group processes were included. The proceedings of the institute were published for the association membership in the *American Journal of Occupational Therapy.*

therapist, and renowned occupational therapist Wilma West (1959) edited the proceedings. Participants made recommendations for the education of the occupational therapist as to:

• The use of group techniques
• The psychodynamics of interpersonal relationships in a group
• Group dynamics
• The therapist's use of self as a therapeutic tool
• Selection of group activities

In keeping with what was becoming state of the art for the provision of psychiatric interventions, "the majority of [occupational therapy] schools felt that teaching group relations is of major and vital importance....that their students need both theory and practice in groups" (West, p. 173).

Papers on group treatment were beginning to emphasize the importance of the interpersonal relationship between the occupational therapist and patient along with the role of activity in fostering patient adjustment (Fidler & Fidler, 1960; Gratke & Lux, 1960; Novick, 1961). This practice also received empirical support. Efron, Marks, and Hall (1959) compared the benefits of an individual-centered activity (called traditional occupational therapy) with those of a group-centered activity (making lawn chairs for the hospital) for patients with schizophrenia. They found no significant difference in benefits between the activities, but stated "... there is some support for the hypothesis that, for the activities studied, the personality of the therapist is more important than the activity per se" (pp. 123/555).

The increased use of group treatment in the 1950s resulted from several factors. After World War II, many veterans needed psychiatric treatment to help them readjust to peacetime. With the availability of medication to control behavior, therapists could design groups to help patients move from hospital life to community living (Feuss & Maltby, 1959; Moss & Stewart, 1959). It is not coincidental that occupational therapists applied concepts from the growing field of group dynamics to their practice. Four major studies on the use of occupational therapy group intervention for community adjustment of patients with psychosis were also conducted in Veterans Administration Hospitals during the 1950s (Bobis, Harrison, & Traub, 1955; Efron, Marks, & Hall, 1959; Levine, Marks, & Hall, 1957; Nelson et al., 1956). Another factor was the interest of social scientists in studying small-group behavior (Mosey, 1971). Additionally, many therapists in the 1950s were more prepared to apply theoretical material to their practice, a result of several schools' standards that required an undergraduate degree prior to admission into an occupational therapy certificate program (Jantzen, 1972) (Box B.6).

By the end of the 1950s, occupational therapy, just as other life sciences, began shifting its focus from a holistic to a reductionist paradigm (Kielhofner & Burke, 1977). This shift resulted from medicine's attempt to achieve scientific status by becoming more of a physical science and its subsequent pressuring of occupational therapy to accept a reductionist model as well (Kielhofner & Burke, 1977). The emphasis on group dynamics and process in occupational therapy group intervention was different from this technical view of patients and treatment models emerging in the late 1950s. Nevertheless, the growth of reductionism in other areas of occupational therapy and in medicine was more influential than the trend toward more holistic occupational therapy group approaches. With the growth of a holistic perspective in occupational therapy group treatment, one may wonder if the occupational therapists who led groups were somehow different from their professional counterparts who did not lead groups. Regardless, given the historically subordinate position of all occupational therapists, this scenario of the medical model hierarchy strongly influencing the occupational therapy profession's shift to reductionistic approaches was predictable. According to Kielhofner and Burke (1977), "By the end of the 1950s, the reductionist model was brought into occupational therapy as the basis of a new paradigm" (p. 682). The reductionist paradigm, they observed, took three forms:

1. The kinesiological model
2. The psychoanalytic, or interpersonal communication, model
3. The sensory integrative, or neurological, model

The three models reflected the attempt to establish a scientific basis for practice.

Box B.6   **Increased Understanding**

Mosey (1971) attributed the changes that occurred in this period to the following developments: occupational therapists' more sophisticated understanding of specific diseases, the development of psychiatric theories that viewed problematic interpersonal relationships as the cause of mental illness, the use of a team approach and medication in the care of psychiatric patients, and the new theoretical perspective of social scientists who were studying small groups.

These models are termed reductionist due to their being strictly channeled to achieve specific ends. Therapists attempted to define narrowly the specific goals to be achieved and to achieve them in a more direct manner. In the psychoanalytic model, occupational therapists attempted to help patients explore the intrapsychic determinants, or psychodynamics, of their maladaptive behavior through a task-oriented group (Box B.7).

Ego Building–Psychodynamic Era: 1962–1969

The 1960s were years of change in many areas. Numerous crises that had major social impacts included the Vietnam war, urban riots, planned obsolescence, campus unrest, rising crime, inflation, and environmental pollution (Diasio, 1971). Balanced against these crises were the more positive trends of the consumer protection movement, peace and civil rights, women's liberation, ecology and community health, desire for community control, and the human potential movement (Diasio, 1971). These social crises and movements affected group treatment. Like other professionals, occupational therapists perceived the need for social and scientific accountability.

Research in this period reflected the growing awareness of the need for long-term concern. In their dynamic "four-phase concept" approach, Linn, Weinroth, and Shamah (1962), two physicians and an occupational therapist, suggested that the occupational therapist provide an "unstructured work situation" so that changes in the patient's psychiatric illness could be detected. They hypothesized that a patient hospitalized for an acute psychiatric illness progressed through four distinct phases: (1) acute emotional decompensation, (2) initial emotional restitution, (3) pre-discharge symptom flare-up, and (4) meaning reaction (following discharge from inpatient treatment). Fidler (1966) described the prototype for occupational therapy group treatment in the psychodynamic era of the 1960s: "These groups are structured for the purpose of providing a group experience wherein members may explore the many and varied problems which arise in the process of task selection and completion such as decision making, accepting responsibility, being productive, and sharing with others. Individual feelings and behavior are discussed in terms of how they impede or enhance group cohesiveness and task accomplishment" (p. 73).

Box B.7   Building Abilities

The occupational therapy group was often aimed at developing ego strengths: the patient's ability to test reality, apply judgment, make decisions, and modify behavior on the basis of self-observation.

This approach supported the concept of milieu therapy. Material brought up in occupational therapy groups was then discussed in verbal psychotherapy and other individual and group therapies.

Occupational therapy groups were guided by two fundamental principles during the psychodynamic period. First, if exposed to a healthy milieu of accepting and cooperative staff and a variety of self-initiated activities with a range of emotional-interpersonal demands, the patient will develop or reconstitute intrapsychic or ego skills necessary for community living (Barker & Muir, 1969; Fidler & Fidler, 1963; German, 1964; Lamb, 1967; Llorens, 1968; Llorens & Johnson, 1966; Llorens & Rubin, 1967; Reilly, 1966; Shannon & Snortum, 1965; Slavson, 1967/1979). Second, if given an interpersonal task in a group, opportunity for the group to develop into a cohesive unit, feedback on the nature of interactions, and modeling of appropriate social skills or responses, the patient can develop ego skills for adapting to interpersonal situations (Fidler, 1966, 1969; Gillette & Mayer, 1968; Howe, 1968; Johnston, 1965; Mosey, 1968, 1969; Owen & Newman, 1965; Rothaus, Hanson, & Cleveland, 1966; Shannon & Snortum, 1965). The goals and methods of occupational therapy groups thus became, in part, like those of psychotherapy groups (Box B.8).

The 1960s were a hallmark period for occupational therapy group intervention. Many papers describing occupational therapy group formats were written, and group work flourished as a form of treatment. Many empirical papers on occupational therapy groups exemplified the concern for a scientific approach. Several studies focused on the effectiveness of activity groups for promoting social interaction (Ellsworth & Colman, 1969; Gralewicz, Hill, & Mackinson, 1968; Pasework & Hornby, 1968; Pearman & Newman, 1968; Werner, Maddigan, & Watson, 1969). The American Occupational Therapy Association (AOTA) responded to its membership's need for a more sophisticated understanding of evaluation methods in terms of planning for and providing intervention for psychiatric patients (Mazer, 1968). In an attempt to encourage participation in the newly developing community mental health programs and to improve professional training in working with individuals with psychiatric impairment, national and regional educational institutes were conducted by the AOTA from 1964 through 1968. These seminars supported psychiatrists' dynamic model of group psychotherapy and adapted it to occupational therapy by introducing an activity process into the group (Gillette & Mayer, 1968).

Box B.8   **Opening Doors**

Through occupational therapy groups, individuals found healthy modes of self-expression, gained improved self-esteem, and found emotional satisfaction of their needs.

The reductionist trend of the 1960s did not last and ultimately left many occupational therapists dissatisfied with their roles as therapists. Kielhofner and Burke (1977) speculated that in the 1960s occupational therapists were concerned with the inadequacy of their theoretical knowledge and were confused about their roles as health professionals. The two researchers surmised, "The problems of social adaptation, for which the medical model was inadequate and which was not addressed by reductionism, are anomalies that earmarked the failure of reductionism in the clinical arena of occupational therapy" (p. 685).

Adaptation Era: 1970s–1990s

The groups described in the literature of the 1970s and 1980s were designed to help patients meet their health needs, cope with skill deficiencies, overcome performance problems, and manage environmental constraints. The advances of medical research in developing drugs to treat a wide range of mental illnesses and expanding understanding of biological and chemical processes did not resolve the problems of living in the world for people coping with day-to-day life. As more types of patients were defined, the limits of medicine—strictly defined—came to be recognized. Medical treatment could not adequately aid the chronically disabled, nonverbal, or those without the capacity for insight to adequately cope with living among people. As practitioners in the field of occupational therapy came to recognize the types of problems still unsolved, they sought forms of group therapy that would address these problems.

The newly developing goals and concerns of the profession were reinforced by external economic factors. During the 1970s, the U.S. economy faced a severe recession, which led to restricted funds, reduced hospital stays, increased demand for quality assurance, and improved cost/benefit ratios. Group treatment flourished in this economic climate. Given the need for serving large numbers of patients at a reduced or maintained cost with fewer personnel, the need for occupational therapy group treatment grew in the 1980s. In the 1980s the Bureau of Labor Statistics of the U.S. Department of Labor predicted a "substantial shortfall of occupational therapy personnel" through 1990 (Acquaviva & Presseller, 1983, p. 79). The number of occupational therapists enrolled in an accredited entry-level master's program increased dramatically. In 1970, for example, 142 students were enrolled in such programs; by 1981, enrollments had increased to 577 students (Dataline, 1982). The importance of group dynamics, self-awareness, and the interdisciplinary team were being emphasized in occupational therapy curricula and practice (Odhner, 1970b; Steiner, 1972).

Additionally, since the 1970s it was required that students be trained in the use of groups as a treatment modality (Delworth, 1972; American Occupational Therapy Association, 1973;

Maynard & Pedro, 1971; Posthuma & Posthuma, 1972). The educational trends of the 1970s were followed by an increase in the use of groups in the 1980s. The direction of the theoretical work had been signaled by Ellsworth and Colman (1969), who proposed that treatment be based on behavior principles, specifically on the behavioral approach of B. F. Skinner, which stressed reinforcement and reward for desired behavior. This theoretical approach allowed therapists to concentrate on helping patients to adapt their behavior to situational needs and goals. Occupational therapy groups focused on patients' skill deficits (Denton, 1982; Fidler, 1984; Goldstein, Gershaw, & Spraflin, 1979; Hersen & Luber, 1977; Hughes & Mullins, 1981; Kramer & Beidel, 1982; Maslen, 1982; Mosey, 1970, 1981; Neistadt & Marques, 1984; Stein, 1982; Talbot, 1983) and social well-being (Mosey, 1973b, 1974). Occupational therapy groups of the Adaptation Era were generally based on one of three factors: (1) diagnosis, (2) role, or (3) setting (Box B.9). The unifying thread in these groups was their concern for helping the patient develop daily living skills and function through adaptation (Box B.10).

It was during this period that the functional group model, on which this book is based, emerged (Howe & Schwartzberg, 1986, 1995, 2001). The functional group model evolved at a period of high interest in groups as an intervention as well as from the need to articulate the aspects of an occupational therapy approach that could address patient needs at multiple levels. Toward the end of the 1980s, an increasing number of occupational therapists were employed in school systems to work with children who had special needs. Goals of treatment were more for habilitation and prevention than for rehabilitation. Service delivery followed a community model rather than the medical model. Policies in school systems varied from community to community. In some schools, children were treated in small groups; in others, occupational therapy was done on a one-to-one basis.

With the increased economic pressures on medical care, more attention was given to documenting the cost-effectiveness of group treatment as compared with individual treatment (Gauthier, Daziel, & Gauthier, 1987; Kurasik, 1967; Trahey, 1991). The group approach to treatment became the most economical for both the patient and the service delivery system. Increased hospital costs and the movement of patients into community programs and home treatment required a behavioral, skills-oriented, learning approach, and this quickly became the paradigm for occupational therapy groups. An outcome-focused approach to groups as well as group leaders who could work as facilitators, consultants, and educators to informal groups in the community also became necessary.

The adaptation approach of the 1970s and 1980s echoed the introduction of occupational therapy groups in the 1920s. In fact, during this period, there were many reports of activity-focused groups (Falk-Kessler & Froschauer, 1978; Fearing, 1978; Goldstein & Collins, 1982; Kiernat, 1979; Rance & Price, 1973; Rider & Gramlin, 1980; Schuman, Marcus, & Nesse, 1973; Schwartzberg, Howe, & McDermott, 1982). These groups, however, were only superficially like the groups of the Project Era of the 1920s and early 1930s. In the Adaptation Era,

Box B.9   **Groups Classified**

During the Adaptation Era (1970–1990), occupational therapy groups were usually described in the literature according to one of three types: patient diagnosis, meaningful role(s), or intervention setting.

Groups based on diagnosis included the following:

- Exercise groups for persons with hemiplegia (Bouchard, 1972)
- Groups for individuals post stroke (Wilson, 1979)
- Emotion identification groups for patients with psychiatric impairments (Angel, 1981)
- Activity groups for hyperactive children (Cermak, Stein, & Abelson, 1973; McKibbin & King, 1983)
- Groups for individuals with Parkinson's disease (Gauthier, Daziel, & Gauthier, 1987)
- Counseling groups for patients with spinal cord injury (Mann, Godfrey, & Dowd, 1973)
- Groups for persons with alcoholism (Lindsay, 1983)
- Groups for elderly patients, diagnosed with psychiatric impairments, demonstrating regressed behavior (Noce, Breuninger, & Noce, 1983; Ross & Burdick, 1978)
- Groups for patients with schizophrena (King, 1974; Linn et al., 1979; Odhner, 1970a; VanderRoest & Clements, 1983)
- Groups for patients diagnosed with borderline personality disorder (Goodman, 1983)
- Range-of-motion groups for persons with arthritis (Van Deusen & Harlowe, 1987)

Groups focusing on roles dealt with the following:

- Adjusting to physical disability (Versluys, 1980)
- Women's identification (Donohue, 1982)
- Fostering intergenerational relationships between elderly and adolescent patients with psychiatric impairment (Mahier & Tachabrun, 1978)
- Peer interactions in children with emotional disorders (Fahl, 1970)
- Community roles for clients with psychiatric impairments (Broekema, Danz, & Schloemer, 1975; Heine, 1975; Webb, 1973)
- Senior occupational therapy students (Botkins, 1979)
- Occupational therapists returning to the job market (Labovitz, 1978)

Groups concerned with the setting included the following:

- Acute care facilities (Corry, Sebastian, & Mosey, 1974; Neville, 1980)
- Psychiatric outpatient clinics (Kuenstler, 1976)
- Extended care facilities (Fearing, 1978)
- Community-based groups for the elderly (Menks, Sittles, Weaver, & Yanow, 1977)
- Geriatric day hospitals (Aronson, 1976; Kiernat, 1976)
- Emergency psychiatric settings (Hyman & Metzker, 1970)

Box B.10   **Adaptable Treatments**

> Whether the group was for treatment of a physical problem or an emotional one, the emphasis seemed to be on social adaptation through structured, graded learning experiences.

groups clearly had a functional aim and a theoretical rationale. Socialization and communication were always goals, as was the use of activity to remediate specific patient factors or to improve members' motor, process, activity, or occupational performance abilities. In the Project Era, the occupational therapy group had been described as a collective. The group was an organized unit, although it did not necessarily have a unified goal or an interdependent task. By the time of the Adaptation Era, the group format was determined according to specific factors related to the patients as well as the type of reimbursement and staffing available.

Wellness Era (1990–Present)

The empowerment of patients to take an active role in health care represents a new era in the design and development of occupational therapy programs and services. Johnson (1986) defines the term "wellness" as follows: "Wellness provides an opportunity for people to seek assistance with their problems of living and adapting and to create new options and solutions without acquiring a diagnostic label in the process of doing so. It also provides an opportunity for people who see themselves as whole complete individuals who, on occasion, have problems and who seek help in a supportive environment" (p. 13). In the Wellness Era, the focus of group work has shifted from diagnosis or pathology to an emphasis on the health of the individual, on the inborn capacity for wholeness and well-being that exists in every person and that can be supported and developed through the use of groups. These groups must be versed in an understanding of occupation, group dynamics, the importance of ego building, and the need for a supportive context for therapeutic and educational change to occur.

With the rapidly changing pattern of the health delivery system, corresponding changes have occurred both for the patients seeking health care and for the professionals providing those services. Duncombe and Howe (1985, 1995) researched the nature and scope of group work in the occupational therapy profession by surveying two random samples of practicing therapists in the United States. A three-part questionnaire, with minor changes, was used for both surveys. Respondents were asked for information about the facility where they worked, whether they used groups as a method of treatment, and, if not, the reason why. In the third part, respondents were requested to provide information on as many as four treatment groups they led and to complete a checklist of the characteristics and goals of the groups. A group was defined as "an aggregate of people who share a common purpose which can be attained only by group members interacting and working together" (Mosey, 1973a, p. 45).

Results from the first survey (120 respondents) provided information from 72 therapists who reported on the 209 groups that they led. In the second survey (188 respondents), 92 therapists who led groups reported leading 233 groups. The descriptions of the groups fell into six major categories; however, there were clearly some areas of overlap in the activities used. Overlapping is characteristic of the flexibility required in occupational therapy practice. The main types of groups were clustered as follows: four types of task groups, two types of discussion groups, exercise groups, self-expression groups, sensorimotor or sensory integration groups, and educational groups. The authors established 10 categories of groups:

1. Cooking
2. Activities of daily living
3. Arts and crafts
4. Special task
5. Self-expression
6. Exercise
7. Feelings-oriented discussion
8. Reality-oriented discussion
9. Sensorimotor and sensory integration
10. Educational (Box B.11)

During the 10-year period when the first and second surveys were completed, the types of groups led by occupational therapists showed little change except for a decrease in the number of self-expression and feelings-oriented discussion groups. In part, this was a result of the medical changes in the treatment of individuals with psychiatric conditions and the changes in the reimbursement guidelines for those types of groups.

Although some things changed, others remained the same. Occupational therapy groups continued to be small groups of 6 to 10 members and continued to include a greater number of activity, as opposed to verbal, groups. Both of these findings were statistically significant ($p < .01$). The most commonly listed group goals were identified as increasing task, cognitive, and physical skills. Although the therapists identified the types of groups that they were leading, often no clear difference existed between categories naming group activities. The identical activities were used for achieving different goals. For instance, both the exercise groups and the sensorimotor/sensory integration groups included similar activities such as exercises, games, and specific gross- and fine-motor activities to increase strength and stimulation.

Overlapping activities were also used in cooking, daily living, and task groups. Again, the activities of these groups were similar in nature but with different purposes or meaning,

Box B.11   **Types of Task Groups**

Duncombe and Howe (1985) developed brief descriptions of 10 types of groups:

1. Cooking Group. Cooking groups usually combined the tasks of planning, shopping for ingredients, cooking, and eating a meal. These groups, having five to eight members, often cooked a meal for a much larger group. A majority of the cooking groups were therapy programs for adult and adolescent mental health patients. Cooking groups were also found in rehabilitation programs for persons with spinal cord injuries, arthritis, and neurological conditions. These short-term, open or closed groups, had the specific goals of facilitating communication and socialization, increasing task skills, sharing information, and educating members.

2. Activities of Daily Living Group. This category contained the largest number of reported groups. Living skills groups were conducted in hospitals, clinics, day-care programs, nursing homes, and rehabilitation programs for adults with psychosocial dysfunctions, head and neurological injuries, and stroke and cardio-vascular conditions. Depending on the settings, these groups shared two distinct sets of goals. Some groups worked on developing living skills or greater independence in self-care within the institution, and other groups worked on pre-discharge living skills and on preparing for independent living in the community. The daily living skills groups were predominantly closed, short-term groups with three to eight members and with specific goals to increase task skills and share information.

3. Arts and Crafts Group. Arts and crafts groups were typically used for the evaluation and treatment of psychosocial disorders. Members worked on individual projects within a group setting. Some of these groups—particularly those concerned with evaluation of existing skills—were small, with fewer than five members. Other groups, concerned with developing leisure skills, had as many as 15 members and were designed to increase task skills and promote socialization and communication between members.

4. Special Task Group. These task groups met to create a product other than a meal. They were used most often in community mental health and developmental disabilities programs for adults as well as in after-school programs for children and adolescents. One type of task group worked on projects such as publishing a newsletter or a yearbook or planning and holding a recreational or social event. Another type of task group concentrated on prevocational or work-related assembly and production projects. Some task groups were small, others as large as 20 members. They were usually long-term, closed groups whose goals were to increase socialization and communication as well as task skills.

5. Self-Expression Group. These groups consisted of therapists working with adults with psychosocial problems. The specific goals were for socialization and communication in small groups of fewer than 10 members. These groups primarily used art modalities to encourage self-expression. At the time the second survey was completed, these groups had been mostly discontinued owing to changes in psychiatric treatment methods and criteria for reimbursement.

Box B.11   **Types of Task Groups** (continued)

6. Exercise Group. Members of exercise groups were involved in doing physical exercise to increase coordination, mobility, and strength. Group activities consisted of games involving ball play such as catch, ping-pong, volleyball, and bowling. Also included were recreational sports and movement activities. Members often participated in these activities from a chair or a wheelchair. Group size varied from 6 to as many as 20, and participants were often adults with psychosocial, physical, or developmental disabilities. The primary goals were to increase physical abilities and to facilitate communication and socialization.

7. Feeling-Oriented Discussion Group. These groups were usually found in mental health programs and were sometimes designated as group psychotherapy. Role-playing, poetry, and fantasy often promoted discussion. These groups were small verbal groups of 6 to 10 adults. Activities included such modalities as self-awareness and self-esteem work, grief work, and anger management. The goals were to provide support, increase communication and socialization, and achieve insight.

8. Reality-Oriented Discussion Group. These groups were designed for adults and the elderly. Topics for discussion included current events, the daily news, and events concerning the program, individual treatment goals, the use of time, and program or discharge planning. Some groups used specific group techniques such as assertiveness training and role-playing. Groups were predominantly verbal, short-term, and open or closed, and the goals were to increase communication and socialization, provide education, and share information.

9. Sensorimotor and Sensory Integration Group. These groups were for preschool through high-school children who were receiving group treatment in school or after-school programs. Problems consisted of learning disabilities, cerebral palsy, developmental disorders, auditory problems, and/or visual problems. Group members participated in gross- and fine-motor activities as well as in touch, taste, and movement activities. Groups were predominantly long-term, and the goals were to develop physical abilities, improve sensory integration, and provide opportunities for communication and socialization.

10. Educational Group. The majority of the educational groups were for parents and families of individuals receiving treatment. Also included were groups that provided information and discussion on medications, joint protection for arthritis, and family effectiveness. These were verbal, short-term groups with goals to provide support and meet health needs, to teach, and to share information.

depending on patients or context. For example, cooking may be seen as a life skill task, a leisure interest or hobby, an emotionally meaningful task, or as a task used to develop work skills. Activities in the task groups were more often leisure- or work-oriented, whereas the activities of daily living groups were more often self-care–oriented. However, all were directed at increasing skills for independent living in the present milieu, be it in a group facility or an independent living arrangement in the community.

The therapists responding to the survey indicated that facilitating communication and socialization were some of the most important goals for their groups. In discussing concepts from socialization theory, Burke (1983) noted: "Socialization offers the useful perspective that persons acquire behavior in the process of being exposed to role models, expectations, demands for performance, and information about performance. Socialization aids development of new and appropriate thinking and behaving throughout the life span" (p. 136).

Clearly, communication is an essential component of group participation, and increased communication contributes to greater learning in the group experience. Socialization also involves the interaction process between individuals and alleviates isolation. Both play an important part in assisting individuals to adjust to new circumstances and to achieve and maintain health.

Occupational therapy is not alone in stressing the value of small support groups in promoting wellness and successful living in the community. The field of medicine has published a number of studies showing that the incidence rates of recovery from illness and prevention of illness were higher among individuals who were involved in socialization and support groups (Ornish, 1998). For individuals with cancer, "group support may be particularly beneficial....People who have been recently diagnosed with cancer may find it hard to get emotional support when they most need it" (p. 57). Dossey (1999) noted a similar finding: "Social contact was proved to be an important factor in resisting all major diseases" (p. 165).

Although the goals of occupational therapy groups have not changed dramatically, the context and the locale where groups are to be found, as well as the role of the occupational therapist and the population served, have expanded considerably. Occupational therapists are working in an expanding number of systems: educational systems, community-based social systems, medical systems, and even in the business arena. A trend in survey responses showed an increase of occupational therapists employed in school programs and in programs labeled "other." These "other" programs included community programs such as home treatment, private practice, outpatient clinics, and early intervention. Concurrently, there was a decrease in the number of therapists working in psychiatric hospitals. This trend paralleled the demographic changes in the profession (American Occupational Therapy Association, 1991; Price, 1993) and reflected a trend away from primarily medical-based practice to a community-based practice. This was of particular interest because it raised the potential for the development of new areas of practice such as groups designed to promote health and wellness for people of all ages (Strickland, 1991).

Streib (1999) published results of a survey of occupational therapy practitioners detailing their employment situations. This study was taken from a self-selected sample of 100 registered occupational therapists and occupational therapy assistants who were asked where they currently work. Many of the respondents indicated that they worked in primarily medical settings such as hospitals, nursing facilities, outpatient treatment, or home health. Others were working for school systems in the community. However, approximately 40% of the respondents checked "other." This study showed a continuing trend toward a greater number of occupational therapy practitioners working in community-based, nonmedical settings.

Scott (1999) identified the following types of settings: "...a shelter for women who were homeless and mentally ill, senior programs for well-elderly persons and persons with mental illness, an in-patient pediatric sickle-cell unit and a university health club with programs for students and staff members" (p. 569) in which occupational therapy students could gain experience working with patient groups in areas of community service and be supervised by occupational therapy faculty. Types of groups included a smoking cessation program, in which the occupational therapy students co-led support groups to "help members cope with the pressures of nicotine withdrawal and lifestyle changes supplemented with deep breathing techniques and relaxation tapes supplied by the American Lung Association" (Scott, p. 570).

Boisvert (2004) described an occupational therapy group program for individuals dealing with substance abuse receiving services in residential and day programming. The residential and day programs aimed to promote wellness to support a lifestyle of sobriety. The focus of occupational therapy group intervention was client-centered and followed a structured program based on the Model of Human Occupation addressing residents' occupations and life roles and instrumental activities of daily living (IADLs). Residents who completed the program demonstrated 78% improvement in Rosenberg Self-Esteem Scale scores, with <.001 statistical significance.

Another day program established parenting groups for substance-dependent women (Knis-Matthews, 2003). The occupational therapists acknowledged the women's need for learning or relearning the IADL of child rearing with effective parenting skills. Groups were structured as modules around the particular member concerns. Toward the end of the 6 consecutive weeks, children joined the biweekly sessions. On completion of the program, some of the women interacted more comfortably with their children and initiated lifestyle changes.

Jackson et al. (1998) described how occupational therapy intervention, on which the well elderly study conducted by Clark et al. (1997) was based, was included as part of a well-elderly program organized in a Los Angeles area for residents 60 years or older living independently in subsidized apartment complexes. Each participant engaged one-on-one for 1 hour per month with the therapist "for developing customized plans for lifestyle redesign in which the participants were encouraged to creatively employ occupation in a personalized way to adapt to the challenges associated with aging" (1998, Jackson et al., p. 327) in addition to a 2-hour weekly group session. In the group sessions, participants joined in a four-part group process consisting of didactic presentations, peer exchanges, direct experience, and personal exploration in a module format, led by an occupational therapist. The elders who joined this program exhibited gains in physical health, physical functioning, social functioning, vitality, mental health, and life satisfaction. The participants in the occupational therapy group modules experienced significant benefits in self-rated perceptions of quality of life satisfaction, physical and social functioning, vitality, and other areas of functioning.

Families occupy an important role in the lives of individuals with disabilities, and therapists need to be aware of this focus (Humphry, Gonzales, & Taylor, 1993). Family and parent groups have long been a part of occupational therapy with infants and children, and a family caregiver role has been extended to the care of aging parents. Support groups can also address mental health concerns; specific health-related problems such as diabetes, AIDS, and cancer; and post–addiction treatment concerns. Some of these groups are organized as leaderless groups; in these, the occupational therapy practitioner may assume the role of an organizing guide. In others, the occupational therapist's role may be to coordinate and lead the group as well as contribute information to the group. The role may vary from consultant to facilitator to group leader. As a participant observer researching helping factors of a peer-developed support group for persons with head injuries, Schwartzberg (1994) noted the positive attributes to be "believing and feeling part of the group because members have a common problem and can validate the effects of the injury by sharing and receiving information in a variety of ways through the group" (p. 297). Just as in many other peer support groups, members shared a common condition, situation, symptoms, and experiences.

The variety of programs in the community where occupational therapy groups enrich the health and quality of life of individual continues to broaden. This in no way implies that what has traditionally been successful in medical and rehabilitation programs should be abandoned. Rather, the profession needs to broaden its scope, vision, and areas of practice. As Fidler stated, "As a profession, our single focus on an identity as a therapy, as a remedial rehabilitation service, has, I believe, significantly hampered our development. This narrow identity has, over many years, hindered our discovery and validation of the rich and broad dimensions of occupation" (Fidler, 2000, p. 99).

Even as its form has changed through the years, professionals remain convinced of the value of the occupational therapy group as an intervention method. Occupational therapy groups have provided services to many people, often in times of severe economic crisis in the United States. During the next few decades, we can expect a deeper understanding of the curative as well as rehabilitative effects of occupational therapy group intervention and a growing interest in its use.

Completed Forms for Chapter 5 Case Studies

Case Study #1:
Open Group on an Inpatient Psychiatry Unit ——————————————

GROUP HISTORY:

Name of group: "Getting It Together"

Leaders: Lauri Levy, OTR/L; Jack Jones, MHC

General status: *How long has the group been in existence? What is its anticipated duration? How often and for how long does the group meet? What is its general stage and level of development? Who has authority over goals and structure of the group?*

This group meets daily for 45 minutes and is an ongoing group that has existed on the psychiatric inpatient unit for over 3 years. It is expected to continue as a part of the unit's occupational therapy program. This is an open group, with the membership changing on a weekly, often daily, basis. Group members may be in the group for anywhere from 3 to 20 days depending on date of discharge, which may be related to disposition issues if the needed level of care upon discharge is not yet available. Because the membership changes, the group is, in a sense, always in the formation stage. However, the group needs to be structured to facilitate proceeding through development and closing (termination) in each session. The chief of psychiatric services, a psychiatrist, has ultimate authority over the goals and structure of any therapies conducted on the unit. The occupational therapist has direct responsibility for designing, implementing, and evaluating groups they conduct.

Leadership and membership criteria: *How was the group leadership and membership determined (i.e., assigned, voluntary or involuntary, referral)? If it is a closed group, what criteria are used to select the members? What was prior group leadership style?*

The group leadership was a collaborative decision between occupational therapy and nursing staff and has been relatively stable for the past year. Leaders established that group members needed to have unit-based privileges and were required to maintain personal safety in the presence of other group members and while using supplies or media as evidenced by self-control of urges to harm self or others. After assessing the needs of the hospital's psychiatric inpatient population, the leaders, in consultation with the interdisciplinary team, determined that at any given time there could be eight patients in need of such a group. The inpatient unit is an acute care psychiatric service with an average length of stay of 3–5 days. The group, generically named the Project Group, aka Getting It Together, has voluntary membership in that patients can choose the group as part of their treatment program. The group leadership style continues to fluctuate between autocratic and democratic, meaning leader-directed to group-centered based on the needs and abilities of the members in each session. Currently, the group follows a cognitive-behavioral frame of reference, as integrated into the therapeutic milieu of the unit, under the direction of the chief of psychiatry. This frame of reference is integrated with the functional group approach in accordance with the functional group model.

Group structure and current membership: *What is the group structure (format, general purpose, methodology)? How stable is the group membership? What is the rate of attendance? Is it an open or closed group? If it is an open group, are there any new members in the group? How long have the new and old members been in the group?*

The group is an open group. Usually, new members join the group or terminate from the group on a daily basis. Group size ranges from 4 to 8 (maximum) members. The general purpose and goals of the group are to increase member ability to engage in meaningful activity and to develop skills to support positive social participation. In past groups, members have been able to use the structure of setting personal goals for each session when cued by the leader.

Outcomes: *What outcomes have the group as a whole accomplished? What have individual members achieved? In what way has the group or leadership been unsuccessful?*

An activity or occupation-based approach has generally been effective in engaging members, depending on their interests and level of group readiness. Setting goals and focusing on peer support have been effective in terms of promoting decision making and social participation. However, processing goal achievement at the close of group sessions has been problematic as members still primarily seek leader feedback about their performance.

Comments: *Are there any other factors pertinent to understanding, assessing, and planning for the group?*

In addition to this group, patients attend daily community meetings, group therapy, individual counseling, and individual occupational therapy sessions. The primary focus of acute inpatient psychiatric treatment is problem identification and symptom management in preparation for discharge to home or the next level of care. Most group members are also being treated with psychiatric medications or are being evaluated for such treatment. The current group time is 4:00–4:45 p.m., right before the diner hour, which can be distracting for some members. Some members' conditions require readmission to the hospital, and therefore some members have attended this group in prior hospitalizations. Other members may have no group experience or have participated in groups in other settings or contexts (i.e., AA, NA, clubhouse model recovery groups, outpatient therapy).

ASSESSMENT OF MEMBERS AND CONTEXT:

Assessment of group members *(client profile, including range of behaviors, why seeking services, desired goals/outcomes):*

General description: Group members are currently receiving care on a 15-bed psychiatric inpatient unit of an urban, private, nonprofit general hospital. Prior to hospitalization, many resided primarily in the urban communities surrounding the hospital area. Some members are currently experiencing homelessness. Culturally, many of the patients identify themselves as Chinese, Irish Catholic, African American, Vietnamese, Puerto Rican, and Russian. English is not the primary language for approximately half the patient population. Socioeconomic status ranges from middle class and upper middle class to unemployed or homeless. Hospitalization costs are being covered through third-party payers. Common patient diagnoses include mood disorders, schizophrenia and other thought disorders, personality disorders, substance use disorders, and eating disorders. Some patients have medical problems, such as cardiac conditions, arthritis, diabetes, and multiple sclerosis, but these conditions are stabilized and secondary to their psychiatric disorder. All patients are between 16 and 70 years of age. Some patients have identified that they tend to sleep during the day; that they take medications when they are available or when they remember or are reminded; and that they spend their time predominantly walking around, watching TV, or on the Internet. Many acknowledged smoking cigarettes or marijuana and drinking as a means to "relax."

General description of members' expected environment: All group members are expected to return to their homes to live alone or with family members in the community or to be discharged to a more suitable living arrangement in the community. In these contexts, members will be expected to resume roles as parents, workers, students, group home residents, or retirees.

DESCRIPTION OF CURRENT OCCUPATIONAL PERFORMANCE:

Education/work: Two members are college students; one is a homemaker; one is retired; three are employed (an office manager, a chef, and a freelance writer); and one has a long-term history of unemployment.

Self-care (ADLs/IADLs): All are independent in basic activities of daily living (ADLs) (bathing, dressing); they have difficulty making decisions, especially when human transactions are involved, or in managing more complex personal hygiene and grooming or in instrumental ADLs (IADLs) such as care of others/pets, and with fiscal, health, and home management (shopping, banking, bill paying, nutrition/exercise, general personal item and household maintenance).

Play/leisure: All members have expressed dissatisfaction with their use of leisure time. Some feel they have few to no interests; others are either all-consumed with work or do not have the resources (people, places, money, and so forth) to participate in volunteer prevocational activities.

Social participation: Most members identify estrangement or conflict in family or peer relationships and avoidance of structured community activities (clubs, church/synagogue, library membership, voting, etc.), which may for some be due to experiencing symptoms such as paranoia, delusions, flashbacks, or phobias, thus resulting in a high degree of isolation, even when around others.

STRENGTHS AND DEFICITS IN MOTOR AND PROCESS SKILLS:

Physical and neuromotor: All members are ambulatory and all have adequate gross- and fine-motor coordination and range of motion to perform routine ADLs. They are all able to maintain balance when performing activities seated or standing, walking or moving about during simple gross-motor activities (simple exercise routines). Many are unable to perform tasks with the strength and endurance required for the members' pre-hospitalization routines; for example, they may take frequent rests or complain of strain or fatigue. Some are experiencing medication side effects such as dry mouth, numbness or stiffness, tremulousness, or motor restlessness, some of which may or may not diminish.

Cognitive: Members are able to understand simple written and verbal instructions and can concentrate on structured tasks for up to 30 minutes. All have grossly intact memory skills for factual information, but some experience cognitive distortions in recalling verbal interactions involving affective material. Members are generally oriented to time, place, and person. Most members have some insight into current difficulties as being related to their mental illness. Some members become anxious and have difficulty sequencing a plan of action when solving problems, whereas others are able to make abstract judgments but have difficulty with simple decisions involved in daily living.

Psychosocial: Members have difficulty recognizing and verbalizing their emotions. Although members are able to imitate behaviors, they have difficulty identifying when a change in action is needed. Some members rely totally on others to fulfill their needs, whereas others are unwilling to accept suggestions or help. Most members are unable to identify their strengths and therefore focus their discussions on limitations. Several members are unable to handle frustration with a task and show their anxiety by not completing the activity, moving about restlessly, or being irritable and devaluing the task. Some members attempt to interact with others in a group by always offering help (often to the exclusion of attending to their own needs), others by demanding assistance and withdrawing if it is not immediately available. Some members vacillate between extreme expressions of affect or relatedness (anger/silliness, poor boundaries, neediness/rejection).

What is the significance of these factors with regard to forming the group, setting individual member goals, and/or planning group session(s)?
Ideally, to promote total participation, the group should be composed of no more than eight members (men and women) and have two leaders (one male and one female). The group will need to be advised on how to select relatively short-term activities with little complexity and minimal opportunity for error. The leaders will need to assume an active role in adapting the activities so that a variety of group membership roles can be assumed. The leaders will also need to observe the group's process, suggest alternative behaviors, and assume group membership and leadership roles when the members are unable to do so. A highly supportive, genuine, and consistent emotional climate must be established and reinforced by the leaders.

ASSESSMENT OF GROUP CONTEXT (THE FACILITY):

General description of program *(mission, administrative structure):* The group is conducted on the 15-bed psychiatric inpatient unit of an urban, private, nonprofit general hospital. The interdisciplinary staff consists of mental health counselors, nurses, an occupational therapist, psychiatrists, a psychologist, and social workers. Staff mix is diverse in terms of age, gender, sexual orientation, and educational level beyond undergraduate education, but many are white. The group will be part of the milieu therapy program offered to patients on the unit. The hospital's occupational therapy staff working on the unit will provide the functional group protocol. Co-leadership will be interdisciplinary (i.e., occupational therapy/nursing staff). The inpatient unit is one of the services offered through the hospital's department of psychiatry. Regulatory bodies include the Joint Commission on Accreditation for Hospital Organizations and the state's Department of Health and Human Services.

General description of physical environment: The unit has a long hallway with six semiprivate rooms and two single rooms. A quiet room; a sensory room, used to provide a calming space; and the nurses' station are at one end; a kitchen/dining area, the occupational therapy room, staff offices, and a community living room are at the other. The occupational therapy room has one long rectangular table, a small circular table, and countertops, and activity supply cabinets are along the walls. The room is painted in soft green; patients' projects are scattered about; and there are many hanging plants by a Plexiglas window over a large work sink.

General description of emotional climate: The emotional climate varies according to the patient population on the unit. At times, the atmosphere is calm and quiet; at other times it is noisy, high-keyed, and energetic. There are occasional outbursts (yelling, crying, screaming, physical or verbal threats) by patients, addressed by staff trained in de-escalation techniques.

Frames of reference, purpose, and objectives: Using a biopsychosocial model coupled with the cognitive-behavioral frame of reference (i.e., that thinking, feeling, and behavior are related), this short-term unit provides a safe environment for patients who present as at risk of harm to self or others. Its primary purposes are evaluation, alleviation of acute symptoms of the patient's psychiatric condition, and referral to longer-term inpatient care or outpatient services in the community.

What is the significance of these factors with regard to forming the group, setting individual member goals, and/or planning group session(s)?
Because of high patient turnover, the session plans must be revised and group held on a daily basis. Leaders should attend morning rounds or community meetings to get a sense of the unit and treatment plan issues that may be affecting members. Closure will have to be structured into every session, as will the opportunity and format for discussion.

ENVIRONMENTAL SUPPORTS AND CONSTRAINTS:

Facilities and materials: A wide range of activities can be conducted in the occupational therapy room and kitchen areas. The unit is not, however, large enough to accommodate group activities that require extensive movement, physical sports equipment, or space.

Scheduling: Because of other treatments, unit-wide meetings, ADL/IADL times, hospital meals, and evening patient visiting hours, the group meeting time is on a fixed schedule and can not be changed.

Group norms and prior therapy group experience (if any): Physically or verbally abusive behaviors are not allowed. Patients who are unable to respect this requirement are provided one-to-one services for their own safety or the safety of others. Patients who do not partici-pate in their treatment program, as established by the individual patients and staff, are transi-tioned to long-term treatment at other facilities.

Do any of the environmental constraints require modification of the group, or could the situation be altered?

Group plans must take into consideration budgetary and physical plant resource issues.

FUNCTIONAL GROUP PROTOCOL:

Name of group: "Getting It Together"

Leaders: Lauri Levy, OTR/L; Jack Jones, MHC

Time/length of meeting(s): Monday–Friday, 4:00–4:45 p.m.

Place: Occupational Therapy Room or other as arranged

Group format: Open

Rationale: This group will meet daily as average length of stay is 3–5 days, with range being 2–20 days.

General group goals:

- To be able to contribute ideas in the group for the selection of a group project.
- To be able to carry out selected aspects of the group project in the presence of others in the group; for example, get and distribute materials to group members.
- To be able to verbally express satisfaction about one's own interaction in the group, con-tribution to the project, and the group's final product
- To be able to assume group maintenance roles such as encourager (i.e., "Let's try it."), compromiser (i.e., "Can we do what some members want to do today and what the rest want to do tomorrow?"), and gatekeeper (i.e., "Let's not pick a theme until we hear every opinion in the group.").
- To be able to assume group task roles, such as asking for information, giving opinions, or expressing wishes.

Rationale for goal selection: On admission, members presented problems such as poor self-esteem; preoccupation with internal stimuli; withdrawal from family, friends, or coworkers; loss of interest in vocational or avocational activities; indecisiveness and disorganization around daily routines and routine decision making; all resulting in an inability to complete tasks required for daily functioning, such as food shopping, meal preparation, physical care of children, and attention to personal hygiene in terms of care of hair, skin, teeth, cosmetics/shaving, etc.

Outcome criteria for successful goal attainment in session(s): At least once every session, each member gives or seeks information; follows through with an action step necessary for the completion of the group project; and displays satisfaction or enjoyment through laughing, joking, or smiling in a manner appropriate to the context.

Group composition and criteria for selecting members: Ideally, the group should include both men and women and a maximum of eight members. In addition, prospective candidates for the group should at minimum be able to communicate verbally in a simple manner; understand simple communications (for example, written and verbal instructions); concentrate on a structured task, in the presence of seven other patients and two therapists, for a minimum of 30 minutes; and understand the goals and methods of the group. It is expected that members will have a variety of problems in areas of occupational performance and may potentially have underlying issues in performance skills or patterns or body structures and functions that affect their participation in some aspects of group activity. Prospective group members' psychiatric conditions may influence their abilities to fulfill social needs; feel masterful or useful; and meet obligations of social roles such as parent, worker, community member, or hobbyist.

Leadership roles and functions: The group has two leaders. Their primary roles and functions are:

- To establish a group structure that encourages a large amount of membership involvement in the group's task and selected processes
- To protect the safety of individual group members and the morale of the group as a whole
- To encourage action within the range of member abilities
- To provide opportunities for members to assess the accuracy of their perceptions of their abilities, as they are able, through group task and verbal feedback
- To act as resource persons for making projects and elements of group process and dynamics; to communicate observations of members' adaptive and maladaptive behaviors to the group members, as appropriate, and unit staff

Characteristics of group contract: Members are expected to attend sessions on a regular basis unless unusual circumstances prevail. Members, if possible, or their designee should notify leaders before the session in question. Members are required to remain in each group session for the 45 minutes or to negotiate with the group or leaders if a special contract or arrangement is necessary because of extenuating circumstances. Material discussed by other group members is not to be shared outside the group unless within the confines of a therapeutic relationship with unit staff or by group leaders in the context of maintaining safety or reporting related to service provision. Physical or verbal abuse is not tolerated in the group. If members are unable to fulfill the requirements of the group contract, they will be asked to leave or be removed from the group.

Group methods and procedures to be employed: Graded, structured activity such as crafts, horticulture, expressive art, and cooking. Leaders will facilitate:

• Group agenda.
• Group process.
• Task engagement, analysis, and adaptation (as needed).
• Social participation, member-to-member interaction (as needed).

SESSION PLAN:

Name of group: "Getting It Together"

Date: June 6

Session activity: "What's in a Name?"—introducing new members to group

Specific goals for the group session: Given a task that is primarily leader-structured and -directed, members will:

• Learn other group members' names.
• Talk to another group member and address comments to the group as a whole.
• Take turns talking in a group.

Specific goals for group members: Gary, Eric, Liz, and Pearl:

• To be able to state their names to new members and make one comment each to a new member, such as: "What I am working on in this group is [task or goal]...."
• To express their feelings and reactions to leaders in a socially appropriate manner about being members of a group that has four new members (e.g., "It is hard for me to learn new members' names," "...to have the group change," etc.).
New group members (Li, John, Betty, Lakisha):
• To verbalize feelings about being in the group and choose to participate in task or conversation with leaders or group members.

Description and rationale for methods and procedures:

• Review and explain group's purpose, goals, and rules per written display board; leader and member roles, group structure, and timeline.
• Describe icebreaker activity ("What's in a name?") in simple and clear fashion.

Rationale: Overall aim of activity is to facilitate introduction of new members into group; help previous members acknowledge change in membership; describe purpose of group; and instill feelings of safety and belonging for all group members.

Description and rationale for leadership role:

• Prepare new members for group by individual pre-group interviews.
• Review session plan among co-leaders; prepare flip chart with simple directions/pictographs.
• Gather supplies necessary for group activity.
• Provide task structure and support.

Rationale: Provide a structured environment that reassures members and maintains safety but not be so directive as to encourage overly dependent behavior.

List material and equipment needed: Paper (lined and unlined)
Fine-tip, colored, nontoxic, erasable markers

Time and sequence outline for sessions, including what you will do and say as leader and what group is expected to do:

• Explain group's purpose, leader and member roles; review rules and expectations. (5 minutes)
• Explain that because so many new members are in the group today, the leaders have planned an activity to help group members get to know one another. Pass around paper, asking members to take a piece of either lined or plain paper and pass pile to person to the left. Place the remaining paper and packs of markers in the center of the table. Ask that everyone choose a marker and write down his or her first and last name across the top of the paper. Explain that they are to write down two things they like about their name and two things they might not like about their name. Tell group members that after they have completed the first part of the activity, each member will share some of what he or she has written with the person sitting to his or her right. Explain that, once everyone has finished talking with the person on their right, members will then take turns introducing that person by saying what he or she said they did and did not like about their name (co-leader will point out simple steps that are outlined on flip chart in both words and simple pictographs). (10 minutes)
• Ask if everyone understands how to proceed or if anyone has questions. Clarify as needed. Explain that group members will be encouraged to talk about the activity afterward and to say what they thought or felt about it at the end of the group. (5 minutes)
• Group will then do the described activities. Leaders will encourage member participation, keep group activity within time limits of session by prompting group to complete various aspects of task, and provide feedback or clarify directions as needed. (15 minutes)
• Leaders will facilitate member discussion concerning task, summarize the purpose of today's session (getting to know one another), discuss potential plans for the following session with group members, and facilitate clean-up as necessary. (15 minutes)

Other information pertinent to this specific session: In this session, half the group will be composed of new members. Hospital translator will be present.

Case Study #2:
Closed Group in an Outpatient Occupational Therapy Clinic————————

GROUP HISTORY:

Name of group: Community Re-entry: "Moving Forward"

Leaders: Russell Lee, MS, OTR/L; Alicia Wright, COTA/L

General status: *How long has the group been in existence? What is its anticipated duration? How often and for how long does the group meet? What is its general stage and level of development? Who has authority over goals and structure of the group?*
This group format has been offered at an outpatient clinic for the past year. The group was started because patients seen in the outpatient clinic expressed a need for more input and support. They found returning home very stressful and complained of strained family and coworker relationships, fatigue, depression, anxiety, and feeling useless. The first group was started as a peer support group, with the consultation of an occupational therapist. The group consists of 8 consecutive 90-minute sessions over 2 weeks. Generally, the group moves through the stages of formation to closure in each session as well as over the 2-week period, with leaders providing a structure that facilitates group development. The director of rehabilitation, an occupational therapist, and chief physiatrist have ultimate authority over the group's goals and structure

Leadership and membership criteria: *How was the group leadership and membership determined (i.e., assigned, voluntary or involuntary, referral)? If it is a closed group, what criteria are used to select the members? What was prior group leadership style?*
The group is voluntary and composed of a maximum of eight members. The members are patients referred from the rehabilitation hospital, 17 years of age or older. Patients referred to the group need help with community re-entry, energy conservation, time management, and adjustment to a disability. Diagnoses generally include: post hip fracture or post total hip replacement (THR)/total knee replacement (TKR), post traumatic brain injury (TBI)/cardiovascular accident (CVA), and post surgery and cardiac conditions. The occupational therapist screens patients on physician, inpatient occupational therapy or physical therapy, or social work referral. Patients must be oriented times three (person, place, time), able to communicate verbally and understand oral instructions, relatively emotionally stable, and able to con-

centrate on group tasks for up to 60 minutes. The group leadership has been predominantly democratic, depending on member needs and abilities. The group was developed according to the functional group model. However, person-environment-occupation and biomechanical frames of reference also inform leader reasoning.

Group structure and current membership: *What is the existing group structure (format, general purpose, methodology)? How stable is the group membership? What is the rate of attendance? Is it an open or closed group? If it is an open group, are there any new members in the group? How long have the new and old members been in the group?*

This is a closed group with required attendance. The group meets 4 times per week for 2 weeks. The structure of the group consists of eight sessions. The group is intended to be educational in regard to self-care and community re-entry while providing a group-centered, cohesive support system. The group leaders, an occupational therapist and occupational therapy assistant, have the power to change the group's structure as long as the goals remain the same in regard to community re-integration.

Outcomes: *What outcomes have the group as a whole accomplished in the past? What have individual members achieved? In what way has the group or leadership been unsuccessful?*

Program evaluation found an outcome to be that the patients required less follow-up care at home.

Comments: *Are there any other factors pertinent to understanding, assessing, and planning for the group?*

Members may have mild to moderate impairments in body structures and body functions that may be affecting motor, process, and communication skills such as balance, mobility, coordination, energy (pacing and endurance), and speech. Pain management and/or sleep disturbance are also concerns. Transportation to and from the clinic has been an issue for some members.

ASSESSMENT OF MEMBERS AND CONTEXT:

Assessment of group members *(client profile, including range of behaviors, why seeking services, desired goals/outcomes):*

General description: Seven adults, ranging from 31 to 66 years of age. There are four women (two had CVAs, one is post hip fracture, and the other is post bilateral TKR secondary to arthritis) and three men (one has a TBI post motor vehicle accident that occurred while driving when intoxicated, one has mild brain injury post anoxia due to a myocardial infarction (MI) resulting in triple bypass surgery, and one is post spinal fusion with chronic pain secondary to ruptured lumbar discs). All are mildly depressed or anxious. All members live in suburban areas and cities within a 90-minute drive.

General description of members' expected environment: All members will return to live at home, alone or with spouses, family members, or children. Two members are retired, two are homemakers, one is unemployed (with plans to return to part-time work), one runs a small family business, and one is a teacher.

DESCRIPTION OF CURRENT OCCUPATIONAL PERFORMANCE:

Education/work: The range of member work skills comprises full to partial homemaking/parenting, full-time employment as a third-grade teacher, unemployed with work potential (for example, one formerly employed full-time as a lawyer, another held maintenance job for 3 years), active in retirement, and retired and completely dependent on family with no interest in work.

Self-care (ADLs/IADLs): Member self-care skills range from complete independence in daily living skills (i.e., grooming and hygiene, feeding/eating, dressing, functional mobility, functional communication) to partial dependence in functional mobility (wheelchair mobility, transfers, ambulation), dressing, grooming/hygiene, and feeding/eating.

Play/leisure: Member leisure skills range from recognition of avocational interests to no ability in identifying activities or social situations that are perceived as leisure pursuits or fun. All members express concern regarding their ability to adapt leisure activities, schedule, or home environment to enable participation in avocational pursuits (civic, social, or leisure). Many members have difficulty identifying community resources available for leisure activities.

Social participation: Members identify experiencing difficulty with transitioning back into social settings, including family routines, spiritual communities, work, and other community venues (grocery store, hairdresser, library, or settings such as health club or community service venues—Rotary club, PTA, etc.). Members indicate that they are uncomfortable or struggling with loss of traditional roles (driver of family car, head of household finances or maintenance, etc.).

STRENGTHS AND DEFICITS IN MOTOR AND PROCESS SKILLS:

Physical and neuromotor: Many members become restless and agitated when expected to perform an activity. Several members have various amounts of physical dysfunction from a stroke, arthritic condition, neuromuscular disorder, chronic pain, general lethargy, or disuse of body. Problems include poor dexterity and incoordination in fine-motor tasks or gait, limited active range of motion, fatigue or strain when using muscular force required for certain activities, poor sensory awareness and postural balance, and poor visual-spatial awareness.

Cognitive: All members are able to concentrate on a task or concept for 30–60 minutes; are oriented to person, place, and time; and have immediate and recent memory. Range of insight varies from excellent to poor. Problem-solving ability ranges from being able to make decisions to total reliance on concrete cues for evaluating decisions and plans.

Psychosocial: Most members seldom initiate conversation with individuals other than the staff or their own family members; all express concern and anxiety over their appearance and ability to be productive or loved.

What is the significance of these factors with regard to forming the group, setting individual member goals, and/or planning group session(s)?
To promote participation, the group should ideally be composed of no more than eight members (mixed gender) and have two leaders (mixed gender). The leaders will need to assume an active role in adapting the activities to facilitate member participation and ensure the members assume a variety of group roles (task and maintenance). The leaders will need to observe the group's process, suggest alternative behaviors, and assume group membership roles when the members are unable to do so. A highly supportive, genuine, and consistent emotional climate must be established and reinforced by the leaders.

ASSESSMENT OF GROUP CONTEXT (THE FACILITY):

General description of program *(mission, administrative structure):* The group is one of the services offered through the occupational therapy department to inpatients of the hospital. The leadership responsibility rotates among the occupational therapy staff of 18 certified occupational therapists and 2 occupational therapy assistants. The director of occupational therapy provides supervision. Consultation is also available from the hospital physicians, nurses, speech-language pathologists, social workers, physical therapists, and neuropsychologist.

General description of physical environment: Large occupational therapy clinic with plinths, mirrors, mats, weights, and pulleys; a single bed; an adapted kitchen; a prevocational area with a Baltimore Therapeutic Equipment (BTE) machine; computers with adaptive keyboards and mice; various tools and an indoor garden; an activity area with tables and chairs; and reception desk and offices in foyer of clinic space.

General description of emotional climate: Cheerful, warm, friendly, relaxed, and supportive. Therapists are approachable and often have interns or student trainees working with them. There is a strong emphasis on open and direct communication with patients and their families.

Frames of reference, purpose, and objectives: Biopsychosocial model; ecological systems model; person, environment, occupation model; rehabilitation and prevention services in a private rehabilitation hospital.

What is the significance of these factors with regard to forming the group, setting individual member goals, and/or planning group session(s)?
Because other therapists treating patients in one-to-one therapies use the clinic space, coordination of use of room, supplies, and equipment with other staff therapists will be necessary.

ENVIRONMENTAL SUPPORTS AND CONSTRAINTS:

Facilities and materials: All materials are within easy access. Audiovisual equipment (laptop, LCD) will be borrowed from rehabilitation department.

Scheduling: The group is scheduled in the morning. Some patients will need transportation assistance to bring them to and from the occupational therapy clinic.

Group norms and prior therapy group experience (if any): Although the group content and curriculum is pre-established, for these members this is a new group forming for the first time.

Do any of the environmental constraints require modification of the group, or could the situation be altered?
The group time might be rescheduled to 4:00 to 5:30 p.m., when the occupational therapy clinic is least crowded and patients have more flexibility in their schedules.

FUNCTIONAL GROUP PROTOCOL:

Name of Group: Community Re-entry: "Moving Forward"

Leaders: Russell Lee, MS, OTR/L; Alicia Wright, COTA/L

Time/length of meeting(s): 10:00–11:30 a.m.; 8 consecutive sessions in 2 weeks

Group format: Closed

Rationale: This group is focused on issues related to community re-entry. It is therefore limited to patients who were referred as part of their disposition planning.

GENERAL GROUP GOALS:

Member objectives:

• To identify changes necessary as a result of current disability status in order to perform aspects of meaningful roles such as family member, friend, self-care, work, or leisure roles.

- To identify changes in living environment and relationships necessary for adaptation to current disability. This includes the need for orthotics, prosthetics, and assistive/adaptive equipment as well as the maintenance of such equipment and involvement of other individuals such as family members.
- To identify potential barriers to adjustment to community living; for example, overindulgence of family members, architectural barriers, physical isolation, limited mobility, or emotional withdrawal of friends, family, lover, and coworkers.
- To discuss strategies for intervening with potential barriers; for example, to be able to ask for and receive help; to plan alternate routes, time frames, and modifications of physical environment so that mobility is increased; to be able to give and receive feedback; to suggest compromises or alternatives.
- To identify a peer support network in the community to aid adjustment to disability.
- To be able to prevent or minimize pain, fatigue, or diminished performance (cognitive or physical) through organizing activities and schedule to minimize energy output.
- To use joint protection and/or body mechanics principles to minimize stress on joints and prevent falls/injury.
- To be able to position self physically so that optimal safety and functioning in life roles are feasible.
- To be able to select, perform, and coordinate activity schedule to maintain a balance between rest, sleep, work, and leisure needs and interests.
- To describe abilities and strengths.

Leader objectives:

- Evaluate performance problems related to occupational behaviors necessary for functioning in life roles.
- Determine needs for patient referral for outpatient/home treatment services.

Rationale: These goals were selected because the members are dealing with community reentry and changes in life roles, which may include asking other people to fulfill some needs (for example, personal care or resumption of usual responsibilities). It is also recognized that although members are expected to meet criteria for functional performance at discharge, there is variation in what clients/families/health-care providers perceive or must regard as return to function. Therefore, clients need strategies and support to maintain themselves physically, emotionally, and socially in the community and to continue to achieve a maximum level of functioning. Similarly, patient education is necessary to prevent further debilitation or disability. As is often the case, patients present as highly dependent on staff/family members to fulfill needs. Families often express concern over being able to cope with the level of impairment and the extent of disability their loved one presents at home.

Outcome criteria for successful goal attainment in session(s) stated in behavioral terms:

• Changes are made in members' home environment to accommodate or prevent further disability; for example, changes in furniture heights; family member available to transport patient to work.

• Members seek and offer assistance; share concerns; seek and offer suggestions in the group.

• Members meet with or phone friends, employer, or family to discuss changes necessary to resuming or modifying role activities.

• Members plan a weekly schedule incorporating units of work, rest, play, and sleep equivalent to energy output level needed to resume valued roles.

• In doing group activities, members position themselves and protect their joints so that they can complete projects with minimal stress and at a maximal level of functioning.

• Members have the telephone numbers of at least two individuals they can call for support.

Group composition and criteria for selecting members: The group is composed of a maximum of eight men and women patients who are 17 years of age or older. Usual diag-noses include neurological disorders (such as stroke, multiple sclerosis, Guillain-Barré syndrome), post surgery, cardiac disease, and comorbid conditions such as arthritis, alcoholism, brain injury, and chronic pain. Members should be oriented times three (person, place, time), be able to concentrate on a task for 30–60 minutes, be able to communicate verbally and understand oral instructions, and be relatively emotionally stable (i.e., not emotionally labile).

Leadership roles and functions: Two leaders will conduct this group. The sessions are planned into eight units, designed and implemented by the group leaders. One leader will have responsibility for screening patient referrals and introductory interviews. The other leader will have responsibility for writing notes in the patients' records and for making discharge plans. The responsibilities for these functions will rotate between the leaders after completion of an eight-unit group.

Characteristics of group contract: Members are required to attend all eight sessions. They must express an interest in sharing their concerns about discharge with other group members and be willing to participate in the group's activities. They must have prior permission and a referral from their attending physician.

Group methods and procedures to be employed:

Session 1: Introduction to the group: a discussion of its purpose, goals, and procedures. Icebreaker exercise.

Session 2: Individual collages: "What I Value"; group discussion.

Session 3: The "Pie of My Life" pre-hospitalization and post-hospitalization: an expressive art activity, group discussion.

Session 4: Energy conservation, adapting activities or environment, pain management: lecture, slide show, demonstration, practice, group discussion.

Session 5: Lifestyle redesign, time management principles: lecture, problem-solving exercises, group discussion.

Session 6: Dealing with human and architectural barriers, identifying community resources: handout with information, discussion, role play, group discussion.

Session 7: Community integration at home, at work, and socially; what is working/what needs work: nominal group process exercise, group discussion.

Session 8: Group closure: conduct review of topics (revisit one or two topics in more depth per members' selection); evaluation of group series, party.

Note: These plans would be modified according to the group's needs. For example, if the group has members of a predominant age, gender, functional impairment, or with common roles, the sessions would focus on issues related to these concerns.

SESSION PLAN:

Name of group: Community Re-entry: "Moving Forward"

Date: December 15, second of eight sessions

Leaders: Russell Lee, MS, OTR/L; Alicia Wright, COTA/L

Activity: Individual collages: "What I Value"; group discussion

Specific goals for the group session: To build group cohesiveness while assisting members with identifying priorities in life as a means to assist with long-term goals of time management, energy conservation, and adjustment to current disability status.

Members will:

- Identify what they value and find meaningful in terms of time/energy devoted to tasks via expressive art (collage) activity
- Share what they value/find meaningful with group and discuss concerns related to being able to participate in valued tasks/roles/activities
- Participate in group process to learn to prioritize and brainstorm ways to address concerns as method of problem solving and to receive group support

Specific goals for group members:

Jim (brain injury post MI): to identify strategies for decreasing time and amount of assistance needed with ADLs

John (TBI post MVA): to increase safety awareness as part of realistic short-term goal setting for activity participation

Steve (lumbar fusion): to identify how to incorporate strategies for pain prevention and management into daily routine and take initiative to obtain work hardening assessment

Jeanette (post CVA): to prioritize homemaking tasks to safely resume aspects of meal preparation and home maintenance roles

Wendy (post THR): to identify strategies to enable return to work

Brenda (post CVA): to organize child care tasks and identify strategies for more fully resuming tasks previously performed in mothering role

Juanita (post hip fracture): to assist with understanding and adjustment to current precautions and disability status

Description of methods and procedures: Expressive art activity and group discussion.

Rationale: To increase trust and member sharing of thoughts/feelings to facilitate sense of universality, and to foster group support, cohesion, problem solving, and goal setting by establishing an environment that encourages free expression of common concerns paired with group support and problem solving about how to address concerns.

Description of leadership role:

• Encourage expression of fears and perceptions in here and now through verbal and nonverbal means.
• Clarify group goals and task.

Rationale: To enable group to establish a balance of individual and group goals and ensure that the group is a safe place to express concerns.

Describe necessary preparations: Gather art materials.

List material and equipment needed:

Magazines/newspapers (including a variety of precut magazine pictures/words representative of work, family member, leisure roles, etc.)

Alphabet stickers

Glue sticks

Scissors

8" × 11" poster board

Time and sequence outline for session:

1. Introduce group to activity: state purpose, goals, and methods. (5 minutes)
2. Encourage group members to create individual collages as a means of identifying what is important to them in terms of time/energy use or describing feelings or concerns they have as they go through the process of community re-entry. (10 minutes)
3. Members make collages with leader assistance/adaptation as necessary. Members are encouraged to help each other and ask for help when needed. (approximately 30 minutes)

4. Encourage members to show collages and share verbally what they identified. Process relationship to group's goals, and identify individual member goals related to any insights gained through activity or group discussion. Summarize common themes in regard to members' values, interests, goals, roles, and concerns. (15 minutes)

Other information pertinent to this specific session *(i.e., any new members, co-leaders, or guests? Is there an unusual tone in the group or event that is about to occur or has occurred that may be affecting members' mood or participation?):* There may be possible effect due to time of year (weather, holiday season).

Case Study #3: Community-Based Group ⸺⸺⸺⸺⸺⸺⸺⸺

GROUP HISTORY:

General status: *How long has the group been in existence? What is its anticipated duration? How often and for how long does the group meet? What is its general stage and level of development? Who has authority over goals and structure of the group?*
This is a new group that is to be formed for the first time. It is to be 10 weeks in duration. The members are to be senior citizens living in the community surrounding the senior center. The director of the center has contracted with an occupational therapist, who will be responsible for designing, overseeing implementation (via weekly supervision with group leaders), and evaluating the group.

Leadership and membership criteria: *How was the group leadership and membership determined (i.e., assigned, voluntary or involuntary, referral)? If it is a closed group, what criteria are used to select the members? What was prior group leadership style?*
The group leaders will be the wellness director of the senior center, who will be assisted by one of the center's volunteers. The membership will be voluntary and composed of members identified as frail elders who currently attend the senior center who might benefit from the additional attention and structure the group will provide. Prospective members will be interviewed and asked to join the group. The group will be a closed group of seven to nine members. It will meet once a week for 90 minutes.

Group structure and current membership: *What is the group structure (format, general purpose, methodology)? How stable is the group membership? What is the rate of attendance? Is it an open or closed group? If it is an open group, are there any new members in the group? How long have the new and old members been in the group?*
Not applicable as this is a new group.

Outcomes: *What outcomes have the group as a whole accomplished? What have individual members achieved? In what way has the group or leadership been unsuccessful?*
Not applicable as this is a new group.

Comments: *Are there any other factors pertinent to understanding, assessing, and planning for the group?*
This group is being designed for center members who may need more support physically or emotionally to engage in center activities. An occupational therapist will be consulting on the design and implementation of the group, providing weekly meetings with group leaders, and occasionally observing group members in order to make specific recommendations concerning group process and means of enhancing members' functioning (i.e., assessment of member functioning, use of adaptive devices, methods of cognitive cuing, leadership strategies).

ASSESSMENT OF MEMBERS AND CONTEXT:

Assessment of group members *(client profile, including range of behaviors, why seeking services, desired goals/outcomes):*

General description: The group meets at the senior center, which is a community center for senior citizens in a suburban neighborhood. Center members are primarily local residents and come to the center from their homes. Education ranges from high school graduate to higher education. The members interviewed for this small group are frail elders who have ongoing medical difficulties, which include various levels of dementia, post stroke, arthritis, diabetes, low vision, and hearing loss. One person has been receiving chemotherapy for cancer, and some are experiencing grief and depression. Ages range from 70 to 95 years. The group is to have five women and two men.

General description of members' expected environment: Participants currently visit the senior center 1 or 2 days a week. Some live independently, others in the home of a relative. Roles include grandparent, parent, friend, community member, and family member.

Description of current occupational performance:

Education/work: Members are retired, and none are participating in volunteer roles outside of center community service activities. None are participating in adult education at this time.

Self-care (ADLs/IADLs): Members demonstrate a range of self-care ability from independent to partially dependent on assistance. Home health aides, relatives, and/or household help assist with bathing, dressing, and other personal needs. Meals are delivered to some members, and others eat with their families. Transportation to the center is provided by friends or relatives and occasionally by taxi or center minibus.

Play/leisure: Information regarding use of leisure time and interests was vague. Family members instigate most leisure activities/outings. Most leisure pursuits are solitary and quiet/passive, including television, reading, crossword/word search puzzles (large print), handicrafts (needlepoint/cross stitch), or card games with family members. Outings generally are to dine out, attend spiritual activities (church, synagogue), or participate in larger gatherings (holiday meals, family reunions, weddings, funerals).

Social participation: Members arrive at the center between 9 and 10 a.m. Some have tea or coffee, which is provided for them by the center volunteers, but few of them participate in center activities.

STRENGTHS AND DEFICITS IN MOTOR AND PROCESS SKILLS:

Physical and neuromotor: Members demonstrate various levels of ambulatory ability. Three use walkers, one a cane. Some have visual or hearing deficits. A few appear to have fine-motor coordination, strength, and range-of-motion deficits. All members appear able to maintain sufficient balance to perform tabletop activities.

Cognitive: Members understood that the purpose of the pre-group interview was to seek membership in the new group. All are oriented to time, place, and person.

Psychosocial: Two members appeared withdrawn at the time of the interview; an accompanying relative gave most of the information. One member seemed confused and appeared to be having trouble with her hearing aid. Others appeared reluctant to initiate conversation, although they appeared to understand the questions asked, and their answers were appropriate.

What is the significance of these factors with regard to forming the group, setting individual member goals, and/or planning group session(s)?
Group leaders will need to provide a group structure with activities as well as a physically and emotionally safe climate while encouraging members to interact in the group. The leaders will have to assume an active role in adapting activities and assume membership and leadership roles when members are unable to do so. A supportive and genuine emotional climate will need to be established and reinforced by the leaders.

ASSESSMENT OF GROUP CONTEXT (THE FACILITY):

General description of program *(mission, administrative structure):* The senior center is a community-based center for senior citizens. It is funded by grant money, city funds, and private funds. There is a board of directors that oversees the administration of the center. There is an administrator who makes policy and administrative decisions in conjunction with the board. The administrator, a social worker, is directly responsible for staff selection and the program. The administrator, in consultation with the board, engaged the occupational therapist to design the new group and negotiated the funds for her consultation fees. The center is assisted by a dedicated group of volunteers who help lead activities and assist in the daily functions of the center.

General description of physical environment: The senior center is a modern, two-story building with a large recreation room, kitchen and eating area, and meeting rooms on the first floor. Offices and additional meeting rooms are located on the second floor. There is a large parking lot in the back that provides direct ground-level entrance. In the room where the group will meet, there are cupboards, a sink, and a rectangular table. The room is well lighted and has a row of windows on one wall. The room is easily accessible for walkers, wheelchairs, etc.

General description of emotional climate: The general climate at the center is friendly and warm. Members are supportive of one another in particular. The objective is to help participants age in place: remaining as independent as possible, living in their home environment where they are happiest and the quality of their lives is maximized.

Frame of reference, purpose, and objectives: The purpose of the center is to meet the ongoing needs of community-dwelling elders from a biopsychosocial perspective.

What is the significance of these factors with regard to forming the group, setting individual member goals, and/or planning group session(s)?
The structure of the senior center allows for the creation of a weekly closed group where the same participants come every Wednesday morning. A review of the group structure and process will be done weekly.

ENVIRONMENTAL SUPPORTS AND CONSTRAINTS:

Facilities and materials: It is possible to carry out a wide range of activities while sitting around the table. Other rooms might be available should more private space be required. Materials are available for the group in the cupboard, and special purchases can be made as needed. An assistant to the group leader will be available from the group of experienced volunteers, and time will be allowed for the volunteer and the leader to plan and discuss the group sessions. The volunteer has agreed to attend the group consistently for 10 weeks.

Scheduling: This group is scheduled to meet on Wednesday mornings from 10:00 to 11:30 a.m. in the activity room. The time allows for transportation to be complete and is an optimal time in terms of member energy levels. The duration has been selected to give participants ample time to complete the short-term activities without feeling hurried.

Group norms and prior therapy group experience (if any): Group participation will be voluntary. Members will be asked to attend weekly and encouraged to participate fully. Physical or verbally abusive behaviors will not be acceptable.

Do any of the environmental constraints require modification of the group, or could the situation be altered?
None at present.

FUNCTIONAL GROUP PROTOCOL:

Name of group: "Time Flies"

Time/length of meeting(s): Wednesday, 10:00–11:30 a.m.

Place: Senior Center Activity Room

Group format: Closed

Rationale: To limit the number of participants and to have a stable group of similar abilities.

General group goals: Members will:

• Interact verbally with other group members.
• Participate actively in the group.
• Contribute ideas to the selection of group activities.
• Find ways to reminisce and enjoy themselves during group activities.

Rationale for goal selection: Members are either at risk of or experience social isolation. Members manifest various levels of decreased role performance as well as decreased ability and competence in the areas of physical, cognitive, and psychosocial skill performance.

Outcome criteria for successful goal attainment in session(s) stated in behavioral terms: During each session, each member will:

• Contribute verbally to the group at least once by expressing his or her thoughts or reminiscences to another group member or commenting about the group activity.
• Take steps to help complete the group activity.
• Show pleasure or increased comfort level in the group by smiling or evidencing signs of decreased irritability or agitation.

Group composition and criteria for selecting members: Group consists of five females and two males. Prospective members must express voluntary desire to join the group.

Leadership roles and functions: The group is composed of a leader and one volunteer; they will plan and evaluate the group sessions together. The leaders will seek suggestions and encourage input from members in planning activities and sessions. Leaders will also model desired group behavior, i.e., listening, participating verbally, showing support, and giving feedback. While maintaining the group structure, the leaders will seek to adapt to the changing needs and dynamics of the group. Leaders will allow the group the freedom to adapt the plans to their needs and preferences within a safe and caring environment.

Characteristics of group contract: Participants, once they have been chosen, are expected to attend and participate in the group activities each week for 10 weeks, sending word via center staff if they will be absent. Leaders and members are expected to keep conversations held in the group confidential when away from the group.

GROUP METHODS AND PROCEDURES TO BE EMPLOYED:

- Structured group tasks within range of member ability.
- Modification of group process and adaptation of task as needed.
- Simple structured interactive activities.
- Crafts, role validation activities, life review/reminiscence activities.
- Leader guidance for discussion and leader assistance with activities as needed.

SESSION PLAN:

Name of group: "Time Flies"

Date: September 7

Session: Making Scrapbook pages; 3rd of 10 sessions

Specific goals for the group session: Members will:

- Share materials and meaningful verbal exchange through activity and reminiscence.
- Participate actively in creating scrapbook pages on verbal or nonverbal level (i.e., stating preferences/likes/dislikes in choice of materials, engaging in conversation about memories of own or other members' life events).
- Express feelings (of enjoyment, sadness, etc.) regarding activity and/or life events in a socially appropriate manner during the group.

Specific goals for group members:
- Sophie: often anxious due to her mild dementia, to demonstrate comfort in the group setting via engaging in scrapbooking task with familiar objects (personal picture or memorabilia) and/or in conversation with leaders or other members about personal memories.
- Agnes: easily fatigued, to attend and remain involved in the activity for the entire session with short rest breaks as needed.
- Tom: to ask for assistance when needed vs. discontinuing the task.
- Betty: to be more open to ideas of others and relate more positively with leaders and members (vs. presenting as negative or hopeless i.e., "beyond needing or being worthy of support").

- Irina: to communicate effectively with leaders and members.
- Clara: to interact more with leaders and members.
- Joe: to focus more on engaging in task and discussion with members (vs. constantly chatting and joking about center staff/volunteers).

Description and rationale for methods and procedures:

- Provide members with an individual task that can facilitate group-centered sharing and discussion as well as leisure interest that can be pursued at home or in senior center outside of group sessions. Leaders will prepare and show scrapbook with pages made of the same materials as a model so that members can have an idea of what their finished product might look like.
- Provide an activity that adapts comfortably to the different skill levels of individual members. The materials for making the scrapbook pages range from applying stickers to gluing on craft store foam, paper, and fabric cutouts/appliqués. Members will be encouraged to ask for help from leaders and other group members should they need help.
- Additional materials will be available to allow members opportunity to engage in making additional scrapbook pages to create their own scrapbook outside of the group or senior center (i.e., at home, with family) should members (or their family/caretaker) identify this activity as a meaningful/enjoyable way to interact and reminisce.

Rationale: Decrease sense of isolation and build group cohesiveness through sharing of memories and materials.

Description of leadership role:

- Help members understand the purpose of the group's activity.
- Encourage and facilitate group members' participation in activity, sharing of materials/memories, and getting to know one another more through conversation.
- Provide cueing as needed and promote group discussion and interaction.

Rationale: To instill feelings of safety and belonging in the group.

Describe necessary preparations: Review session plan with co-leader.
Purchase scrapbook supplies necessary for group activity. Prepare four different sample scrapbook pages. Remind members, in person the afternoon prior and via follow-up phone call on morning of the group, of the activity plan and that they are to try to bring at least one photo or memorabilia item (postcard, newspaper clipping) for scrapbook activity.

List material and equipment needed:
Scrapbook pages of several colors so that group members can choose a color
     Old issues of *Time/Life/Newsweek* or travel magazines; precut magazine pictures

Postcards of local attractions

Scrapbook appliqués, stickers, photo corners, etc.,

Craft glue, glue sticks, markers, scissors, cropping tools (i.e., pinking shears to cut artful edges)

Sample completed scrapbook pages/scrapbook

Time and sequence outline for sessions, including what you will do and say as leader and what group is expected to do:

- Greetings and distribution of member name tags. (10 minutes)
- Introduction to group activity, purpose, goals, and methods, with visual cueing. Show model of scrapbook pages and point out how different materials were used. (10 minutes)
- Members choose scrapbook materials, with assistance as needed, from bins passed around, which are then placed around the table as space permits. (10 minutes)
- Members assemble scrapbook page with assistance of leaders and adaptations in approach to task as per occupational therapy consultant's recommendations as necessary (i.e., table-top magnifying lens, securing project to table with dycem, encouraging use of both hands, adapted scissors, etc.). Leaders assume task and maintenance roles as needed to facilitate group members' participation in task and/or discussion about feelings, memorabilia, memories, or scrapbook supplies. Members are encouraged to help each other and to ask for help and feedback about page arrangement as needed. (40 minutes)
- Bring activity to closure. Reassure any members who have yet to complete their page that there will be opportunities to do so, either within or outside of group. Ask members to rate their satisfaction or dissatisfaction with the scrapbook activity or group session (rate on a scale of 1 = satisfied to 10 = dissatisfied) and to discuss their ratings as member is able or time allows.

Other information pertinent to this specific session *(any new members, co-leaders, or guests? Is there an unusual tone in the group or event that is about to occur or has occurred that may be affecting members' mood or participation?):*
Occupational therapy consultant will be observing as part of contractual arrangement for feedback and supervision/mentoring of group leaders. Leaders will introduce consultant and briefly address her role as observer at beginning of session.

Completed Forms for Chapter 6 Case Studies

Case Study #1:
Open Group on an Inpatient Psychiatry Unit

SESSION EVALUATION:

Name of group: "Getting It Together"

Session activity: Icebreaker: "What's in a Name?"

Date: Monday, June 6

Leaders: Lauri Levy, OTR/L; Jack Jones, MHC

Were the goals accomplished? (*state outcome and give rationale in terms of whether the session was helpful in addressing group and individual member goals*):
Partially. Gary had difficulty taking turns speaking in the group and interrupted several times while other group members were talking. Betty, a new group member who was sitting to Gary's right, remained in the group for 10 minutes and departed, saying she was too "nervous" to sit any longer. Jack paired off with Gary for the remainder of the session and worked on providing feedback to Gary concerning how he felt when Gary kept interrupting him and other members in the group. All other members accomplished the session goals. Eric was able to explain ground rules to new members. Liz suggested another idea (anagrams of first name) for learning about others' names and how they would describe themselves. Betty has displayed inability to attend other groups on the unit, so it was good that she stayed for at least the introduction phase.

Do you have any information that indicates the session(s) has/have been helpful to the members' functioning (adaptation) outside of the group? *(explain):*

Yes. The leaders observed group members chatting informally on the unit at dinner immediately after the group session.

Was the group structure adequate for accomplishing the goals? *(give rationale, taking into consideration: leadership; time/length of meeting; open- vs. closed-group format; sequence, methods, and procedures; media/modalities/techniques employed; norms/behaviors reinforced implicitly or explicitly; methods of reinforcement; and stage of group's development):*

Partially. For most of the group members, the structure established a nonthreatening climate. Leaders provided modeling and cues to group as a whole to acknowledge Betty's departure and thanking her for coming as well as stating her reason for leaving. Leaders indicated to Betty that they understood being in a group was challenging for her and that they looked forward to her joining them for a little longer next session. Jack (co-leader) wondered aloud if Gary realized he had interrupted others and shared with group how he did not feel heard by Gary when Gary interrupted him, as a means of modeling feedback. Leaders need to reconsider planned use of subgrouping, especially if Betty is in attendance. It appeared to make Betty more anxious and overwhelm her further due to a fairly sudden demand for interaction and with a male group member.

Did the structure provide for "optimal experience" or a "flow state" to occur? *(explain):*

For the most part, members seemed absorbed in the activity and to generally converse or interact in a spontaneous manner when paired with another member. However, the leaders needed to take a more directive role during group discussions, cuing members to share what was learned and to use strategies of referring to what was written down to help remind themselves about what peers said they liked or disliked about their name. Discussion regarding how members felt about activity was more difficult, requiring more leader structure of dialogue as well.

Did the structure provide optimal purposeful, self-initiated, spontaneous, and group-centered action to allow meaningful interaction, enhanced performance skills, and/or adaptation to occur through "occupation"? *(explain):*

Given the group's being in a formation stage of development, the structure did encourage members to interact and enabled them to learn something about each other's names. With leader input, seven of the eight members completed the structured group task and participated in some aspect of group discussion.

Did the structure provide for new learning or reinforcement of current level of functioning or occupational performance, or did it reinforce functioning below current level of ability? *(explain):*

The structure seemed to encouraged all members to see the value of putting forth one's best effort and to use the support of others in a group. Strategies of written expression to identify feelings or assist with remembering information were also practiced. Except for Betty, the range of group processes enabled members to participate at a parallel through cooperative level.

Did the structure provide an opportunity for evaluation and feedback regarding the group procedures, process, and member progress? *(explain):*
Yes. Members were encouraged to discuss their reactions to the session and ideas for future sessions. The leaders had ample opportunity to observe member behavior/reactions to varying amounts of task structure.

What changes would you make regarding group goals and structure for the next session or if you were to lead this session again?
Betty might be offered increased female leader support, and/or she might avoid activities that require subgroup pairings to increase her sense of safety in the group. Also, considerations need to be given to extra time needed when translation is needed.

Were you adequately prepared for the session? *(give rationale, taking into consideration time, place, materials, and physical and emotional environment):*
Partially. Knowing there would be four new members was essential to the preparations, including planning a structured exercise to learn names. Perhaps an alternate agreement ("contract") for Betty would have been more empowering for her to identify when to leave (i.e., after 10 minutes).

How did you function as leader? *(How did your behavior and role affect the group? What did you do that was effective? Were there opportunities for leader intervention that may have been missed? What did you learn about yourselves as group leaders?):*
When Gary had difficulty taking turns and Betty said she was leaving the group, Jack had to assume more group task roles and therefore felt he was working too hard to consciously try to model group maintenance roles through his interactions with Gary (risking rift in therapeutic rapport). However, members responded by imitation and began to encourage each other to listen and share. This was effective because it helped to model group norms and encouraged group-centered participation, but it inadvertently created a sense of more authority in Lauri's role as "leader" and "mother." Transferences about Lauri being "good enough" seem to have emerged. Lauri remembers thinking about this when responding to Betty's departure and in wondering about how to respond to group members' perceptions of her as reflected in some of their comments/jokes (i.e., "Yes, mother"; "You sound like my wife/mother"; "What are you, my mother?").

Was the group interaction as you anticipated? *(explain; if problems occurred, what can you identify as a basis for understanding the problems?):*

We did not anticipate the effect that Betty's leaving would have on the group. The expectation that she remain in the group for 45 minutes was unrealistic and appeared to overwhelm her. We did not feel prepared to address the transferences and issues of rejection that emerged in conversation at that point, as well as the now obvious symbolic connection of activity to parental figures. Accepting Liz's suggestion of anagram of name as an alternate approach to task seemed to help shift member focus back to "getting to know one another."

In the future, what might you do differently as group leaders? *(give rationale):*
We might make alternate agreements ("contracts") with patients who need to grade the amount of time spent in the group to decrease other members' sense of rejection. For example, Betty could have been told she could try contracting to stay in the group for 10 minutes the first time, 15 minutes the second, and so on, thereby encouraging success and establishing helpful limits. We need to more carefully consider symbolic level of icebreaker activities as well as effect of one co-leader assuming increased member role to consider how to keep co-leader balance. Co-ed co-leadership does afford opportunities to explore some of the transferences; however, nature of hospitalization is short-term and focus is problem identification. Therefore, issues that lead to member regression need to be reframed as something worthy of considering when in an appropriate context and member feels ready/strong enough emotionally to do so. More frequent reminders to members of group name ("Getting It Together") as being linked to working together as a group to support one another in increasing one's ability to function (vs. falling apart emotionally and/or decreasing one's ability to manage day to day) may be worthwhile. This may also serve as a helpful cognitive reframe for members.

Case Study #2:
Closed Group in an Outpatient Occupational Therapy Clinic

SESSION EVALUATION:

Name of group: Community Re-entry: "Moving Forward"

Date: December 15, second of eight sessions

Session: "What I Value" (prioritizing concerns and time/energy use)

Leaders: Russell Lee, MS OTR/L; Alicia Wright, COTA/L

Were the goals accomplished? *(state outcome and give rationale):*
Partially. Members expressed their individual frustrations and fears about discharge from treatment and a pervading sense of loss. However, only one or two members saw the value of the group as a means of support, asking questions such as: "How will talking about this

change anything?" One member expressed dislike of collage activity, wanting instead to write out list of member concerns on dry erase board.

Was the session helpful in addressing short- and long-term group and individual member goals?

Partially. Some members were able to identify a feeling of belonging to the group in that there were common themes to members' fears, frustrations, and concerns. However, several still questioned "What will being in this group do?" and yet seemed to need increased support around their feelings of loss. This tension seemed to suggest a need for individual member needs and goals and group goals to be further negotiated and tested in order for the group as a whole and individual members to experience a balance between the two in the group.

Do you have any information that indicates the session(s) has/have been helpful to the members' functioning (adaptation) outside of the group? *(explain):*

Not at this time. One member identified that she would like to learn more about getting assistance in her home e.g., getting a home health aide was mentioned as a possible way to address concerns during brainstorming).

Was the group structure adequate for accomplishing the goals? *(give rationale, taking into consideration: leadership; time/length of meeting; open- vs. closed-group format; sequence, methods, and procedures; media/modalities/techniques employed; norms/behaviors reinforced implicitly or explicitly; methods of reinforcement; and stage of group's development):*

The benefit of the group activity was not easily apparent to members. A more structured goal-setting activity might be preferable for this early stage of the group's formation.

Did the structure provide for "optimal experience" or a "flow state" to occur? *(explain):*

No. Many members did not appear comfortable with the expressive art activity format and stated they needed more time to talk about their individual concerns and feelings of loss.

Did the structure provide optimal purposeful, self-initiated, spontaneous, and group-centered action to allow meaningful interaction, enhanced performance skills, and/or adaptation to occur through "occupation"? *(explain):*

No. As typical of a group in the formation stage, members appeared to have difficulty assuming responsibility for the group, questioning purpose of the group, and seemed to need more structure or leader approval or input when making group decisions.

Did the structure provide for new learning or reinforcement of current level of functioning or occupational performance, or reinforcement of functioning below current level of ability? *(explain):*

Members initially seemed overwhelmed with lack of structure in expressive art task as a way of identifying issues related to community re-entry, because of re-emergence of feelings of loss of meaningful tasks roles assumed prior to illness/injury. However, with validation, support, and encouragement, members were able to verbalize their individual concerns regarding managing life tasks and roles. By being encouraged to share these concerns, members began to talk about what they wanted rather than what their family and friends wanted. Once leaders identified common themes, members were able to acknowledge some commonalities in feelings and experiences.

Did the structure provide an opportunity for evaluation and feedback regarding the group procedures, process, and member progress? *(explain):*
Yes. Members were actively encouraged to give the leaders feedback verbally and in writing via session feedback form. Members identified what they wanted from leaders and areas they hoped to address in future sessions (e.g., community mobility).

What changes would you make regarding group goals and structure for the next session or if you were to lead this session again?
Offer more choices in terms of activity (e.g., art vs. journal worksheet), with the specific aim of airing member concerns to allow more opportunities for discussion prior to goal setting. Offer more group-centered visuals (dry erase posters/board) with some preset structure to allow room for broadening to members' input.

Were you adequately prepared for the session? *(give rationale, considering such elements as time, place, materials, and physical and emotional environment):*
We were not prepared for the extent to which members wanted to talk about their feelings of loss/anger. Collage activity seemed to serve more to remind them of losses in roles, opportunities, body image, etc., than was anticipated or intended.

How did you function as leaders? *(How did your behavior and role affect the group? What did you do that was effective? Were there opportunities for leader intervention that may have been missed? What did you learn about yourselves as group leaders?)*
Although the value of the group as a means of intervention and support is apparent to leaders, members seemed to need more time for discussion to learn what value it holds for them and how it will be helpful.

Was the group interaction as you anticipated? *(explain; if problems occurred, what do you hypothesize as a basis for understanding the problems?):*
We expected more group-centered action and member readiness to take initiative than was realistic this early in the group's formation stage. Members' personalities and circumstances suggest that they need more time and support to adjust and feel empowered to make changes necessary to improve their quality of life. Building member trust, increasing group cohesion, and finding activities that allow members to recognize elements of univer-

sality in their experiences as well as instilling hope about what is possible by talking together in the group seems indicated.

In the future, what might you do differently as group leaders? *(give rationale):*
Consider devoting a session or part of a session to issues of loss and change, perhaps with a guest speaker in a group session. Create a task structure that is more readily adapted to individual members' comfort with expression. This can allow us to facilitate group members feeling more empowered to make choices as a part of "moving forward" and thus promote a balance in members assuming group task and maintenance roles.

Case Study #3: Community-Based Group

SESSION EVALUATION:

Name of group: "Time Flies"

Date: September 7, 3rd of 10 sessions

Session: Scrapbooking

Leaders: Mary Munroe, Wellness Director; Sage Stilton, Volunteer

Consultant: Jacki Wright, OTD, OTR/L

Were the goals accomplished? *(state outcome and give rationale):*

• Member interaction: Members shared materials, and there was discussion about where to place individual items on scrapbook pages. Some members expressed their opinions regarding the activity and gave each other feedback.

• Group-centered activity: The activity was the idea of a group participant (suggested by Betty in the second session), and all members agreed to this choice of activity. Leaders were supportive of the group's ability to carry out the task by providing needed materials and guidance. Some members needed cuing to get started, but all participated to the level of their ability. Some members showed enjoyment of this activity by smiling, and a few expressed feeling satisfied with their finished product and a desire to continue the activity in future group sessions, with family member, or volunteer outside of group sessions.

Was the session helpful in addressing individual member and group goals?
Yes. Sophie appeared less confused about the task. She kept looking at the sample as she decided how to assemble her page. It seemed to present a concrete guide for her. Agnes stayed in the room during the entire session. This is the first time she has been able to do so. She

participated in the activity for the entire session, with rest breaks every 15 minutes. Tom was able to ask Betty to cut out a picture from a magazine for him. He also asked her for approval as to where to mount the picture on the page. Betty responded to Tom's request for help and gave him the reassurance that he seemed to need. Additionally, many members commented on similarity in experiences or feelings about past events. One member acknowledged feeling surprised to learn things about each other and feeling glad to be getting to know each other better. Others members were quiet but task-focused and receptive to peers feedback/comments.

Do you have any information that indicates the session(s) has/have been helpful to the members' functioning (adaptation) outside of the group? *(explain):*
We have noticed some members congregating during the morning coffee hour (while awaiting arrival of other center members and beginning of morning group).

Was the group structure adequate for accomplishing the goals? *(give rationale, taking into consideration: leadership; time/length of meeting; open- vs. closed-group format; sequence, methods, and procedures; media/modalities/techniques employed; norms/behaviors reinforced implicitly or explicitly; methods of reinforcement; and stage of group's development):*
A closed-group format seems to be helping members to get to know each other. Socialization is an important goal of this group. The duration of this group is adequate for accomplishing goals. Time was needed for the members to gather personal memorabilia, greet each other, remember each other's names, and orient themselves to the task at hand. Time will continue to be needed to review activities done to date, topics discussed, and the decisions made at the previous meeting for members who are experiencing memory loss. The sequence, methods, and procedures for the activity were well established. Presenting the model of a scrapbook with completed pages using the same materials seemed to help convey the concept of making scrapbooks together as a way to reminisce and get to know each other better, which also served to clarify the activity goal. In this session, it became evident that this group appears to be well into the formation stage of group development.

Did the structure provide for "optimal experience" or a "flow state" to occur? *(explain):*
The flow state was slow in starting, but eventually all members became so involved in the activity that leaders had to cue them about time remaining in the session.

Did the structure provide optimal purposeful, self-initiated, spontaneous, and group-centered action to allow meaningful interaction, enhanced performance skills, and/or adaptation to occur through "occupation"? *(explain):*
The activity was requested by a group member and also purposeful in terms of facilitating interaction and reminiscence. It also involved self-initiated action in choices of page color, appliqués and placement of items. Spontaneous action was evident in members'

responses in conversation, emotional reactions, and recollections of past events or experiences. Group-centered action was demonstrated by a number of members through their comments to the group as a whole and active discussion about what to do in future sessions.

Did the structure provide for new learning or reinforcement of current level of functioning or occupational performance, or reinforcement of functioning below current level of ability? *(explain):*
The structure of the activity promoted reinforcement of skills, with an added task and emotional element to gently challenge the current level of functioning of the members. It enabled members to participate at a parallel through cooperative group level. The activity helped to reinforce life roles of the past or present. The group structure and task also facilitated member participation in group task and maintenance roles, such as the role of help/opinion-giver in support of others seeking help or feedback. Members were able to express concerns about absence of one member, which suggests the group members are beginning to see themselves as a group rather than a collection of individuals working on a similar task.

Did the structure provide an opportunity for evaluation and feedback regarding the group procedures, process, and member progress? *(explain):*
We provided ongoing positive feedback to members regarding their efforts and productivity. Feedback was directed to individuals as well as the group as a whole. A separate processing period was included in the session plan as well as a verbal structure by which we could obtain direct feedback from the members regarding this activity. We were also able to observe member reactions to and comments about the various parts of the task.

What changes would you make regarding group goals and structure for the next session or if you were to lead this session again?
The following changes may facilitate members more readily engaging in scrapbooking task:

• Mark some of the blank scrapbook pages with guidelines for where materials can be placed if members wish to copy sample (thus providing more structure for those members in this step of the task). Making these decisions seemed a difficult step for some in regard to the "flow" of the activity.
• Use more precut images of themes, such as classic cars, historical people or events, period fashions, etc., as leafing through the magazines proved a distraction for some members.
• Provide small containers for members to take some materials (glue sticks, appliqués, etc.) to promote continued involvement in activity at home or center if desired.

Were you adequately prepared for the session? *(give rationale, considering such elements as time, place, materials, and physical and emotional environment):*
Yes. Given that this was the third session of the group, we felt more aware of the type of structure needed for the group to engage in more group-centered activity.

How did you function as leaders? *(How did your behavior and role affect the group? What did you do that was effective? Were there opportunities for leader intervention that were missed? What did you learn about yourselves as group leaders?)*

We functioned effectively as group leaders during this session. We were attentive to cues from group members and used those cues to direct or redirect the group and particular members. As leaders, we had carefully discussed with the occupational therapist consultant how we could work together in this group. As suggested, modeling collaborative behavior encouraged members to help each other. Sage took the role of being primarily involved with the task of the group, whereas Mary focused more on the physical and emotional needs of members to balance group task and maintenance functions within the group process. Although we had planned well for the group session, we continue to try to be flexible with the structure and follow the group's lead to support self-initiated and group-centered action whenever possible.

Was the group interaction as you anticipated? *(explain; if problems occurred, what do you hypothesize may be a basis for understanding the problems?):*

We did not anticipate members' concern about the absent member and wish we had created a "get well card" or something on which they could concretely convey their expressions of concern directly to her. However, expression of concern indicates a sense of group identity not previously manifested and suggests the group is becoming more cohesive and cooperative, on the whole, than in previous sessions.

In the future, what might you do differently as group leaders? *(give rationale):*

Perhaps be willing to take greater risk with allowing discussion around loss of friends and loved ones to support members with dealing with these ongoing issues and feelings of grief at different stages of life. With this group, we need to keep the activities positive and the tone of the group hopeful. Some members have said they feel they do not have the energy to be creative or productive at this stage of their lives. Therefore, leaders need to provide structured opportunities for creative expression and feeling productive. This can serve as a means for members to give and receive support as well as encouragement and a way to reality-test their perceptions about what they are, in fact, still capable of doing.

Completed Forms for Chapter 7 Case Studies

Case Study #1:

Open Group on an Inpatient Psychiatry Unit

SESSION EVALUATION:

Name of group: "Getting It Together"

Session Activity: Creating items for annual hospital flea market fundraiser

Date: Wednesday, June 8

Were the goals accomplished? (*state outcome and give rationale in terms of whether the session was helpful in addressing group and individual member goals*):

Yes. Liz was able to talk about fears and anger concerning losing leaders' attention. Maggie was able to express anxiety verbally as well. Eric was open regarding his mixed feelings about the group, and Gary was able to tolerate reality testing his wish for the leaders to do more for him. Lakisha was able to acknowledge her improved ability to make decisions as related to her readiness to return to work. Li was able to assist Eric by decorating the wood projects Eric built but, because the hospital translator was absent, could not participate in or benefit from discussion. All members participated in creating craft projects for the fundraiser, some completed items individually while Pearl, Maggie, and Betty worked in pairs or generally assisted others, resulting in 12 items being produced.

Do you have any information that indicates the session(s) has/have been helpful to the members' functioning (adaptation) outside of the group? (*explain*):

Lakisha has been actively addressing returning to work as part of her disposition plan.

Was the group structure adequate for accomplishing the goals? *(give rationale, taking into consideration: leadership; time/length of meeting; open- vs. closed-group format; sequence, methods, and procedures; media/modalities/techniques employed; norms/ behaviors reinforced implicitly or explicitly; methods of reinforcement; and stage of group's development):*

The group structure and format seemed to allow for a balance of group processing and group product/task focus. The members were able to tolerate leaders reinforcing their ability to make decisions and function more interdependently. Members seemed empowered to address individual and group needs and goals via the variety of choices and potential roles the arts and crafts media allowed. The group norms of participation and verbalizing feelings seem to be facilitating more member self-expression and allowing the group to function at times at an egocentric-cooperative level. The group seemed to be more cohesive, providing a supportive and containing environment.

Did the structure provide for "optimal experience" or a "flow state" to occur? *(explain):*

Yes. The diversity of media allowed for members to engage in "helping," either symbolically (for fundraiser) or literally via their role in task production. Betty remaining the entire session was a significant outcome/achievement likely related somewhat to the group structure providing her (as well as other members) "just the right challenge" in terms of amount of verbal processing and hands-on elements.

Did the structure provide optimal purposeful, self-initiated, spontaneous, and group-centered action to allow meaningful interaction, enhanced performance skills, and/or adaptation to occur through "occupation"? *(explain):*

Yes. Again, the media allowed for each member to identify and initiate those tasks they found meaningful and then engage in them in a group-centered way through the context of the purposeful nature of the tasks and overall group goal (products for fundraiser).

Did the structure provide for new learning or reinforcement of current level of functioning or occupational performance, or did it reinforce functioning below current level of ability? *(explain):*

Somewhat. All members were able to engage on some level in social participation. Lakisha was able to make the connection between what she is accomplishing in terms of decision making and her upcoming return to her work role. Eric was able to speak to the variability in his level of comfort with the group context and content. Betty appeared to contain her anxiety via participation in activity to remain the entire session. Pearl and Gary were able to work together; however, some caution needs to be taken to avoid possible codependency in their pairing. Liz and Maggie were able to openly address positive and negative emotions without becoming regressed.

Did the structure provide an opportunity for evaluation and feedback regarding the group procedures, process, and member progress? *(explain):*

Yes. We were able to reality-test member perceptions of our role and close the group in a manner that identified the group's and individual members' accomplishments. There was an increase of initiative in member participation in directing the closing ritual (i.e., Liz identifying she feels she has developed bonds with other group members).

What changes would you make regarding group goals and structure for the next session or if you were to lead this session again?

As the group identifies a sense of cohesion and interdependence, we will need to work more actively on addressing upcoming transitions/discharges. Also, monitoring the pairing of Gary/Pearl will be important so as to not overlook potential subgrouping that could become dysfunctional or disruptive to the group process.

Were you adequately prepared for the session? *(give rationale, taking into consideration time, place, materials, and physical and emotional environment):*

Yes. The choice and setup of arts-and-crafts materials (beading, birdhouses, bookends) proved realistically achievable within the time frame of the session. The added emotional component of doing a "service" for the children's unit appeared highly motivating to all members.

How did you function as leaders? *(How did your behavior and role affect the group? What did you do that was effective? Were there opportunities for leader intervention that may have been missed? What did you learn about yourselves as group leaders?):*

Jack was better able to balance his leader/member role, and Lauri was not so dominant because group activity and structure possibly provided containment for member's anxieties, projections, and transferences. There were likely potential opportunities missed to elicit verbal participation from Betty and to increase independent participation from Pearl. However, due to the fact that previous sessions have been somewhat conflict-laden and emotionally charged, we opted to give members time to increase their sense of safety and build trust with each other. It seemd that Lauri gave more process commentary and Jack provided more support with tasks or via redirection.

Was the group interaction as you anticipated? *(explain; if problems occurred, what can you identify as a basis for understanding the problems?):*

The group seemed more interactive than we anticipated. One hypothesis may be that Gary's medication is helping to mitigate his mania. Therefore, Gary was able to process the feedback he has received from Jack and other members concerning the effect of his manic symptoms on them and his ability to participate in meaningful activities.

In the future, what might you do differently as group leaders? *(give rationale):*

Our redirection/limit setting may need to be more directed at cuing clients to problem-solve tasks before asking us to help.

Case Study #2:
Closed Group in an Outpatient Occupational Therapy Clinic——————

SESSION EVALUATION:

Name of group: Community Re-entry: "Moving Forward"

Session activity: Energy conservation, adapting activities or environment, pain management

Date: December 17; fourth of eight sessions

Leaders: Russell Lee, MS, OTR/L; Alicia Wright, COTA/L

Were the goals accomplished? *(state outcome and give rationale):*
Yes. Members were able to express concerns about being dependent on their families and their anger toward leaders for not allowing the group to continue beyond eight sessions. Members were able to demonstrate some energy conservation techniques.

Was the session helpful in addressing short- and long-term group and individual member goals?
Yes. As members articulated their feelings, they were able to acknowledge fear of losing support of leaders. Once feelings were validated, members were able to move on to set realistic goals for remaining sessions.

Do you have any information that indicates the session(s) has/have been helpful to the members' functioning (adaptation) outside of the group? *(explain):*
Yes. Some members identified that written instructions in a handout would be helpful in terms of implementing strategies at home.

Was the group structure adequate for accomplishing the goals? *(give rationale, taking into consideration: leadership; time/length of meeting; open- vs. closed-group format; sequence, methods, and procedures; media/modalities/techniques employed; norms/behaviors reinforced implicitly or explicitly; methods of reinforcement; and stage of group's development):*
The pace seemed too rushed due to time constraints, multiple media/energy conservation stations, and members' ongoing needs for processing feelings. The group has developed some cohesion and become more group-centered; thus, the didactic portion was too leader-centered.

Did the structure provide for "optimal experience" or a "flow state" to occur? *(explain):*
Not consistently due to variability of format and differing amounts of member comfort with didactic portion and work task simulations. More opportunity was needed for problem solving and practice.

Did the structure provide optimal purposeful, self-initiated, spontaneous, and group-centered action to allow meaningful interaction, enhanced performance skills, and/or adaptation to occur through "occupation"? *(explain):*

No. More group problem solving and open-ended time for member identification of problem situations for more meaningful simulations would have been helpful to more fully engage members during practice of techniques.

Did the structure provide for new learning or reinforcement of current level of role functioning or occupational performance, or did it reinforce functioning below current level of ability? *(explain):*
Partially. All members attempted to practice the techniques and discussed how and why they felt the procedures would or would not work at home.

Did the structure provide an opportunity for evaluation and feedback regarding the group procedures, process, and member progress? (e*xplain):*
Yes. The work simulation gave members an opportunity to give each other feedback and practice exercises and gave the leaders a chance to observe.

What changes would you make regarding group goals and structure for the next session or if you were to lead this session again?
Elicit suggestions in the third session regarding situations that members find difficult due to decreased energy, mobility issues, or pain. Rework didactic to be more group-centered and engaging.

Were you adequately prepared for the session? *(give rationale, taking into consideration time, place, materials, and physical and emotional environment):*
Not fully. The goals were unrealistic for the time allotted and different materials would have been helpful for more meaningful work simulations.

How did you function as leader? *(How did your behavior and role affect the group? What did you do that was effective? Were there opportunities for leader intervention that may have been missed? What did you learn about yourselves as group leaders?)*
We were effective in providing information and support through structure and allowed for group-centered support and problem solving to emerge by classifying common themes, issues, and highlighting members' suggestions regarding alternative approaches to tasks. As leaders we are still too reliant on our plans, possibly fearing we will not "educate" our members enough. This may be related to our own frustrations with the limited time we have to spend with our clients (i.e., system/institutional transference regarding health-care limits on us as providers).

Was the group interaction as you anticipated? *(explain; if problems occurred, what can you identify as a basis for understanding the problems?):*
The group members were somewhat angrier than expected. This may be because of the holiday season and related feelings regarding residual loss in functioning and impending discharge from outpatient services as loss of support system through group.

In the future, what might you do differently as group leaders? *(give rationale):*
Divide group into two subgroups for practice session to increase member time for sharing and
decrease time required for work simulations. Consider ways to openly address feelings of frustration regarding limits posed on leaders and members by reality of health-care system.

Case Study #3: Community-Based Group

SESSION EVALUATION:

Name of group: "Time Flies"

Session activity: Greeting cards; part II: collaborative verse

Date: October 12, 6th of 10 sessions

Leaders: Mary Munroe, Wellness Director; Sage Stilton, Volunteer

Consultant: Jacki Wright, OTD, OTR/L

Were the goals accomplished? *(state outcome and give rationale):*
Partially. The reminiscence experience did not encourage the expression of thoughts and feelings in the "here and now"; however, members did express feelings about the activity in the
"here and now" discussion at the end of the session. All members participated in the activity,
but Tom required leaders support to find a way to participate in collaborative verse construction (reading topics aloud). Betty and Irina said they did not enjoy it. They were encouraged
to take a more active role in the planning of activities in the future.

Was the session helpful in addressing individual member and group goals?
Partially. Tom practically reverted to nonparticipation in the task. Activity dragged somewhat
and felt very leader-directed. Betty and Irina needed redirection at times concerning subgrouping. Clara was able to share her feelings about level of task difficulty. Sophie demonstrated progress in her initiative in passing out name tags. Because Joe assisted Agnes, this
seemed to facilitate his being much more engaged with his peers. Many members were able
to share reminiscences about special occasions and greeting cards.

**Do you have any information that indicates the session(s) has/have been helpful to the
members' functioning (adaptation) outside of the group?**
Partially. Some members are continuing to meet for coffee before the group, and today Joe
suggested they eat lunch together after the group.

Was the group structure adequate for accomplishing the goals? *(give rationale, taking into
consideration: leadership; time/length of meeting; open- vs. closed-group format; sequence,*

*methods, and procedures; media/modalities/techniques employed; norms/behaviors rein-
forced implicitly or explicitly; methods of reinforcement; and stage of group's development):*
Yes. However, some members were only superficially involved in the writing. All members
of the group did get involved in reminiscence, brainstorming, or constructing the final product, owing in part to the group norm that has developed in which all group members participate in the activity and verbal discussion at some level. Group leaders, as well as some
members, have reinforced this norm.

Did the structure provide for "optimal experience" or a "flow state" to occur? *(explain):*
Partially. This was evident in the less structured brainstorming aspect of the activity (round
robin) and the final construction of the cards (Tom). Some members found it difficult to contribute to the actual verse writing.

**Did the structure provide optimal purposeful, self-initiated, spontaneous, and group-
centered action to allow meaningful interaction, enhanced performance skills, and/or
adaptation to occur through "occupation"?** *(explain):*
Somewhat. However, more progress needs to be made. Members need to be more involved in
thinking through the activity selection and decision making needed to best meet the particular interests of the group.

**Did the structure provide for new learning or reinforcement of current level of func-
tioning or occupational performance, or did it reinforce functioning below current level
of ability?** *(explain):*
The overall group structure did provide for an expression of positive and negative feelings
about the group activity. Some members did learn that their opinions were respected and welcomed and that they could influence the group planning process and thereby increase the
amount of group satisfaction.

**Did the structure provide an opportunity for evaluation and feedback regarding the
group procedures, process, and member progress?** *(explain)*
Yes. The structured processing time at the end of the session assisted members' involvement
in evaluating member participation and the group's process.

**What changes would you make regarding group goals and structure for the next session
or if you were to lead this session again?**
We need a format that ensures members contribute to the selection of group tasks in a way
that reassures them that their ideas are welcome and supported. We need to reinforce that
members do possess the skills necessary to complete the task successfully and that it is fine
to ask for help from other members. Some members seem hesitant or fearful to test skills that
they may not have used recently. We also tried to emphasize that the group can assert more

control in changing or adapting the activity selection when it is not meeting their needs or maintaining their interest.

Were you adequately prepared for the session? *(give rationale, taking into consideration time, place, materials, and physical and emotional environment):*
Yes. The meeting started on time, leaders were prepared, materials were at hand, and there was a supportive and consistent emotional environment.

How did you function as leader? *(How did your behavior and role affect the group? What did you do that was effective? Were there opportunities for leader intervention that may have been missed? What did you learn about yourselves as group leaders?):*
We have an effective procedure for starting the group session. Sophie gave each person, including leaders, their name tags. We greeted everyone and asked how members were doing as an important event (Olga announced going to hospice) had happened in our last meeting. A review of the last session followed (including the process of selecting the activity for today). This opening part of the group session seems to be effective in creating a mutually helping and safe, caring environment, creating a feeling of group cohesiveness. However, some members still seem to require time to readjust to the environment and climate of the group, and additional comments or possible changes to the plan need to be encouraged. We need to allow time for that to happen before starting the group activity, especially because today the activity required them to be involved at more of a project level. We need to also try to sense the pace of the group members, more explicitly observe when task/process seems not to be working, and help the group adjust the plan accordingly during the session. At the end of the session, enough time remained for the members to share their observations and feelings.

Was the group interaction as you anticipated? *(explain; if problems occurred, what can you identify as a basis for understanding the problems?):*
Some members were more outspoken than anticipated about their dislike of the activity. Creativity in the abstract nature of writing seemed a difficult and uncomfortable process for these members who still do not feel confident in their skills. We encouraged them to become more involved in future discussions of activity selection; acknowledged that everyone has likes and dislikes, strengths and challenges; and encouraged members to talk about these with the group.

In the future, what might you do differently as group leaders? *(give rationale):*
We need to spend more time helping members describe what they have in mind when they suggest doing a particular activity at the next session. It is not clear whether all members understood what writing a group verse would entail.

Completed Forms for Chapter 8 Case Studies

Case Study #1:
Open Group on an Inpatient Psychiatry Unit

SESSION EVALUATION:

Name of group: "Getting It Together"

Session Activity: Mural painting

Date: Friday, June 10

Leaders: Lauri Levy, OTR/L; Jack Jones, MHC

Were the goals accomplished? *(state outcome and give rationale):*

Yes. All group members participated in the painting of a mural. The theme selected was "New Beginnings." Members shared positive feelings, negative reactions, and memories about the group and their hospital experience.

Was the session helpful in addressing individual member and group goals?

Yes. Betty and Maggie were able to remain involved with the group the entire session and verbalize their feelings instead of leaving or demonstrating decreased performance. Eric was able to state he would miss Liz (soon to be discharged) and her creativity, and Pearl made an insightful suggestion for a mural theme and a supportive comment to Lakisha about her returning to work. Li was able to communicate via translator more about himself and his wish for the support of friendships. Liz joked about "Out with the old and in with the new" and discussed her upcoming discharge early next week.

Do you have any information to suggest that the session(s) has/have been helpful to the members' functioning (adaptation) outside of the group? *(explain):*
Partially. Liz and Eric were able to acknowledge that the group has been helpful, stating they wished for a similar group in the community as they transition to new living arrangements and back to their school environments.

Was the group structure adequate for accomplishing the goals? *(give rationale, taking into consideration: leadership; time/length of meeting; open- vs. closed-group format; sequence, methods, and procedures; media/modalities/techniques employed; norms/ behaviors reinforced implicitly or explicitly; methods of reinforcement; and stage of group's development):*
Yes. It seemed to reinforce group members actively assuming group member roles (task and maintenance).

Did the structure provide for "optimal experience" or a "flow state" to occur? *(explain):*
At times. During the mural painting, group members appeared to lose track of time because they were so engaged in their individual and collaborative processes. Members readily engaged in the mural activity and conversation at a level that matched their capabilities with minimal prompting.

Did the structure provide optimal purposeful, self-initiated, spontaneous, and group-centered action to allow meaningful interaction, enhanced performance skills, and/or adaptation to occur through "occupation"? *(explain):*
Yes. By having the group members select a mural theme, they were challenged to express their feelings. However, in the next session the group members should be encouraged to select the activity modality so that they can further examine their decision-making process and tendency to rely on or seek approval from group leaders.

Did the structure provide for new learning or reinforcement of current level of functioning or occupational performance, or did it reinforce functioning below current level of ability? *(explain):*
The structure did provide for new learning. Members learned that rather than heightening a sense of anxiety and fear, expressing their thoughts and emotions enabled them to acknowledge feelings of loss or sadness and opportunities that may arise via change. Having a structured process time at the beginning and end of the session gave the members the opportunity to be heard and their progress/performance in the group acknowledged by both leaders and peers.

What changes would you make regarding group goals and structure for the next session or if you were to lead this session again?

In the next session, members should be urged to make more task decisions; then sequence a plan of action and cue to help members detect when a change in action is needed.

Were you adequately prepared for the session? *(give rationale, taking into consideration time, place, materials, and physical and emotional environment):*
Yes. All the necessary materials were available, and the leaders provided a supportive, enthusiastic, environment while providing consistent feedback regarding member performance.

How did you function as leader? *(How did your behavior and role affect the group? What did you do that was effective? Were there opportunities for leader intervention that may have been missed? What did you learn about yourselves as group leaders?):*
We effectively established the group's procedures for the session, encouraged members to participate in the task by asking for their opinions and feelings, and reality tested members' behavior or ideas by exploring possible cognitive distortions that may be part of the relationship between member thoughts and feelings and behavior. We believe this was effective in bringing about a feeling of cohesiveness and safety in the group and that members became aware of similarities in their reactions. We learned that we are gaining comfort with exploring member reactions when the group is involved in an expressive art activity.

Was the group interaction as you anticipated? *(explain; if problems occurred, what can you identify as a basis for understanding the problems?):*
As anticipated, members initially relied on the leaders for task structure and emotional support. Expressing feelings remains difficult for the members, especially in light of facing the loss of two active members due to their success resulting in their upcoming discharge from the hospital.

In the future, what might you do differently as group leader? *(give ratuionale):*
To reinforce the idea of member choice and responsibility, we suggest a choice among three forms of mural techniques (i.e., collage, montage, or painting).

Case Study #2:
Closed Group in an Outpatient Occupational Therapy Clinic————

SESSION EVALUATION:

Name of group: Community Re-entry: "Moving Forward"

Date: December 20, last of eight sessions

Leaders: Russsell Lee, MS, OTR/L; Alicia Wright, COTA/L

Were the goals accomplished? *(state outcome and give rationale):*
Yes. Members prepared food for party, expressed their sadness about group coming to a close, and commented on accomplishments in the group. Members were able to complete feedback forms and identify residual theme of wanting "more time." Leaders were able to process members' wish and plans for reunion.

Was the session helpful in accomplishing group and individual member goals?
Yes. Each member was able to identify aspects of his or her progress toward specific goals set at the outset of group series. Members were supportive and worked collaboratively on food preparation and clean-up. Jim and Juanita took leadership roles, including taking initiative to follow up on members' wish to continue meeting (trying for a "reunion" after the holidays).

Do you have any information that indicates the session(s) has/have been helpful to the members' functioning (adaptation) outside of the group?
Yes. Members' reports are specific in terms of resuming meaningful tasks and roles as well as finding community resources to support their continued progress (i.e., AA meetings, work hardening evaluation, home health aide).

Was the group structure adequate for accomplishing the goals? *(give rationale, taking into consideration: leadership; time/length of meeting; open- vs. closed-group format; sequence, methods, and procedures; media/modalities/techniques employed; norms/ behaviors reinforced implicitly or explicitly; methods of reinforcement; and stage of group's development):*
Yes. Food preparation was very useful in highlighting some of group themes and member goals. The discussion allowed for processing of members' desire to continue meeting as well as for members to assert leadership roles in negotiating their transition from leader-led to member-led per their initiative. Members were able to process in face-to-face context the reality of this group ending in a manner that suggested they understood but were desirous of seeking continued support from each other in a community context.

Did the structure provide for "optimal experience" or a "flow state" to occur? *(explain):*
Yes. Members laughed and talked spontaneously. They also all contributed to the food preparation task led by another member with minimal leader input.

Did the structure provide optimal purposeful, self-initiated, spontaneous, and group-centered action to allow meaningful interaction, enhanced performance skills, and/or adaptation to occur through "occupation"? *(explain):*
Yes. Food preparation and sharing a snack together as well as the format of the evaluation process allowed members to share what they learned in both words and action as well as share and process with leaders their feelings about the group's termination.

Did the structure provide for new learning or reinforcement of current level of functioning or occupational performance, or did it reinforce functioning below current level of ability? *(explain):*

For the most part, it appears members have learned that they can get more support and goal achievement by sharing and initiating action. This, however, has resulted in their wish to remain together, which may or may not be realistic or adaptive in the long run. The session was planned and structured to focus on termination and evaluation; thus, members were prepared for the fact that this was the final session and engaged in tasks to symbolize and support the feedback exchange.

What changes would you make regarding group goals and structure for the next session or if you were to lead this session again?

The member feedback suggested that a more concrete transitional object would be useful (collated resource notebook of all previous handouts). Perhaps a "more time" theme could be integrated into this object similar to a "goodbye" scrapbook/yearbook.

Were you adequately prepared for the session? *(give rationale, taking into consideration time, place, materials, and physical and emotional environment):*

For the most part, yes, but our wish to make the group more "natural" via "party" (having food preparation and eating together in the kitchen) may have added to members' reluctance to "end" their group.

How did you function as leader? *(How did your behavior and role affect the group? What did you do that was effective? Were there opportunities for leader intervention that may have been missed? What did you learn about yourselves as group leaders?):*

Our laissez-faire leadership allowed members to take more initiative, be group-centered, and interact with each other. We may have missed an opportunity to address resistance to ending the group that was evident in the members congregating in the lobby and needing reminders to come to the group, resulting in a late start. We still struggle with our own wish to work with clients, especially when the group has reached this stage of development, which may come through subconsciously in our choice of activity or avoidance of limit setting in the final session.

Was the group interaction as you anticipated? *(explain; if problems occurred, what can you identify as a basis for understanding the problems?):*

In some ways the group interaction was better than anticipated. John's identifying Alcoholics Anonymous meetings as a means to keep safe pleasantly surprised us. However, Jim's asserting leadership in regard to suggesting the group continue meeting outside of the treatment context came as a surprise and may be a sign of recovery but may also suggest a return to his premorbid maladaptive tendencies to overcommit. Jeanette's offering her home may also be potentially maladaptive as a way to avoid her discomfort with being "seen" out in the community.

In the future, what might you do differently as group leaders? *(give rationale):*
Resist temptation of moving group to kitchen. Offer simpler refreshments, and focus more time on review and evaluation of group series, with each member assembling own resource notebook according to his or her own needs, adding a member feedback page on which he or she can record feedback to each other.

Case Study #3: Community-Based Group ——————

SESSION EVALUATION:

Name of group: "Time Flies"

Date: October 27, final session of a closed group

Leaders: Mary Munroe, Wellness Director; Sage Stilton, Volunteer (Jacki Wright, OTD, OTR/L, Supervising Consultant)

Were the goals accomplished? *(state outcome and give rationale):*
In general, all the goals were accomplished, although the charged atmosphere of the group (because of Joe's initial absence) made the process seem more disorganized and regressed. However, Joe's absence, in conjunction with the activity, stimulated conversation and socialization between group members and increased their initiative and interest in the activities. Although somewhat disjointed and disrupted by Joe's late arrival, members discussed the activity and reflected on their growth and change over the 10 weeks. The activity as well as the outcome of the group processing as possible reasons for Joe's behavior (not telephoning) helped members to address the group experience and their feelings about termination.

Was the session helpful in accomplishing group and individual member goals?
Partially. Sophie and Agnes were quiet and withdrawn from the group at times. However, Tom exceeded our expectations, as did Irina and Betty in their ability to confront one another with their observations and feelings about the changes they had noted in each other over the course of the group meetings. All members were able to address the issue of termination of the group series on some level (task and/or emotional).

Do you have any information that indicates the session(s) has/have been helpful to the members' functioning (adaptation) outside of the group? *(explain):*

Yes. Families have reported increased involvement and initiative in family matters. Group members often have lunch together after the morning group and sit together or encourage each other to attend other group activity at the center.

Was the group structure adequate for accomplishing the goals? *(give rationale, taking into consideration: leadership; time/length of meeting; open- vs. closed-group format; sequence, methods, and procedures; media/modalities/techniques employed; norms/ behaviors reinforced implicitly or explicitly; methods of reinforcement; and stage of group's development):*

Partially. The activity and methods were adequate in terms of addressing termination. We were unrealistic in terms of how much we could accomplish and did not anticipate Joe's absence/late arrival and its subsequent effect on the group members. Once we regrouped, it seemed that the group norms of participation and positive pairing to assist each other with tasks became an effective way to complete the activity. The group seems to have developed to a cooperative level in that the regression seemed more in response to the stress/tension of Joe's coming late than the termination of the group per se. Members were also able to tolerate and work through their moments of conflict and confrontation with minimal leader input.

Did the structure provide "optimal experience" or a "flow state" to occur? *(explain):*

Partially. The collage had moments in which members seemed to be involved enough in the activity that their anxieties and inhibitions were lessened. However, the disjointed nature of the session in terms of group process, addressing termination, and interpersonal issues seemed to detract from members having an optimal experience.

Did the structure provide optimal purposeful, self-initiated, spontaneous, and group-centered action to allow meaningful interaction, enhanced performance skills, and/or adaptation to occur through "occupation"? *(explain):*

Yes. Making the collage and focusing on this being our last session seemed meaningful to the members and elicited a large amount of self-initiated input from Tom, Betty, and Irina. All members spontaneously shared reminisces with each other. This allowed leaders to facilitate group-centered activity and discussion.

Did the structure provide for new learning or reinforcement of current level of functioning or occupational performance, or did it reinforce functioning below current level of ability? *(explain):*

Yes, all the members seemed to have learned that if they take more initiative in the activity sessions and help each other work successfully as a group, they get to know one another better and their overall sense of well-being improves. This structure also supported the group's overall goal of reinforcing members' realizing their true capacities and maximizing their current level of individual functioning.

Did the structure provide an opportunity for evaluation and feedback regarding the group procedures and member progress? *(explain):*

No. There was not enough time at the end of the session for careful feedback and evaluation of group and member progress. The collage did allow for some discussion of the level of enjoyment and satisfaction that members experienced in their favorite sessions.

Were you adequately prepared for the session? *(give rationale, taking into consideration time, place, materials, and physical and emotional environment):*

Partially, as this session was planned to focus on termination, we question if we were really prepared to deal with members' feelings about the group's coming to an end. We seemed to over-plan the task nature of the group with too much "to do" in our effort to provide a transitional object (individually framed reproductions of group collages). This may be about our own discomfort with losses/endings.

What changes would you make regarding group goals and structure for the next session or if you were to lead this session again?

We might consider making the collages and decorating the individual frames in the previous session. We could assemble the group collage in the larger tri-frame and then hang the group collage as part of the close of the final session. In the final session, we could pass out the individual digital copies and place them in the members' frames. This would allow for more focused times for discussion and reflection.

How did you function as leader? *(How did your behavior and role affect the group? What did you do that was effective? Were their opportunities for leader intervention that may have been missed? What did you learn about yourselves as group leaders?):*

Our leadership style was democratic and supportive, which seemed to empower the members to complete the task and share their feelings about termination. We avoided confronting Joe in terms of his remark about his doctor's appointment. We became more focused on the task-related issues, likely due to our own discomfort with confrontation and questioning if it was appropriate at this point because of the lack of time and this being our last group.

Was the group interaction as you anticipated? *(explain; if problems occurred, what can you identify as a basis for understanding the problems?):*

No, we had hoped for a more relaxed final session. In retrospect, we were likely more anxious and disappointed than we realized about Joe's being late and then appearing flippant in his remark about doctor's appointment. When we became aware of Sophie's increased agitation and Agnes' withdrawal, it seemed important to reassure members of the group that it was safe for them to express their feelings. Mary modeled this by expressing her own feelings that endings were difficult for her to deal with to validate the losses members may be experiencing.

In the future, what might you do differently as group leaders? *(give rationale):*
We should continue the procedure of making phone calls the morning of our final session to confirm that members will be in attendance. By spending the last two sessions on the collage, this will allow more time to address issues of closure and focus on the group process versus the task. It will also allow Sage time to digitally photograph the group collages and pre-print the individual copies for members to frame.

References

Acquaviva, F.A. & Presseller, S. (1983). Nationally speaking: Occupational therapy manpower. American Journal of Occupational Therapy 37(2): 79–81.

Agazarian, Y. & Gantt, S. (2003). Phases of group development: Systems-centered hypotheses and their implications for research and practice. Group Dynamics: Theory, Research, and Practice 7(3), 238–252.

American Occupational Therapy Association. (1955). Institute: Theme interpersonal relationships. American Journal of Occupational Therapy 9(5): 212–223, 230–232.

American Occupational Therapy Association (1991). Member Data Survey 1990 (1991). Rockville, MD: American Occupational Therapy Association.

American Occupational Therapy Association. (2002). Occupational therapy practice framework: Domain and process. American Journal of Occupational Therapy 56(6), 609–639.

Anderson, C.L. (1936). Project work: An individualized group therapy. Occupational Therapy and Rehabilitation 15(4): 265–269.

Angel, S.L. (1981). The emotion identification group. American Journal of Occupational Therapy 35(4): 256–262.

Aronson, R. (1976). The role of an occupational therapist in a geriatric day hospital setting—Maimonides Day Hospital. American Journal of Occupational Therapy 30(5): 290–292.

Atkinson, J.W. & Feather, N. (1966). A Theory of Achievement Motivation. New York: John Wiley & Sons.

Back, K. (1951). Influence through social communication. Journal of Abnormal Psychology 46(3), 9–23.

Bales, R. (1950). Interaction Process Analysis. Reading, MA: Addison-Wesley.

Bales, R.F. (1955). Adaptive and integrative changes as sources of strain in social systems. In A.P. Hare, E.F. Borgatta, & R.F. Bales (eds.), Small Groups. New York: Knopf.

Bales, R.F. & Borgatta, E.F. (1962). Size of group as a factor in the interaction profile. In A.P. Hare, E.F. Borgatta, & R.F. Bales (eds.), Small Groups, 2nd ed. New York: Knopf.

Barker, P. & Muir, A.M. (1969). The role of occupational therapy in a children's inpatient psychiatric unit. American Journal of Occupational Therapy 23(5): 431–436.

Barnes, M.A. & Schwartzberg, S.L. (2000). Activity analysis of group process. Journal of Psychotherapy in Independent Practice 1(2), 21–32.

Barnes, M.A. & Schwartzberg, S.L. (2003). A case study: An occupational therapy approach. In S. Simon Fehr (ed.), Introduction to Group Therapy: A Practical Guide, 2nd ed. Binghamton, NY: Haworth Press.

Barris, R., Kielhofner, G., & Hawkins, J.H. (1983). Psychosocial Occupational Therapy Practice in a Pluralistic Arena. Laurel, MD: Ramsco.

Bem, D., Wallach, M., & Kogan, N. (1965). Group decision making under risk of aversive consequences. Journal of Personal and Social Psychology 1: 453–460.

Benne, K.D. & Sheats, P. (1978). Functional roles of group members. In L.P. Bradford (ed.), Group
Development, 2nd ed. La Jolla, CA: University Associates, 52–61.

Bennis, W.G. (1989). On Becoming a Leader. Reading, MA: Addison-Wesley.

Bennis, W.B. & Shepard, H.A. (1956). A theory of group development. Human Relations 9(4):
415–457.

Bernard, H.S. (2005). Commentary countertransference: The evolution of a construct. International
Journal of Group Psychotherapy 55(1), 151–160.

Berne, E. (1963). The Structure and Dynamics of Organizations and Groups. New York: Grove Press.

Bickes, M.B., DeLoache, S.N., Dicer, J.R., et al. (2001). Effectiveness of experiential and verbal
occupational therapy groups in a community mental health setting. Occupational Therapy in
Mental Health 17(1), 51–72.

Billow, R. & Gans, J.S. (2005). A sinking depression. In L. Motherwell & J. J. Shay (eds.),
Complex Dilemmas in Group Therapy: Pathways to Resolution. New York: Brunner-Routledge,
143–151.

Bing, R.K. (1981). Occupational therapy revisited: A paraphrastic journey. American Journal of Occupational Therapy 35(8): 499–518.

Bion, W.R. (1959). Experiences in Groups. New York: Basic Books.

Blackman, N. (1940). Experiences with a literary club in the group treatment of schizophrenia. Occupational Therapy and Rehabilitation 19(5): 293–303.

Bober, S.J., McLellan, E., McBee, L., et al. (2002). The feelings art group: A vehicle for personal
expression in skilled nursing home residents with dementia. Journal of Social Work in Long Term
Care 1(4), 73–87.

Bobis, B.R., Harrison, R.M., & Traub, L. (1955). Activity group therapy. American Journal of Occupational Therapy 9(1): 19–21, 50.

Bockoven, J.S. (1971). Occupational therapy—an historic perspective: Legacy of moral treatment—
1800s to 1910. American Journal of Occupational Therapy 25(5): 223–225.

Boisvert, R.A. (2004). Enhancing substance dependence intervention. OT Practice 9(10):11;6.

Borg, B. & Bruce, M.A. (1991). The Group System: The Therapeutic Activity Group in Occupational
Therapy. Thorofare, NJ: Slack.

Botkins, S. (1979). A peer discussion group of senior occupational therapy students. American Journal
of Occupational Therapy 33(2): 123–125.

Bouchard, V.C. (1972). Hemiplegic exercise and discussion group. American Journal of Occupational
Therapy 26(7): 330–331.

Brabender, V. & Fallon, A. (1996). Termination in inpatient groups. International Journal of Group
Psychotherapy, 46(1), 81–98.

Bradford, L.P. (1978). Group formation and development. In L.P. Bradford (ed.), Group Development,
2nd ed. La Jolla, CA: University Associates, 4–12.

Bradford, L., Stock, D., & Horwitz, M. (1978). How to diagnose group problems. In L.P. Bradford
(ed.), Group Development, 2nd ed. La Jolla, CA: University Associates, 62–78.

Broekema, M.C., Danz, K.H., & Schloemer, C.U. (1975). Occupational therapy in a community aftercare program. American Journal of Occupational Therapy 29(1): 22–27.

Bronfenbrenner, U. (1979). The Ecology of Human Development: Experiments by Nature and Design.
Cambridge, MA: Harvard University Press.

Brooker, D. & Duce, L. (2000). Well-being and activity in dementia: A comparison of group reminiscence therapy, structured goal-directed activity, and unstructured time. Aging and Mental Health
4(4): 354–358.

Brown, N.W. (2003). Conceptualizing process. International Journal of Group Psychotherapy 53(2), 225–244.

Burke, J.P. (1983). Defining occupation: Importing and organizing interdisciplinary knowledge. In G. Kielhofner (ed.), Health Through Occupation: Theory and Practice in Occupational Therapy. Philadelphia: F.A. Davis, 125–138.

Canton, E.L. (1923). Psychology of occupational therapy. Archives of Occupational Therapy 2(5): 347–357.

Cartwright, D. & Zander, A. (1960). Group Dynamics: Research and Theory, 2nd ed. New York: Harper & Row, 69–92.

Cartwright, D. & Zander, A. (1968). Motivational processes in groups: Introduction. In D. Cartwright & A. Zander (eds.), Group Dynamics Research and Theory, 3rd ed. New York: Harper & Row, 401–417.

Castore, G.F. (1962). Number of verbal interrelationships as a determinant of group size. Journal of Abnormal Social Psychology 64: 456–457.

Cermak, S.A., Stein, F., & Abelson, C. (1973). Hyperactive children and an activity group therapy model. American Journal of Occupational Therapy 26(6): 311–315.

Chafe, W.H. (1972). The American Woman: Her Changing Social, Economic, and Political Roles, 1920–1970. New York: Oxford University Press.

Clark, F., Azen, S.P., Zemke, R., et al. (1997). Occupational therapy for independent-living older adults: A randomized controlled trial. Journal of the American Medical Association 278: 1321–1326.

Clark, F.A., Carlson, M., Jackson, J., & Mandel, D. (2003). Lifestyle redesign improves health *and* is cost-effective. OT Practice 8(2):9–13.

Cohen, A.M. & Smith, R.D. (1976). The Critical Incident in Growth Groups: Theory and Technique. La Jolla, CA: University Associates.

Cohn, E.S. & Czycholl, C. (1991). Facilitating a foundation for clinical reasoning. In E.B. Crepeau & T. LeGuard (eds.), Self-Paced Instruction for Clinical Educators and Supervisors. Rockville, MD: American Occupational Therapy Association.

Cole, M.B. (2005). Group Dynamics in Occupational Therapy: The Theoretical Basis and Practice Application of Group Intervention, 3rd ed. Thorofare, NJ: Slack.

Combs, M.H. (1959). An activities program in a custodial care group. American Journal of Occupational Therapy 13(1): 5–8, 26–27.

Cooley, C.H. (1909). Social Organization: A Study of the Larger Mind. New York: Scribner's.

Corey, G. & Corey, M.S. (1977). Groups: Process and Practice. Monterey, CA: Brooks/Cole.

Corey, G. & Corey, M.S. (1982). Groups: Process and Practice, 2nd ed. Monterey, CA: Brooks/Cole.

Corry, S., Sebastian, V., & Mosey, A.C. (1974). Acute short-term treatment in psychiatry. American Journal of Occupational Therapy 28(7): 401–406.

Csikszentmihalyi, M. (1975). Beyond Boredom and Anxiety: The Experience of Play in Work and Games. San Francisco: Jossey-Bass.

Csikszentmihalyi, M. (1990). Flow: The Psychology of Optimal Experience. New York: Harper Collins.

Dataline. (1982). Occupational Therapy Newspaper 36(11): 3.

DeCarlo, J.J. & Mann, W.C. (1985). The effectiveness of verbal versus activity groups in improving self-perceptions of interpersonal communication skills. American Journal of Occupational Therapy 39(1): 20–27.

Delworth, U.M. (1972). Interpersonal skill development for occupational therapy students. American Journal of Occupational Therapy 26(1): 27–29.

Denton, P.L. (1982). Teaching interpersonal skills with videotape. Occupational Therapy in Mental Health 2(4): 17–33.

Deutsch, M. (1960). The effects of cooperation and competition upon group process. In D. Cartwright & A. Zander (eds.), Group Dynamics: Research and Theory, 2nd ed. New York: Harper & Row, 461–482.

Diasio, K. (1971). Occupational therapy—A historical perspective: The modern era—1960 to 1970. American Journal of Occupational Therapy 25(5): 237–242.

Dion, K.L., Miller, N., & Magnan, M. (1970). Cohesiveness and Social Responsibility as Determinants of Group Risk Taking. Proceedings of the Annual Convention of the American Psychological Association, 335–336.

Donohue, M.V. (1982). Designing activities to develop a women's identification group. Occupational Therapy in Mental Health 2(1), 1–19.

Donohue, M.V. (2003). Group profile studies with children: Validity measures and item analysis. Occupational Therapy in Mental Health 19(1), 1–23.

Dossey, L. (1999). Reinventing Medicine. New York: HarperCollins.

Duncombe, L. & Howe, M.C. (1985). Group work in occupational therapy: A survey of practice. American Journal of Occupational Therapy 39(3), 163–170.

Duncombe, L. & Howe, M.C. (1995). Group treatment: Goals, tasks, and economic implications. American Journal of Occupational Therapy 49, 199–205.

Dunton, W.R. (1937). Quilt making as a socializing measure. Occupational Therapy and Rehabilitation 16(4): 275–278.

Efron, H.Y., Marks, H.K., & Hall, R. (1959). A comparison of group-centered and individual-centered activity programs. Archives of General Psychiatry 1(5):552–555.

Egan, G. (1975). The Skilled Helper. Monterey, CA: Brooks/Cole.

Eklund, M. (1997). Therapeutic factors in occupational group therapy identified by patients discharged from a psychiatric day centre and their significant others. Occupational Therapy International 4(3): 198–212.

Eklund, M. (1999). Outcome of occupational therapy in a psychiatric day care unit for long-term mentally ill patients. Occupational Therapy in Mental Health 14(4): 21–45.

Ellsworth, P.D. & Colman, A.D. (1969). A model program: The application of operant conditioning principles to work group experience. American Journal of Occupational Therapy 23(6): 495–501.

Fahl, M.A. (1970). Emotionally disturbed children: Effects of cooperative and competitive activity on peer interaction. American Journal of Occupational Therapy 24(1): 31–33.

Falk-Kessler, J. & Froschauer, K.H. (1978). The soap opera: A dynamic group approach for psychiatric patients. American Journal of Occupational Therapy 32(5): 317–319.

Fearing, V.G. (1978). An authors' group for extended care patients. American Journal of Occupational Therapy 32(8): 526–527.

Festinger, L. & Thibaut, J. (1951). Interpersonal communication in small groups. Journal of Abnormal and Social Psychology 16: 92–99.

Feuss, C.D. & Maltby, J.W. (1959). Occupational therapy in the community. American Journal of Occupational Therapy 13(1): 9–10, 25.

Fidler, G. (2000). Beyond the therapy model: Building a future. American Journal of Occupational Therapy 54(1): 99–101.

Fidler, G.S. (1966). A second look at work as a primary force in rehabilitation and treatment. American Journal of Occupational Therapy 20(2): 72–74.

Fidler, G.S. (1969). The task-oriented group as a context for treatment. American Journal of Occupational Therapy 23(1): 43–48.

Fidler, G.S. (1984). Design of Rehabilitation Services in Psychiatric Hospital Settings. Laurel, MD: Ramsco.

Fidler, G.S. & Fidler, J.W. (1954). Introduction to Psychiatric Occupational Therapy. New York: Macmillan.

Fidler, G.S. & Fidler, J.W. (1960). Introduction to Psychiatric Occupational Therapy, 2nd ed. New York: Macmillan.

Fidler, G.S. & Fidler, J.W. (1963). Occupational Therapy: A Communication Process in Psychiatry. Macmillan: New York.

Fidler, G.S. & Fidler, J.W. (1978). Doing and becoming: Purposeful action and self-actualization. American Journal of Occupational Therapy 32(5): 305–310.

Fidler, G.S. & Fidler, J.W. (1983). Doing and becoming: The occupational therapy experience. In G. Kielhofner (ed.), Health Through Occupation: Theory & Practice in Occupational Therapy. Philadelphia: F.A. Davis, 267–280.

Fiedler, F. (1967). A Theory of Leadership Effectiveness. New York: McGraw-Hill.

Fieldsteel, N.D. (1996). The process of termination in long-term psychoanalytic group therapy. International Journal of Group Psychotherapy 46(1): 25–39.

Frank, J.D. (1957). Some determinants, manifestations, and effects of cohesiveness in therapy groups. International Journal of Group Psychotherapy 7: 53–63.

Froehlich, J. & Nelson, D.L. (1986). Affective meanings of life review through activities and discussion. American Journal of Occupational Therapy 40(1): 27–33.

Galigor, J. (1977). Perceptions of the group therapist and the dropout from group. In A. R. Wolberg & M. L. Aronson (eds.), Group Therapy 1977: An Overview. New York: Stratton Intercontinental Medical Book Corporation.

Gans, J.S. & Alonso, A. (1998). Difficult patients: Their construction in group therapy. International Journal of Group Psychotherapy 48(3): 311–326.

Garland, J.A. & Frey, L.A. (1970). Application of stages of group development to groups in psychiatric settings. In S. Bernstein (ed.), Further Explorations in Group Work. Boston: Boston University School of Social Work, 1–28.

Garland, J.A., Jones, H.E., & Kolodny, R. (1965). A model for stages of development in social work groups. In S. Bernstein (ed.), Explorations in Group Work. Boston: Boston University School of Social Work.

Garland, J.A., Jones, H.E., & Kolodny, R.L. (1973). A model for stages of development in social work groups. In S. Bernstein (ed.), Explorations in Group Work: Essays in Theory and Practice. Boston: Milford House, 17–71.

Gauthier, L., Dalziel, S., & Gauthier, S. (1987). The benefits of group occupational therapy for patients with Parkinson's disease. American Journal of Occupational Therapy 41: 360–365.

German, S.A. (1964). A group approach to rehabilitation occupational therapy in a psychiatric setting. American Journal of Occupational Therapy 18(5): 209–214.

Gibb, J. & Gibb, L. (1967). Humanistic elements in group growth. In J. Bugenthal (ed.), Challenges of Humanistic Psychology. New York: McGraw-Hill.

Gibb, J.R. (1958). The occupational therapist works with groups. American Journal of Occupational Therapy 12(4): 205–214.

Gillette, N. & Kielhofner, G. (1979). The impact of specialization on the professionalization and survival of occupational therapy. American Journal of Occupational Therapy 33(1): 20–28.

Gillette, N.P. & Mayer, P.R. (1968). The group method in occupational therapy. In J.L. Mazer (Project Director), Final Report Rehabilitation Services Administration Grant Number 123-T-68 for Field Consultant in Psychiatric Rehabilitation. New York: American Occupational Therapy Association.

Gleave, G.M. (1947). Occupational therapy in children's hospitals and pediatric services. In H. S. Willard & C. S. Spackman (eds.), Principles of Occupational Therapy. Philadelphia: J.B. Lippincott.

Goldstein, A.P., Gershaw, N.J., & Spraflin, R.P. (1979). Structured learning therapy: Development and evaluation. American Journal of Occupational Therapy 33(10): 635–639.

Goldstein, N. & Collins, T. (1982). Making videotapes: An activity for hospitalized adolescents. American Journal of Occupational Therapy 36(8): 530–533.

Goodman, G.B. (1983). Occupational therapy treatment: Interventions with borderline patients. Occupational Therapy in Mental Health 3(3): 19–31.

Gralewicz, A., Hill, B., & Mackinson, M. (1968). Restoration therapy: An approach to group therapy for the chronically ill. American Journal of Occupational Therapy 22(4): 294–299.

Gratke, B. E. & Lux, P. A. (1960). Psychiatric occupational therapy in a milieu setting. American Journal of Occupational Therapy 14(1): 13–16.

Halle, L. & Landy, A. (1948). The integration of group activity and group therapy. Occupational Therapy and Rehabilitation 27(4): 286–298.

Hare, A.P. (1962). Handbook of Small Group Research. New York: Free Press of Glencoe.

Heine, D.B. (1975). Daily living group: Focus on transition from hospital to community. American Journal of Occupational Therapy 29(10): 628–630.

Henry, A., Nelson, D., & Duncombe, L. (1984). Choice making in group and individual activity. American Journal of Occupational Therapy 38(4): 245–251.

Hersen, M. & Luber, R.F. (1977). Use of group psychotherapy in a partial hospitalization service: The remediation of basic skill deficits. International Journal of Group Psychotherapy 27(3): 361–376.

Hersey, P., Blanchard, K.H., & Johnson, D.E. (2001). Management of organizational behavior: Leading human resources, 8th ed. Saddle River, NJ: Prentice Hall.

Homans, G. (1950). The human group. New York: Harcourt, Brace.

Hopkins, H., Smith, H., & Tiffany, E.G. (1983). Therapeutic application of activity. In H. Hopkins & H. Smith (eds.), Willard & Spackman's Occupational Therapy, 6th ed. Philadelphia: J.B. Lippincott.

Hopkins, H.L. (1978). An historical perspective on occupational therapy. In H.L. Hopkins & H.D. Smith (eds.), Willard and Spackman's Occupational Therapy, 5th ed. Philadelphia: J.B. Lippincott, 3–23.

Howe, M. (1968a). A review of selected professional literature describing four youth groups to determine structure with reference to psychiatric occupational therapy. Unpublished master's thesis, San Jose State University, San Jose, CA.

Howe, M.C. (1968b). An occupational therapy activity group. American Journal of Occupational Therapy 22(3): 176–179.

Howe, M. & Schwartzberg, S.L. (1986). A Functional Approach to Group Work in Occupational Therapy. Philadelphia: J.B. Lippincott.

Howe, M. & Schwartzberg, S.L. (1995). A Functional Approach to Group Work in Occupational Therapy, 2nd ed. Philadelphia: J.B. Lippincott.

Howe, M. & Schwartzberg, S.L. (2001). A Functional Approach to Group Work in Occupational Therapy, 3rd ed. Philadelphia: Lippincott Williams & Wilkins.

Hughes, P.L. & Mullins, L. (1981). Acute Psychiatric Care: An Occupational Therapy Guide to Exercises in Daily Living Skills. Thorofare, NJ: Slack.

Humphry, R., Gonzalez, S., & Taylor, E. (1993). Family involvement in practice: Issues and attitudes. American Journal of Occupational Therapy 47: 587–593.

Hurwitz, J.I., Zander, A., & Hymovitch, B. (1960). Some effects of power on the relations among group members. In D. Cartwright & A. Zander (eds.), Group Dynamics: Research and Theory, 2nd ed. New York: Harper & Row, 291–297.

Hyde, R.W., York, R., & Wood, A.C. (1948). Effectiveness of games in a mental hospital. Occupational Therapy and Rehabilitation 27(4): 304–308.

Hyman, M. & Metzker, J.R. (1970). Occupational therapy in an emergency psychiatric setting. American Journal of Occupational Therapy 24(4): 280–283.

Jackson, J., Carlson, M., Mandel, D., et al. (1998). Occupation in lifestyle redesign: The well elderly study occupational therapy program. American Journal of Occupational Therapy 52(5): 326–336.

Jantzen, A.C. (1972). Some characteristics of female occupational therapists, 1970, Part III: A comparison: Faculty and clinical practitioners. American Journal of Occupational Therapy 26(3): 150–154.

Johnson, D.W. (1972). Reaching Out: Interpersonal Effectiveness and Self-Actualization. Englewood Cliffs, NJ: Prentice-Hall.

Johnson, D.W. & Johnson, F.P. (2003). Joining Together: Group Theory and Group Skills, 8th ed. Boston: Pearson Allen & Bacon.

Johnson, D.W. & Johnson, F.P. (2006). Joining Together: Group Theory and Group Skills, 9th ed. Boston: Pearson Allen & Bacon.

Johnson, J.A. (1986). Wellness: A Context for Living. Thorofare, NJ: Slack.

Johnston, N. (1965). Group reading as a treatment tool with geriatrics. American Journal of Occupational Therapy 19(4): 192–195.

Jourard, S. (1964). The Transparent Self. Princeton: Van Nostrand Company.

Kielhofner, G. & Burke, J.P. (1977). Occupational therapy after 60 years: An account of changing identity and knowledge. American Journal of Occupational Therapy 31(10): 674–689.

Kiernat, J.M. (1976). Geriatric day hospitals: A golden opportunity for therapists. American Journal of Occupational Therapy 30(5): 285–289.

Kiernat, J.M. (1979). The use of life review activity with confused nursing home residents. American Journal of Occupational Therapy 33(5): 306–310.

King, L.J. (1974). A sensory-integrative approach to schizophrenia. American Journal of Occupational Therapy 28(9): 529–536.

King, L.J. (1978). Toward a science of adaptive responses. American Journal of Occupational Therapy 32(7): 429–437.

Klein, A.F. (1972). Effective Group Work: An Introduction to Principle and Method. New York: Association Press.

Klein, R.H. (1996). Introduction to special section on termination and group therapy. International Journal of Group Psychotherapy 46(1): 1–4.

Klyczek, J.P. & Mann, W.C. (1986). Therapeutic modality comparisons in day treatment. American Journal of Occupational Therapy 40(9): 606–611.

Knis-Matthews, L. (2003). A parenting program for women who are substance-dependent. AOTA Mental Health Special Interest Section Quarterly 26(1): 1–4.

Knowles, M. & Knowles, H. (1959). Introduction to Group Dynamics. New York: Association Press.

Knowles, M. & Knowles, H. (1972). Introduction to Group Dynamics (rev. ed.). New York: Association Press.

Knowles, M.S. (1970). The Modern Practice of Adult Education. New York: Association Press.

Kouzes, J. & Posner, B. (2003). The leadership challenge. San Francisco: Jossey-Bass.

Koven, B. & Shuff, F.L. (1953). Group therapy with the chronically ill. American Journal of Occupational Therapy 7(5): 208–209, 219.

Kramer, L.W. & Beidel, D.C. (1982). Job seeking skills groups: A review and application to a chronic psychiatric population. Occupational Therapy in Mental Health 2(2): 37–44.

Kremer, E., Nelson, D., & Duncombe, L. (1984). Effects of selected activities on affective meaning in psychiatric patients. American Journal of Occupational Therapy 38(8): 522–528.

Kuenstler, G. (1976). A planning group for psychiatric outpatients. American Journal of Occupational Therapy 30(10): 634–639.

Kurasik, S. (1967). Group dynamics in rehabilitation of hemiplegic patients. Journal of the American Geriatic Society 15: 852–855.

Labovitz, D.R. (1978). The returning therapist: A group approach. American Journal of Occupational Therapy 32(9): 580–585.

Lamb, R.H. (1967). Chronic psychiatric patients in the day hospital. Archives of General Psychiatry 17: 615–621.

Leuret, F. (1840/1948). On the moral treatment of insanity. In S. Licht (ed. & trans.), Occupational Therapy Source Book. Baltimore: Williams & Wilkins. (Article originally written in 1840.)

Levine, D., Marks, H.K., & Hall, R. (1957). Differential effect of factors in an activity therapy program. American Journal of Psychiatry 114: 532–535.

Lewin, K. (1951). Field Theory in Social Science. New York: Harper & Row.

Lewin, K., Lippitt, R., & White, R. (1939). Patterns of aggressive behavior in experimentally created social climates. Journal of Social Psychology 10: 271–299.

Lieberman, M., Yalom, I., & Miles, M. (1973). Encounter Groups: First Facts. New York: Basic Books.

Lifton, W.M. (1961). Working with Groups: Group Process and Individual Growth. New York: John Wiley & Sons.

Lindsay, W.P. (1983). The role of the occupational therapist in treatment of alcoholism. American Journal of Occupational Therapy 37(1): 36–43.

Linn, L., Weinroth, M.D., & Shamah, R. (1962). Occupational Therapy in Dynamic Psychiatry: An Introduction to the Four-Phase Concept in Hospital Psychiatry. Washington, DC: The American Psychiatric Association.

Linn, M.W., Caffey, E.M., Klett, C.J., et al. (1979). Day treatment and psychotropic drugs in the aftercare of schizophrenic patients. Archives of General Psychiatry 36: 1055–1066.

Lippitt, G.L. (1961). How to get results from a group. In L.P. Bradford (ed.), Group Development. La Jolla, CA: University Associates, pp. 31–36.

Llorens, L.A. (1968). Changing methods in treatment of psychosocial dysfunction. American Journal of Occupational Therapy 22(1): 26–29.

Llorens, L.A. & Johnson, P.A. (1966). Occupational therapy in an ego-oriented milieu. American Journal of Occupational Therapy 20(4): 178–181.

Llorens, L.A. & Rubin, E.Z. (1967). Developing Ego Functions in Disturbed Children: Occupational Therapy in Milieu. Detroit: Wayne State University Press.

Lockerbie, L. & Stevenson, G.H. (1947). Socialization through occupational therapy. Occupational Therapy and Rehabilitation 26(3): 142–145.

Loeser, L.H. (1957). Some aspects of group dynamics. International Journal of Group Psychotherapy 7(1): 5–19.

Lundgren, C.C. & Persechino, E.L. (1986). Cognitive group: A treatment program for head-injured adults. American Journal of Occupational Therapy 40(6): 397–401.

Mackenzie, K.R. (1996). Time-limited group psychotherapy. International Journal of Group Psychotherapy 46(1), 41–60.

Mahier, S.H. & Tachabrun, B.R. (1978). Experience and youth group: For elderly and adolescent psychiatric patients. American Journal of Occupational Therapy 32(2): 115–117.

Mandel, D.R., Jackson, J.M., Zemke, R., et al. (1999). Lifestyle Redesign: Implementing the Well Elderly Program. Bethesda, MD: American Occupational Therapy Association.

Mann, W., Godfrey, M.E., & Dowd, E.T. (1973). The use of group counseling procedures in the rehabilitation of spinal cord injured patients. American Journal of Occupational Therapy 27(2): 73–77.

Markowitz, G.E. & Rosner, D. (1979). Doctors in crisis: Medical education and medical reform during the Progressive Era, 1895–1915. In S. Reverby & D. Rosner (eds.), Health Care in America: Essays in Social History. Philadelphia: Temple University Press.

Marsh, L.C. (1936). Group treatment of relatives of psychotic patients. Occupational Therapy and Rehabilitation 15(1): 1–17.

Maslen, D. (1982). Rehabilitation training for community living skills: Concepts and techniques. Occupational Therapy in Mental Health 2(1): 33–49.

Maslow, A. (1962). Toward a Psychology of Being. Princeton: Van Nostrand.

Maslow, A.H. (1970). Motivation & Personality, 2nd ed. New York: Harper & Row.

Mattingly, C. & Fleming, M.H. (1994). Interactive reasoning: Collaborating with the person. In C. Mattingly & M. H. Fleming (eds.), Clinical Reasoning: Forms of Inquiry in a Therapeutic Practice. Philadelphia: FA Davis, 178–196.

Maynard, M. & Pedro, D. (1971). One day experience in group dynamics in an occupational therapy assistant course. American Journal of Occupational Therapy 25(3): 170–171.

Mazer, J.L. (Project Director) (1968). Final Report Rehabilitation Services Administration Grant Number 123-T-68 for Field Consultant in Psychiatric Rehabilitation. New York: American Occupational Therapy Association.

McKibbin, E. & King, J. (1983). Activity group counseling for learning-disabled children with behavior problems. American Journal of Occupational Therapy 37(9): 617–623.

Menks, F., Sittles, S., Weaver, D., et al. (1977). A psychogeriatric activity group in a rural community. American Journal of Occupational Therapy 31(6): 376–384.

Meyer, A. (1922/1977). The philosophy of occupational therapy. American Journal of Occupational Therapy 31(10): 639–642. (Article originally written in 1922.)

Miles, M.B. (1981). Learning to Work in Groups: A Practical Guide for Members and Trainers, 2nd ed. New York: Teachers College Press.

Mosey, A.C. (1968). Recapitulation of ontogenesis: A theory for practice of occupational therapy. American Journal of Occupational Therapy 22(5): 426–432.

Mosey, A.C. (1969). Dependency and integrative skill as they relate to affinity for and acceptance by an assigned group. American Journal of Occupational Therapy 23(4): 348–349.

Mosey, A.C. (1970a). The concept and use of developmental groups. American Journal of Occupational Therapy 24(4): 272–275.

Mosey, A.C. (1970b). Three Frames of Reference for Mental Health. Thorofare, NJ: Slack.

Mosey, A.C. (1971). Occupational therapy: An historical perspective. Involvement in the rehabilitation movement—1942–1960. American Journal of Occupational Therapy 25(5): 234–236.

Mosey, A.C. (1973a). Activities Therapy. New York: Raven Press.

Mosey, AC. (1973b). Meeting health needs. American Journal of Occupational Therapy 27(1): 14–17.

Mosey, A.C. (1974). An alternative: The biopsychosocial model. American Journal of Occupational Therapy 28(3): 137–140.

Mosey, A.C. (1981). Occupational Therapy: Configuration of a Profession. New York: Raven Press.

Moss, F.B. & Stewart, G. (1959). A program for geriatric patients from hospital to community. American Journal of Occupational Therapy 13(6): 268–271.

Napier, R. & Gershenfeld, M.K. (1973). Groups: Theory and Experience. Boston: Houghton Mifflin.

Napier, R.K. & Gershenfeld, M.K. (1983). Making Groups Work: A Guide for Group Leaders. Boston: Houghton Mifflin.

Neistadt, M.E. & Marques, K. (1984). An independent living skills training program. American Journal of Occupational Therapy 38(10): 671–676.

Nelson, A., Mackenthun, D., Bloesch, M., et al. (1956). A preliminary report on a study in group occupational therapy. American Journal of Occupational Therapy 10(5): 254–258, 262–263, 271.

Nelson, D.L. (1997). Why the profession of occupational therapy will flourish in the 21st century. American Journal of Occupational Therapy 51(1): 12.

Nelson, D.L., Peterson, C., Smith, D.A., et al. (1988). Effects of project versus parallel groups on social interaction and affective responses in senior citizens. American Journal of Occupational Therapy 42(1): 23–29.

Neville, A. (1980). Temporal adaptation: Application with short-term psychiatric patients. American Journal of Occupational Therapy 34(5): 328–331.

Nitsun, M. (1996). The anti-group: Destructive forces in the group and their creative potential. New York: Routledge.

Nitsun, M. (2000). The future of the group. International Journal of Group Psychotherapy, 50(4): 455–472.

Noce, S.F., Breuninger, P.L., & Noce, J.S. (1983). A piagetian-based approach for the assessment and occupational therapy treatment of cognitive deficits in process schizophrenic and psychogeriatric patients. In W.E. Kelly (ed.), The Changing Role of Rehabilitation Medicine in the Management of the Psychiatric Patient. Springfield, IL: Charles C. Thomas, 107–121.

Novick, L.J. (1961). Occupational therapy and social group work in the home for the sick aged: A comparison. American Journal of Occupational Therapy 15(5): 198–203, 211.

Odhner, F. (1970a). A study of group tasks as facilitators of verbalization among hospitalized schizophrenic patients. American Journal of Occupational Therapy 24(1): 7–12.

Odhner, F. (1970b). Group dynamics of the interdisciplinary team. American Journal of Occupational Therapy 24(7): 484–487.

Ormont, L. (1990). The craft of bridging. International Journal of Group Psychotherapy 40(1): 3–17.

Ormont, L. (2004). Drawing the isolate into the group flow. Group Analysis 37(1): 65–76.

Ornish, D. (1998). Love and Survival. New York: Harper Collins.

Orsulic-Jeras, S., Schneider, N.M., & Camp, C.J. (2000). Montessori-based activities for long-term care residents with dementia. Topics in Geriatric Rehabilitation 16(1): 78–91.

Owen, C. & Newman, N. (1965). Utilizing films as a therapeutic agent in group interaction. American Journal of Occupational Therapy 19(4): 205–207.

Pasework, R. & Hornby, R. (1968). The effect upon social interaction patterns of a short-term stimulation program for psychiatric geriatric patients. American Journal of Occupational Therapy 22(3): 195–196.

Pearman, H. E. & Newman, N. (1968). Work-oriented occupational therapy for the geriatric patient. American Journal of Occupational Therapy 22(3): 203–208.

Perls, F., Hefferline, R.E., & Goodman, P. (1971). Gestalt Therapy. New York: Bantam.

Perrins-Margalis, N.M., Rugletic, J., Schepis, N.M., et al. (2000). The immediate effects of a group-based horticulture experience on the quality of life of persons with chronic mental illness. Occupational Therapy in Mental Health 16(1): 15–31.

Persson, D. (1996). Play and flow in an activity group: A case study of creative occupations with chronic pain patients. Scandinavian Journal of Occupational Therapy 3:33–42.

Posthuma, B.W. & Posthuma, A.B. (1972). The effect of a small-group experience on occupational therapy students. American Journal of Occupational Therapy 26(8): 415–418.

Price, S. (1993). The issue is: New pathways for psychosocial occupational therapy. American Journal of Occupational Therapy 47: 557–560.

Rance, C. & Price, A. (1973). Poetry as a group project. American Journal of Occupational Therapy 27(5): 252–255.

Raven, B.H. & Rietsema, J. (1957). The effects of varied clarity of group goal and group path upon the individual and his relation to his group. Human Relations 10: 29–44.

Reed, K.L. (1984). Models of Practice in Occupational Therapy. Baltimore: Williams & Wilkins.

Reed, K.L. & Sanderson, S.R. (1983). Concepts of Occupational Therapy, 2nd ed. Baltimore: Williams & Wilkins.

Reilly, M. (1966). A psychiatric occupational therapy program as a teaching model. American Journal of Occupational Therapy 20(2): 61–67.

Rerek, M.D. (1971). Occupational therapy: A historical perspective: The Depression years—1929 to 1941. American Journal of Occupational Therapy 25(5): 231–233.

Rice, C.A. (2006). Premature termination of group therapy: A clinical perspective. International Journal of Group Psychotherapy, 46(1): 5–23.

Rider, B.B. & Gramlin, J.T. (1980). An activities approach to occupational therapy in a short-term acute mental health unit. Rockville, MD: American Occupational Therapy Association Mental Health Specialty Section Newsletter 3(4).

Rogers, C. (1959). Theory of therapy-personality and interpersonal relationships. In S. Koch (ed.), Psychology: A Study of a Science, vol. 3. New York: McGraw-Hill.

Rogers, C. (1961). On Becoming a Person. Boston: Houghton Mifflin.

Rogers, C. (1969). Freedom to Learn. Columbus, OH: Merrill.

Rose, S.R. (1989). Members leaving groups: Theoretical and practical considerations. Small Group Behavior 20(4): 534–535.

Rosenthal, L. (1987). Resolving Resistance in Group Psychotherapy. Lanham, MD: Jason Aronson.

Rosner, D. (1979). Business at the bedside: Health care in Brooklyn, 1890–1915. In S. Reverby & D. Rosner (eds.), Health Care in America: Essays in Social History. Philadelphia: Temple University Press.

Ross, M. & Burdick, D. (1978). A Sensory Integration Training Manual for Regressed and Geriatric Patients. Middletown, CT: Department of Rehabilitation Services, Connecticut Valley Hospital.

Rothaus, P., Hanson, P.G., & Cleveland, S.E. (1966). Art and group dynamics. American Journal of Occupational Therapy 20(4): 182–187.

Rothman, D.J. (1980). Conscience and Convenience: The Asylum and Its Alternatives in Progressive America. Boston: Little, Brown & Company.

Sampson, E., & Marthas, M. (1981). Group Process for the Health Professions, 2nd ed. New York: John Wiley & Sons.

Schiffer, M. (1979). The genealogy of group psychotherapy. In S.R. Slavson (au.) & M. Schiffer (ed.), Dynamics of Group Psychotherapy. New York: Jason Aronson.

Schulz, C.H. (1994). Helping factors in a peer-developed support group for persons with head injury, Part 2: Survivor interview perspective. American Journal of Occupational Therapy 48(4): 305–309.

Schuman, S.H., Marcus, D., & Nesse, D. (1973). Puppetry and the mentally ill. American Journal of Occupational Therapy 27(8): 484–486.

Schutz, W.C. (1960). FIRO: A three-dimensional theory of interpersonal behavior. New York: Rinehart, Winston.

Schutz, W.C. (1967). Joy: Expanding human awareness. New York: Grove Press.

Schwartzberg, S.L. (1993). Tools of practice: Group process. In H.L. Hopkins & H.D. Smith (eds.), Willard & Spackman's Occupational Therapy, 8th ed. Philadelphia: J.B. Lippincott, 275–280.

Schwartzberg, S.L. (1994). Helping factors in a peer-developed support group for persons with head injury, Part 1: Participant observer perspective. American Journal of Occupational Therapy 48(4): 297–304.

Schwartzberg, S.L. (1998). Group process. In M.E. Neistadt & Crepeau, E.B. (eds.), Willard and Spackman's Occupational Therapy, 9th ed., 120–131. Philadelphia: J.B. Lippincott.

Schwartzberg, S.L. (1999). The use of groups in the rehabilitation of persons with head injury: Reasoning skills employed by the group facilitator. In C. Unsworth, Cognitive and Perceptual Dysfunction: A Clinical Reasoning Approach to Evaluation and Intervention. Philadelphia: F.A. Davis, 455–471.

Schwartzberg, S.L. (2002). Interactive Reasoning in the Practice of Occupational Therapy. Upper Saddle River, NJ: Prentice Hall.

Schwartzberg, S.L., & Abeles, J. (1991). Occupational therapy. In L. I. Sederer (ed.), Inpatient Psychiatry: Diagnosis and Treatment, 3rd ed. Baltimore: Williams & Wilkins, 298–319.

Schwartzberg, S.L., Howe, M.C., & McDermott, A. (1982). A comparison of three treatment group formats for facilitating social interaction. Occupational Therapy in Mental Health 2(4): 1–16.

Scott, A.H. (1999). Wellness works: Community service health promotion groups led by occupational therapy students. American Journal of Occupational Therapy 53(6): 566–574.

Shaffer, J.B. & Galinsky, M.D. (1974). Models of Group Therapy and Sensitivity Training. Englewood Cliffs, NJ: Prentice-Hall.

Shannon, P.D. & Snortum, J.R. (1965). An activity group's role in intensive psychotherapy. American Journal of Occupational Therapy 19(6): 344–347.

Shapiro, E.L. & Ginzberg, R. (2002). Parting gifts: Termination rituals in group therapy. International Journal of Group Psychotherapy 52(3): 319–336.

Siegel, D.J. (2001). Toward an interpersonal neurobiology of the developing mind: Attachment relationships, "mindsight," and neural integration. Infant Mental Health Journal 22(1–2): 67–94.

Slagle, E.C. (1922). Training aides for mental patients. Archives of Occupational Therapy 1(1): 11–17.

Slavson, S.R. (1950). Analytic Group Psychotherapy With Children, Adolescents and Adults. New York: Columbia University Press.

Slavson, S.R. (1967/1979). Vita-Erg therapy with long-term, regressed psychotic women. In S. R. Slavson (au.) & M. Schiffer (ed.), Dynamics of Group Psychotherapy. New York: Jason Aronson. (Article originally written in 1967.)

Smuts, R.W. (1959). Women and Work in America. New York: Columbia University Press.

Springfield, F.B. & Tullis, L.H. (1958). An intensive activities program for chronic neuropsychiatric patients. American Journal of Occupational Therapy 12(5): 247–249.

Steffan, J.A. & Nelson, D.L. (1987). The effects of tool scarcity on group climate and affective meaning within the context of a stenciling activity. American Journal of Occupational Therapy 41(7): 449–453.

Stein, F. (1982). A current review of the behavioral frame of reference and its application to occupational therapy. Occupational Therapy in Mental Health 2(4): 35–62.

Steiner, J. (1972). Reflections on the encounter group and the therapist. American Journal of Occupational Therapy 26(3): 130–131.

Stogdill, R.M. (1948). Personality factors associated with leadership: A survey of the literature. Journal of Psychology 25: 3–71.

Streib, P. (1999). Survey: Most practitioners holding their own. OT Week 13(10): 8–10.

Strickland, R. (1991). Nationally speaking: Directions for the future—occupational therapy practice then and now, 1949–the present. American Journal of Occupational Therapy 45: 105–107.

Talbot, J.F. (1983). An inpatient adolescent living skills program. Occupational Therapy in Mental Health 3(4): 35–45.

Teasdale, T.W., Christensen, A.L., & Pinner, E.M. (1993). Psychosocial rehabilitation of cranial trauma and stroke patients. Brain Injury 7: 535–542.

Tickle-Degnen, L. (2002). Communicating evidence to clients, managers, and funders. In M. Law (ed.), Evidence-Based Rehabilitation: A Guide to Practice. Thorofare, NJ: Slack, 221–254.

Tickle-Degnen, L. & Bedell, G. (2003). Evidence-based practice forum: Heterarchy and hierarchy: A critical appraisal of the "levels of evidence" as a tool for clinical decision making. American Journal of Occupational Therapy 57(2): 234–237.

Trahey, P.J. (1991). A comparison of the cost-effectiveness of two types of occupational therapy services. American Journal of Occupational Therapy 45: 397–401.

Trombley, C.A. (1995). Occupation: Purposefulness and meaningfulness as therapeutic mechanisms. American Journal of Occupational Therapy 49(10): 960–972.

Truax, C. & Mitchell, K. (1971). Research on certain therapist intrapersonal skills in relation to process and outcome. In A. Bergin & S. Garfield (eds.), Handbook of Psychotherapy and Behavior Change. New York: John Wiley & Sons.

Tuckman, B.W. (1965). Developmental sequence in small groups. Psychological Bulletin 63: 384–399.

Tuckman, B.W., & Jensen, M.A. (1977). Stages of small-group development revisited. Group and Organization Studies 2(4): 419–427.

Van Deusen, J., & Harlowe, D. (1987). The efficacy of the ROM dance program for adults with rheumatoid arthritis. American Journal of Occupational Therapy 41(2): 90–95.

VanderRoest, L.L. & Clements, S.T. (1983). Sensory Integration: Rationale and Treatment Activities for Groups. Grand Rapids, MI: South Kent Mental Health Services.

Versluys, H. (1980). The remediation of role disorders through focused group work. American Journal of Occupational Therapy 34(9): 609–614.

Vivero-Chong, R. (2002). Reminiscence therapy: The group approach in long-term care. Canadian Nursing Home 13(3): 5–12.

Von Bertalanffy, L. (1968). General Systems Theory: Foundations, Development, Application (rev. ed). New York: George Braziller.

Ward, J.D. (2003). The nature of clinical reasoning with groups: A phenomenological study of an occupational therapist in community mental health. American Journal of Occupational Therapy, 57(6): 625–634.

Wardi, D. (1989). The termination phase in the group process. Group Analysis 22: 87–98.

Webb, L.J. (1973). The therapeutic social club. American Journal of Occupational Therapy 27(2): 81–83.

Weber, R.L. & Gans, J.S. (2003). The group therapist's shame: A much undiscussed topic. International Journal of Group Psychotherapy 53(4): 395–416.

Werner, V., Maddigan, R.F., & Watson, C.G. (1969). A study of two treatment programs for chronic mentally ill patients in occupational therapy. American Journal of Occupational Therapy 23(2): 132–136.

West, W.L. (ed.). (1959). Changing Concepts and Practices in Psychiatric Occupational Therapy. Dubuque, IA: William C. Brown.

White, C.V. (1953). Group projects with psychiatric patients. American Journal of Occupational Therapy 7(6): 253, 270.

White, R.W. (1959). Motivation reconsidered: The concept of competence. The Psychological Review 66: 297–333.

White, R.W. (1971). The urge towards competence. American Journal of Occupational Therapy 25(6): 271–274.

Wiebe, R.H. (1967). The Search for Order 1877–1920. New York: Hill & Wang.

Wilson, L.G. (1979). The use of a stroke group treatment program on an extended care unit. Canadian Journal of Occupational Therapy 46(1): 19–20.

Winnicott, D.W. (1958). Transitional objects and transitional phenomena. In D.W. Winnicott. Collected Papers: Through Pediatrics to Psychoanalysis. London: Tavistock, 229–242.

Woodside, H.H. (1971). Occupational therapy—an historical perspective: The development of occupational therapy 1910–1929. American Journal of Occupational Therapy 25(5): 226–230.

Yager, J.A., & Ehmann, T.S. (2006). Untangling social function and social cognition: A review of concepts and measurement. Psychiatry 69(1): 47–68.

Yalom, I.D. (1970). The Theory and Practice of Group Psychotherapy. New York: Basic Books.

Yalom, I.D. (1975). The Theory and Practice of Group Psychotherapy, 2nd ed. New York: Basic Books.

Yalom, I.D. (1983). Inpatient Group Psychotherapy. New York: Basic Books.

Yalom, I.D. (1985). The Theory and Practice of Group Psychotherapy, 3rd ed. New York: Basic Books.

Yalom, I.D. & Leszcz, M. (2005). The Theory and Practice of Group Psychotherapy, 5th ed. New York: Basic Books.

Yerxa, E.J. (1967). Authentic occupational therapy. American Journal of Occupational Therapy 21(1): 1–9.

Zander, A. & Havelin, A. (1960). Social comparison and intergroup attraction. Human Relations 13: 21–32.

Bibliography

Abras, T.D. (1999). Meeting the mental health needs of adolescents. OT Week May 13, 8–9.

Adelstein, L.A. & Nelson, D.L. (1985). Effects of sharing versus non-sharing on affective meaning in collage activities. Occupational Therapy in Mental Health 5(2): 29–45.

Allen, C.K. (1985). Occupational Therapy for Psychiatric Diseases: Measurement and Management of Cognitive Disabilities. Boston: Little, Brown & Company.

American Occupational Therapy Association. (1975). Essentials of an accredited educational program for the occupational therapist. American Journal of Occupational Therapy 29(8): 485–496.

Amini, D. (1999). Patients heal each other. Advance for Occupational Therapy Practitioners May 17: 5, 33.

Asch, S.E. (1960). Effects of group pressure upon the modification and distortion of judgments. In D. Cartwright & A. Zander (eds.), Group Dynamics: Research and Theory, 2nd ed. Evanston, IL: Row, Peterson, 189–200.

Bales, R.F. (1955). The equilibrium problem in small groups. In A.P. Hare, E.F. Borgatta, & R.F. Bales (eds.), Small Groups. New York: Knopf.

Bandura, A. (1969). Principles of Behavior Modification. New York: Holt Reinhart & Winston.

Banning, M.R. & Nelson, D.L. (1987). The effects of activity-elicited humor and group structure on group cohesion and affective responses. American Journal of Occupational Therapy 41(8): 510–514.

Barnes, M.A. & Schwartzberg, S.L. (1999). A case study: An occupational therapy approach. In S. Simon Fehr (ed.), Introduction to Group Therapy: A Practical Guide. Binghamton, NY: The Haworth Press.

Benjamin, A. (1978). Behavior in Small Groups. Boston: Houghton Mifflin.

Brinson M. & Kannenberg, K.R. (1996). Mental Health Service Delivery Guidelines. Bethesda, MD: American Occupational Therapy Association.

Brown, T. (1990). Drama and occupational therapy. In J. Creek (ed.), Occupational Therapy and Mental Health. New York: Churchill Livingstone, 211–227.

Bruce, M.A. (1988). Occupational therapy in group treatment. In D.W. Scott & N. Katz (eds.), Occupational Therapy in Mental Health Principles in Practice. Philadelphia: Taylor & Francis, 116–132.

Bruce, M.A. & Borg, B. (1993). Psychosocial Occupational Therapy Frames of Reference for Intervention, 2nd ed Thorofare, NJ: Slack.

Buckley, W. (ed.). (1968). Modern Systems Research for the Behavioral Scientist. Chicago: Aldine.

Cara, E. & MacRae, A. (1998). Psychosocial Occupational Therapy: A Clinical Practice. Albany, NY: Delmar.

Cohn, B.R. (2005). Creating the group envelope. In L. Motherwell & J.J. Shay, (eds.), Complex Dilemmas in Group Therapy: Pathways to Resolution. New York: Brunner-Routledge, 3–11.

Cole, M.B. (1993). Group Dynamics in Occupational Therapy: The Theoretical Basis and Practice Application of Group Treatment. Thorofare, NJ: Slack.

Cole, M.B. (1998). Group Dynamics in Occupational Therapy: The Theoretical Basis and Practice Application of Group Treatment, 2nd ed. Thorofare, NJ: Slack.

Cole, M.B. & Greene, L.R. (1988). A preference for activity: A comparative study of psychotherapy groups vs. occupational therapy groups for psychotic and borderline inpatients. Occupational Therapy in Mental Health 8(3): 53–67.

Corsini, R. & Rosenberg, B. (1955). Mechanisms of group psychotherapy: Process and dynamics. Journal of Abnormal and Social Psychology 15: 406–411.

Cottrell, R.P.F. (ed.). (1993). Psychosocial Occupational Therapy: Proactive Approaches. Rockville, MD: American Occupational Therapy Association.

Donigian, J., & Malnati, R. (1997). Systemic Group Therapy: A Triadic Model. Pacific Grove, CA: Brooks/Cole.

Dressler, J. & MacRae, A. (1998). Advocacy, partnership and client-centered practice in California. Occupational Therapy in Mental Health 14(1/2).

Eklund, M. (1996). Occupational Therapy Group in a Psychiatric Day Care Unit for Long-Term Mentally Ill Patients: Ward Atmosphere, Treatment Process and Outcome. Department of Psychology, Lund University, Lund, Sweden.

Falk-Kessler, J., Momich, C., & Perel, S. (1991). Therapeutic factors in occupational therapy groups. American Journal of Occupational Therapy 45(1): 59–66.

Fine, S.B. (1998). Surviving the health care revolution: Rediscovering the meaning of "good work." Occupational Therapy in Mental Health 14(1/2): 14.

Fleming, M.H. & Mattingly, C. (1994). Action and inquiry: Reasoned action and active reasoning. In C. Mattingly & M.H. Fleming (eds.), Clinical Reasoning: Forms of Inquiry in a Therapeutic Practice. Philadelphia: FA Davis, 316–342.

Galinsky, M.J. & Schopler, J.H. (1974). The social work group. In J.B. Shaffer & M.D. Galinsky (eds.), Models of Group Therapy and Sensitivity Training. Englewood Cliffs, NJ: Prentice-Hall, 19–48.

Glass, T.A., Mendes de Leon, C., & Berkman, L.F. (1999). Population-based study of social and productive activities as predictors of survival among elderly Americans. British Medical Journal 319: 478–483.

Greene, L.R., & Cole, M.B. (1991). Level and form of psychopathology and the structure of group therapy. International Journal of Group Psychotherapy 41(4): 499–521.

Haiman, S. (1990). Selecting group protocols: Recipe or reasoning. In D. Gibson (ed.), Group Protocols: A Psychosocial Compendium. Binghamton, NY: The Haworth Press, 1–14.

Hemphill, B.J. (ed.). (1982). The evaluative process in psychiatric occupational therapy. Thorofare, NJ: Slack.

Holm, M.B. (2000). Our mandate for the new millennium: Evidence-based practice. American Journal of Occupational Therapy 54(6): 575–585.

Holm, M.B. (2001). Our mandate for the new millennium: Evidenced-based practice. AOTA continuing education article. OT Practice July 2001: CE 1–8.

Horwitz, M. (1960). The recall of interrupted group tasks: An experimental study of individual motivation in relation to group goals. In D. Cartwright & A. Zander (eds.), Group Dynamics: Research and Theory, 2nd ed. New York: Harper & Row, 444–460.

Kaplan, K. (1986). The directive group: Short-term treatment for psychiatric patients with a minimal level of functioning. American Journal of Occupational Therapy 40(7): 474–481.

Kaplan, K.L. (1988). Directive Group Therapy: Innovative Mental Health Treatment. Thorofare, NJ: Slack.

Kielhofner, G. (1992). Conceptual Foundations of Occupational Therapy. Philadelphia: F.A. Davis.

Kielhofner, G. (1997). Conceptual Foundations of Occupational Therapy, 2nd ed. Philadelphia: F.A. Davis.

Knis, L.L. (1995). The play's the thing. OT Week August 31: 18–19.

Lakin, M. & Dray, M. (1958). Psychological aspects of activity for the aged. American Journal of Occupational Therapy 12(4): 172–175, 187–188.

Lee, B. & Nantais, T. (1996). Use of electronic music as an occupational therapy modality in spinal cord injury rehabilitation: An occupational performance model. American Journal of Occupational Therapy 50(5): 362–369.

Licht, S. (ed.). (1948). Occupational Therapy Source Book. Baltimore: Williams & Wilkins.

Lillie, M. & Armstrong, H. (1982). Contributions to the development of psychoeducational approaches to mental health service. American Journal of Occupational Therapy 36(7): 438–443.

Locascio, J. (1995). Involving families in psychiatric treatment. OT Week August 24: 24–25.

MacKenzie, K.R. (Spring 1999). Professional ethics and the group psychotherapist. The group solution. Newsletter of the National Registry of Certified Group Psychotherapists.

Margolis, R.L., Harrison, S.A., Robinson, H.J., et al. (1996). Occupational therapy task observation scale (OTTOS): A rapid method for rating task group function of psychiatric patients. American Journal of Occupational Therapy 50(5): 380–385.

Marmer, L. (1995). Group treatment works well in stroke recovery. Advance for Occupational Therapists October 2: 13.

McConchie, S.D. (December 1989). Establishing support and advocacy groups. Mental Health Special Interest Section Newsletter, 5–6, 8. Rockville, MD: American Occupational Therapy Association.

McDermott, A.A. (1988). The effect of three group formats on group interaction patterns. Occupational Therapy in Mental Health 8(3): 69–89.

Morris, P.A., Andreassi, E., & Lichtenberg, P. (1994). Preparing for community living. OT Week August 25: 20–21.

Mumford, M.S. (1974). A comparison of interpersonal skills in verbal and activity groups. American Journal of Occupational Therapy 28(5): 281–283.

Peterson, E.W. (2003). Evidence-based practice case example: A matter of balance. OT Practice 8(3): 12–14.

Polimeni-Walker, I., Wilson, K.G., & Jewers, R. (1992). Reasons for participating in occupational therapy groups: Perceptions of adult psychiatric inpatients and occupational therapists. Canadian Journal of Occupational Therapy 59(5): 240–247.

Posthuma, B.W. (1989). Small Groups in Therapy Settings: Process and Leadership. Boston: Little, Brown & Company.

Posthuma, B.W. (1996). Small Groups in Counseling and Therapy Process and Leadership, 2nd ed. Needham Heights, MA: Allyn & Bacon.

Rabinovitch, S. (1999). An experiment with MOHO: OT uses model to reverse school's approach to disability. Advance for Occupational Therapy Practitioners August 9: 9.

Rogers, C. (1967). The process of the basic encounter group. In J. Bugental (ed.), Challenges of Humanistic Psychology. New York: McGraw-Hill, 270.

Rogers, C. (1970). Carl Rogers on Encounter Groups. New York: Harper & Row.

Ross, M. (1987). Group Process Using Therapeutic Activities in Chronic Care. Thorofare, NJ: Slack.

Ross, M. (1991). Integrative Group Therapy: The Structured Five-Stage Approach, 2nd ed. Thorofare, NJ: Slack.

Ross, M., & Burdick, D. (1981). Sensory Integration: A Training Manual for Therapists and Teachers for Regressed, Psychiatric and Geriatric Patient Groups. Thorofare, NJ: Slack.

Rutan, S. (2005). Treating difficult patients in groups. In L. Motherwell & J.J. Shay (eds.), Complex Dilemmas in Group Therapy: Pathways to Resolution. Brunner-Routledge: New York, 41–49.

Sacenti, L. (1988). Mastery and levels of participation in members of two groups for chronic pain: Self-help and professionally led. Unpublished master's thesis, Tufts University–Boston School of Occupational Therapy, Medford, MA.

Solomon, A.P. & Fentress, T.L. (1947). A critical study of analytically oriented group psychotherapy utilizing the technique of dramatization of the psychodynamics. Occupational Therapy and Rehabilitation 26(1): 23–46.

Sorenson, J.R. (1971). Task demands, group interaction and group performance. Sociometry 34: 483–495.

Spitz, H. (Summer 1999). Brief group psychotherapy and managed care: Integration or disconnection? The Group Solution. Newsletter of the National Registry of Certified Group Psychotherapists.

Stahl, C. (1995). Cognition and social competence. Advance for Occupational Therapists August 7: 19.

St. Clair, M., & Wigren, J. (2004). Object Relations and Self Psychology: An Introduction, 4th ed. Boston: Thompson.

Steffan, J.A. (1990). Productive occupation in small task groups of adults: Synthesis and annotations of the social psychology literature. In A.C. Bundy, N.D. Prendergast, J.A. Steffan, et al. (eds.), Review of Selected Literature on Occupation and Health. Rockville, MD: American Occupational Therapy Association, 175–281.

Stein, F. & Tallant, B. (1988). Applying the group process to psychiatric occupational therapy, Part 1: Historical and current use. Occupational Therapy in Mental Health 8(3): 9–28.

Tallant, B. (1998). Applying the group process to psychosocial occupational therapy. In F. Stein & S. Cutler (eds.), Psychosocial Occupational Therapy: A Holistic Approach. San Diego: Singular, 327–349.

Tannenbaum, R. & Schmidt, W.H. (1958). How to choose a leadership pattern. Harvard Business Review 36 (March–April): 95–101.

Tennstedt, S., Howland, J., Lachman, M.E., et al. (1998). A randomized, controlled trial of a group intervention to reduce fear of falling and associated activity restriction in older adults. Journal of Gerontology Psychological Sciences 53B, 383–394.

Tickle-Degnen, L. (2000). Evidence-based practice forum: Communicating with clients, family member, and colleagues. American Journal of Occupational Therapy 54, 341–343.

Tickle-Degnen, L. (2000). Gathering current research evidence to enhance clinical reasoning. American Journal of Occupational Therapy 54(1), 102–105.

Tubbs, S. (1984). A Systems Approach to Small Group Interaction. New York: Random House.

Tziner, A. & Eden, D. (1985). Effects of crew composition on crew performance: Does the whole equal the sum of its parts? Journal of Applied Psychology 70: 85–93.

Wall, V.D. & Nolan, L.L. (1986). Perceptions of inequity, satisfaction, and conflict in task-oriented groups. Human Relations 39: 1033–1052.

Webster, D. (1988). Patients' perceptions of therapeutic factors in occupational therapy groups. Unpublished master's thesis, Tufts University–Boston School of Occupational Therapy, Medford, MA.

Webster, D. & Schwartzberg, S.L. (1992). Patients' perception of curative factors in occupational therapy groups. Occupational Therapy in Mental Health 12(1): 3–24.

Weinberg, W. (2000). Group Process and Group Phenomena on the Internet. American Group Psychotherapy Association Conference, Los Angeles, February 2000.

Weinstein, E. (1990). The role of the group in the treatment of chronic pain. Occupational Therapy Practice 1(3): 62–68.

Womack, J. & Farmer, P. (1999). Strong roots, flexible branches. OT Practice 4(10): 17–21.

Glossary

ADL: Activities of daily living

Altruism: Doing something for the good of others.

Autocratic: Leader behavior that is a highly structured approach to group.

Catharsis: Letting go of emotions and healing through verbal release.

Closure: The process of bringing a group to an end; concluding a group or group session.

Consensual validation: A comparison of one's own interpersonal assessment with those of others in the group.

Corrective recapitulation: Therapeutic value to re-experiencing emotional attachment and conflict, with healthy interpersonal interactions to promote growth.

Counterdependence: Acting out wishes to be dependent through acts of resistance to authority or withholding.

Countertransference: The leader's psychological world, unconscious or conscious, felt in reaction to the group process, members, and co-leader, which needs to be examined so as to be in leader's awareness.

CVA: Cerebrovascular accident or stroke.

Existential: A belief system derived from existential philosophy of valuing living in the moment and directing one's life within the here and now.

Facilitating environment: Setting, relationships, and objects that promote emotional growth.

Feedback: Stating or demonstrating nonverbally your reaction to another person's behavior.

Flow state: A match between skills and opportunities for action in the environment (Csikszentmihalyi, 1975, 1990).

Frame of reference: A theoretical perspective that influences ways of perceiving observations, information, and methods of intervening in therapeutic and natural settings.

Group maintenance roles: Group member roles that focus on building social-emotional aspects of group process (Benne & Sheats, 1978).

Group task roles: Group member roles that help a group complete specified task goals (Benne & Sheats, 1978).

Holding environment: An interpersonal and object relationship that feels secure enough to contain strong emotions.

Humanistic: A belief system derived from a philosophy of valuing individuals as inherently good.

IADL: Instrumental activities of daily living, such as care of others (family members, pets); using telephones, computers, and writing to communicate with others; health, home, and financial management; shopping, meal preparation, and maintaining safety.

Individual roles: Group member roles that are centered around individual member needs and not relevant to the group's goals (Benne & Sheats, 1978).

Internal stimuli: Mental preoccupations or thought processes that remove an individual's attention from what is happening in the present.

Interpersonal: Interactions between individuals.

Intrapersonal: Internal psychological processes within an individual.

Laissez-faire: Leader behavior that is open-ended and encourages members to do as they wish.

Meaning attribution: Explaining, clarifying, interpreting, providing a cognitive framework for change; translating feelings and experiences into ideas.

MI: Myocardial infarction.

MVA: Motor vehicle accident.

Pairing: Form of subgrouping in response to anxiety (Bion, 1959).

Phenomenological: A narrative based subjective view of a person's life story.

PICO question: A structured process to define a research question to investigate an intervention; consists of person, intervention, condition, and outcome.

Psychological world: A person's internal thoughts and affective states such as wishes, fears, fantasies, drives, motivations, intersubjective reactions, and projections.

Reality testing: A process by which one's understanding of a situation is shared and reviewed with others.

Self-disclosure: Verbalizing one's feelings, stories, and narrative.

Sociogram: An instrument that provides data on the communication pattern in the group, charting specifically who talks to whom.

TBI: Traumatic brain injury.

Termination: A transition to another stage in the life of the individuals involved.

TKR: Total knee replacement.

Transference: A group member's projection of his or her inner world of feelings, conflicts, and associations onto others.

Transitional object: A person or thing that enables a person to feel secure; often symbolic of early developmental object attachment.

Universality: Of common human experience and interest.

Index

Note: Page numbers followed by "f" and "t" indicate figures and tables, respectively.